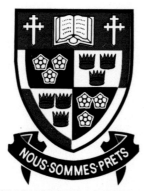

TRYPTOPHAN

Biochemical and Health Implications

CRC SERIES IN MODERN NUTRITION
Edited by Ira Wolinsky and James F. Hickson, Jr.

Published Titles

Manganese in Health and Disease, Dorothy J. Klimis-Tavantzis

Nutrition and AIDS: Effects and Treatments, Ronald R. Watson

Nutrition Care for HIV-Positive Persons: A Manual for Individuals and Their Caregivers,
   Saroj M. Bahl and James F. Hickson, Jr.

Calcium and Phosphorus in Health and Disease, John J.B. Anderson and
   Sanford C. Garner

Edited by Ira Wolinsky

Published Titles

Practical Handbook of Nutrition in Clinical Practice, Donald F. Kirby
   and Stanley J. Dudrick

Handbook of Dairy Foods and Nutrition, Gregory D. Miller, Judith K. Jarvis,
   and Lois D. McBean

Advanced Nutrition: Macronutrients, Carolyn D. Berdanier

Childhood Nutrition, Fima Lifschitz

Nutrition and Health: Topics and Controversies, Felix Bronner

Nutrition and Cancer Prevention, Ronald R. Watson and Siraj I. Mufti

Nutritional Concerns of Women, Ira Wolinsky and Dorothy J. Klimis-Tavantzis

Nutrients and Gene Expression: Clinical Aspects, Carolyn D. Berdanier

Antioxidants and Disease Prevention, Harinda S. Garewal

Advanced Nutrition: Micronutrients, Carolyn D. Berdanier

Nutrition and Women's Cancers, Barbara Pence and Dale M. Dunn

Nutrients and Foods in AIDS, Ronald R. Watson

Nutrition: Chemistry and Biology, Second Edition, Julian E. Spallholz,
   L. Mallory Boylan, and Judy A. Driskell

Melatonin in the Promotion of Health, Ronald R. Watson

Nutritional and Environmental Influences on the Eye, Allen Taylor

Laboratory Tests for the Assessment of Nutritional Status, Second Edition,
   H.E. Sauberlich

Advanced Human Nutrition, Robert E.C. Wildman and Denis M. Medeiros

Handbook of Dairy Foods and Nutrition, Second Edition, Gregory D. Miller,
   Judith K. Jarvis, and Lois D. McBean

Nutrition in Space Flight and Weightlessness Models, Helen W. Lane
   and Dale A. Schoeller

Eating Disorders in Women and Children: Prevention, Stress Management, and Treatment, Jacalyn J. Robert-McComb

Childhood Obesity: Prevention and Treatment, Jana Pařízková and Andrew Hills

Alcohol and Coffee Use in the Aging, Ronald R. Watson

Handbook of Nutrition in the Aged, Third Edition, Ronald R. Watson

Vegetables, Fruits, and Herbs in Health Promotion, Ronald R. Watson

Nutrition and AIDS, Second Edition, Ronald R. Watson

Advances in Isotope Methods for the Analysis of Trace Elements in Man, Nicola Lowe and Malcolm Jackson

Nutritional Anemias, Usha Ramakrishnan

Handbook of Nutraceuticals and Functional Foods, Robert E. C. Wildman

The Mediterranean Diet: Constituents and Health Promotion, Antonia-Leda Matalas, Antonis Zampelas, Vassilis Stavrinos, and Ira Wolinsky

Vegetarian Nutrition, Joan Sabaté

Nutrient–Gene Interactions in Health and Disease, Naïma Moustaïd-Moussa and Carolyn D. Berdanier

Micronutrients and HIV Infection, Henrik Friis

Tryptophan: Biochemicals and Health Implications, Herschel Sidransky

Forthcoming Titles

Handbook of Nutraceuticals and Nutritional Supplements and Pharmaceuticals, Robert E. C. Wildman

Insulin and Oligofructose: Functional Food Ingredients, Marcel B. Roberfroid

Nutritional Aspects and Clinical Management of Chronic Diseases, Felix Bronner

CRC Series in MODERN NUTRITION

TRYPTOPHAN
Biochemical and Health Implications

Herschel Sidransky

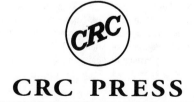

CRC PRESS

Boca Raton London New York Washington, D.C.

Library of Congress Cataloging-in-Publication Data

Sidransky, Herschel, 1925-
  Tryptophan : biochemical and health implications / Herschel Sidransky.
    p. ; cm. -- (CRC series in modern nutrition)
  Includes bibliographical references and index.
  ISBN 0-8493-8568-7 (alk. paper)
    1. Tryptophan. I. Title. II. Modern nutrition (Boca Raton, Fla.)
    [DNLM: 1. Tryptophan--metabolism. QU 60 S569t 2001]
  QP562.T7 S565 2001
  612'.01575—dc21
                                                              2001043170
                                                                    CIP

Visit the CRC Press Web site at www.crcpress.com

No claim to original U.S. Government works
International Standard Book Number 0-8493-8568-7
Library of Congress Card Number 2001043170
Printed in the United States of America 1 2 3 4 5 6 7 8 9 0
Printed on acid-free paper

Series Preface

The CRC Series in Modern Nutrition is dedicated to providing the widest possible coverage of topics in nutrition. Nutrition is an interdisciplinary, interprofessional field par excellence. It is noted by its broad range and diversity. We trust the titles and authorship in this series will reflect that range and diversity.

Published for a scholarly audience, the volumes in the CRC Series in Modern Nutrition are designed to explain, review, and explore present knowledge and recent trends, developments, and advances in nutrition. As such, they will also appeal to the educated general reader. The format for the series will vary with the needs of the author and the topic, including, but not limited to, edited volumes, monographs, handbooks, and texts.

Contributors from any bona fide area of nutrition, including the controversial, are welcome.

We welcome the contribution *Tryptophan: Biochemical and Health Implications* written authoritatively by Dr. Herschel Sidransky. He is a well-known expert who has spent a large portion of his research career on the varied, and often controversial, aspects of the metabolism of the amino acid tryptophan.

Ira Wolinsky, Ph.D.
University of Houston
Series Editor

Preface

The author has been interested in selected aspects of L-tryptophan for many years, including the effects of tryptophan deficiency and of the regulatory effects of tryptophan upon protein synthesis. These interests stimulated the author to attempt to obtain a comprehensive view of the role of L-tryptophan in nutrition, biology, biochemistry, physiology, pharmacology, and toxicology. The subject proved to be a major undertaking, and this book is the culmination of this project. The chapters have been selected to present major areas of the current knowledge of L-tryptophan's role in biology and medicine. Each chapter presents an important aspect of how L-tryptophan, an important indispensable amino acid, may act. Overall, it becomes apparent that L-tryptophan and its metabolites are active and important compounds that make major contributions to the vital functions and actions of cells of a variety of tissues and organs. The role of L-tryptophan in health and disease has become apparent from numerous investigative studies. Much is known, yet there is much to discover. This book is designed to offer a comprehensive overview of the subject and to stimulate others to contribute further advances in this exciting area of biology and medicine.

Author

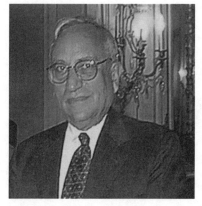

Herschel Sidransky is Professor Emeritus of Pathology at George Washington University Medical Center, Washington, D.C. He earned his B.S. and M.S. degrees in Biochemistry from Tulane University, and an M.D. and training in pathology from Tulane University and Charity Hospital of Louisiana in New Orleans. Dr. Sidransky's research interests have focused on nutritional deficiency diseases, experimental chemical carcinogenesis, toxic liver disease, and tryptophan metabolism. He has authored more than 200 papers and 95 abstracts in these areas. Dr. Sidransky has served on the editorial boards of several leading medical journals and has been a member of the American Society for Investigative Pathology, the American Society for Nutritional Sciences, the American Society for Clinical Nutrition, the American Association for Cancer Research, the Society of Experimental Biology and Medicine, and the United States and Canadian Academy of Pathology.

Dedication and Acknowledgments

This book is dedicated to my co-worker of 40 years, Ms. Ethel Verney. Her able and conscientious contributions to our investigative team have enabled the research on tryptophan in my laboratory to progress and yield publications. Her long-standing contributions and devotion to research are hereby acknowledged.

I also desire to acknowledge the support and encouragement of my wife, Evelyn, and my children, Ellen and David, who have been understanding and considerate during the years that I have devoted to teaching and research. Their support was welcome and indeed vital.

Contents

1

Tryptophan: A Unique Entity

CONTENTS

1.1 Historical Perspectives

Our knowledge of tryptophan began some 100 years ago. In 1901 Hopkins and Cole[1] isolated tryptophan from a pancreatic digest of casein. Its structure was established in 1907 by Ellinger and Flamand,[2] who synthesized a substance that was identical to the tryptophan isolated by Hopkins and Cole. It is noteworthy that about 50 years prior to the discovery of tryptophan by Hopkins and Cole,[1] aspects of tryptophan metabolism began to appear in the research literature, when in 1853 Liebig discovered kynurenic acid in dog urine.[3] Subsequently, kynurenine, a tryptophan metabolite, was identified,[4,5] and the relationship of kynurenic acid to tryptophan was understood. A brief review on the discovery of tryptophan has been described by Curzon.[6]

Although several other amino acids had been described before tryptophan, it was the first demonstrated to be indispensable. Because tryptophan is destroyed by acid hydrolysis of protein, tryptophan-deficient diets were readily formulated, and this led to the demonstration that it was required for growth of animals. In related nutritional studies, Willcock and Hopkins[7] in 1906 observed that mice failed to grow and even died if their sole source of dietary protein was zein. When tryptophan was added to the ration, the lives of the animals were prolonged. A few years later, Osborne and Mendel[8] demonstrated that zein plus tryptophan and lysine promoted normal growth in rats, and they thus established that these two amino acids were essential nutrients. Subsequently, in the 1950s, Rose et al.[9] demonstrated that L-tryptophan was an essential dietary component for humans. Further interest in tryptophan expanded when it was reported that tryptophan could serve as a precursor of the vitamin niacin and NAD[10,11] and of the neurotransmitter serotonin.

Early experimentation with tryptophan dealt with animals exposed to tryptophan-deficient diets. These nutritional studies served to stress the importance of tryptophan in the diet in relation to disturbances in growth and to observed pathologic changes. A few examples are presented below. They reveal that tryptophan caught the interest of nutritionists, pathologists, and clinicians, and they stress its nutritional role in medicine.

Early experiments with mice[7] and with rats[8] showed that tryptophan deficiency leads to a disturbance in growth. This amino acid is also necessary for the maintenance of nitrogen equilibrium in mature rats,[12] mice,[13] pigs,[14] and dogs.[15] A variety of pathological changes in experimental animals have been ascribed to tryptophan deficiency. Cataracts[16,17] and corneal vascularization[18] have been reported in animals subjected to tryptophan deficiency. Indeed, the only authenticated and reproducible example of experimental cataracts caused by dietary deficiencies was that produced in guinea pigs and rats by feeding a diet deficient in or devoid of tryptophan.[19,20] Hematological manifestations of anemia,[21] reduction in plasma proteins,[22] fatty liver,[22-27] and pancreatic atrophy[27] have been reported in tryptophan-deficient rats. Scoliosis has been reported after feeding fish a tryptophan-deficient diet.[28,29]

As a result of discussions during a tryptophan conference in 1971, an international organization was formed with the purpose of furthering tryptophan research by improving communication and collaboration among workers through regular international meetings. The history of this organization, the International Study Group for Tryptophan Research (ISTRY), has been compiled.[30] Its most recent meeting, the ninth international meeting, was held in Hamburg, Germany, in 1998; subsequent meetings are held every three years. Many of these meetings have led to publications, which have served as valuable reviews of the current status of research in tryptophan.[31-39] These publications deal with historical events relating to tryptophan during the past 30 years. They merit review for past and recent accomplishments in tryptophan research involving metabolism, neurochemistry, nutrition, toxicology, and pathology.

1.2   Occurrence in Nature

1.2.1   Occurrence and Requirements

Tryptophan is probably the indole derivative most widely distributed in nature. It is converted into many compounds of important biological significance. Compounds biogenetically related to tryptophan include nicotinic acid (a vitamin), serotonin (a neurohormone), indoleacetic acid (a phytohormone), some pigments formed in the eyes of insects, and a number of alkaloids.

Tryptophan is the least abundant amino acid in most proteins,[40] accounting, on the average, for 1 to 1.5% of the total amino acids in typical plant (1%) and animal (1.5%) proteins. A number of foodstuffs, such as corn, are deficient or limited in tryptophan. Because it is present in low concentrations in most tissue proteins, the requirement of tryptophan in the diet is low compared to that of the other amino acids, particularly the other indispensable (essential) amino acids. In human infants, the requirement for growth is roughly 12 to 40 mg/kg. In adult humans, the minimum daily requirement has been estimated to be 250 mg/d in males and 160 mg/d in females.[41] Considering the recommended daily allowance for protein is 56 g/d for an adult man and 44 g/d for an adult woman, then this amount would supply between 500 and 700 mg/d of tryptophan, assuming that the protein was of high quality. A typical western diet may supply approximately 600 to 1200 mg L-tryptophan from protein intake.[42]

Despite the scarcity of tryptophan in dietary proteins, it rarely appears to be the limiting amino acid for maintenance or growth when the dietary amino acid source is from naturally occurring proteins. An example is the corn protein zein, which is nearly devoid of tryptophan, yet lysine is limiting for growth in this protein since the lysine content in zein in relation to its requirement is the lowest of the indispensable (essential) amino acids. However, since tryptophan may not be limiting for growth in some poor quality proteins, its supply may be insufficient for the normal functioning of the many pathways that depend on an adequate supply or level of tryptophan. One prominent view or belief has been that tryptophan, being present in low levels in proteins, is an important rate-limiting amino acid for many metabolic functions.

Schurr et al.[43] reported the amino acid concentrations in various tissues of the rat. Using these data to calculate tissue-to-plasma ratios, it becomes apparent that the relative availability of plasma tryptophan to tissues is much less than that of other amino acids. The finding, described elsewhere, that tryptophan in serum or plasma can be present as free and bound (to plasma albumin) is unique among amino acids,[44] and this further limits or controls the availability of tryptophan from the blood to organs or tissues, especially the brain. Tryptophan differs from other amino acids in that its concentration in plasma of rats increases (30 to 40%) after fasting, after insulin administration, or after consuming a carbohydrate meal.[45]

1.2.2 Synthesis

Originally, L-tryptophan was first isolated from solutions of tryptic casein hydrolysate by Hopkins and Cole in 1901.[1] Early studies utilized L-tryptophan derived from natural sources. About 48 years later, in 1949, the first successful chemical synthesis of L-tryptophan was achieved.[46] In the early 1980s, chemical synthesis was fully replaced by fermentation methods.[47] With fermentation methods, one differentiates between enzymatic processes and *de novo* synthesis utilizing normal or modified metabolism of microorganisms.[48] Microbiological biosynthesis gained industrial importance following the development of efficient new strains through recombinant DNA technology. In these processes, glucose, ethanol, or anthranilic acid were used as the principle substrates, and L-tryptophan could be obtained in yields of 10 g/l fermentation broth.[48] Thus, L-tryptophan derived in this manner has become available on the world market and is used for foodstuff additives and for pharmacological uses. The significance of this shift from obtaining L-tryptophan from natural sources to commercially derived sources has had important consequences. One has been the reduction in world market price, allowing the increased use of tryptophan in foodstuffs and for pharmaceutical uses. Another has been the undesirable complication or side effect of the development of a significant human disease, eosinophilia myalgia syndrome, due to ingestion of L-tryptophan commercially manufactured by a Japanese company, Showa Denko. This effect is covered in Chapter 11.

1.2.3 Chemistry

Tryptophan is exceptional in the diversity of its biological functions, which are covered throughout this book. It is appropriate to give limited attention to the chemistry of tryptophan. Many complex transformations of tryptophan in foods can occur. Also, a great diversity of derivatives can be formed, some of which conceivably have antinutritional and toxic manifestations. For details concerning such aspects of tryptophan, the reader is referred to sources that cover these aspects in detail.[49,50] The following selected aspects are cited to emphasize some important chemical reactions that may affect humans.

Many studies have been conducted on the stability of free or protein-bound tryptophan during processing and storage. In general, chemical transformations of tryptophan are essentially a function of the temperature and the duration of treatments. Specific modifications can be induced by the presence of oxygen, water,[51] food oxidizing lipids,[52] vitamins,[53] reducing sugars,[54] carbonyl compounds,[55] nitrites,[56] sulfites,[57] halogens,[58] and radiation.[59]

The reactivity of the indole ring of tryptophan[60] has attracted much interest and attention. This aromatic, electron-rich nucleus is susceptible to oxidative cleavage and to substitutions by a number of reagents. It can react as an electron donor with aldehydes or carbocations.

Hydrophobic tryptophan residues present in the interior of food protein molecules contribute to the optical and fluorescent properties of proteins. Their spectral characteristics are considered to be important contributors in the study of protein conformation.[61]

Severe treatments of tryptophan are required to cause a significant degradation of tryptophan. In the absence of oxidizing agents, tryptophan is a stable amino acid, even in strongly basic or acid conditions. During heat treatment, such as industrial or home cooking in the presence of air or steam sterilization, both free and bound tryptophan are relatively stable. However, carboline formation occurs in the presence of carbonyl compounds or/and at high temperatures (above 200°C, as in grill-cooking of meat or fish). Carbolines (α-, β- and γ-) have been identified from the basic fraction of the pyrolysates.[62] Aspects of tryptophan reactions relating to Trp-P-1 (3-amino-1,4-dimethyl-5H-pyrido-(4,3-b)indole) and Trp-P-2 (3-amino-1-methyl-5H-pyrido-(4,3-b)indole) in relation to carcinogenesis are considered in Chapter 6. Also, tryptophan-derived nitroso compounds, considered as potential carcinogens, are attributed to the reaction of tryptophan with nitrite, a meat-curing compound.[56]

For a concise review of the chemistry, see References 49, 50, and 63.

References

1. Hopkins, F. G. and Cole, S. W., A contribution to the chemistry of proteids. Part I. A preliminary study of a hitherto undescribed product of tryptic digestion, *J. Physiol.*, 27, 48, 1901.
2. Ellinger, A. and Flamand, C., Uber Syntetisch Gewonnenes Tryptophan und Einige Seiner Derivate, *Hoppe-Seyle's Z. Physiol. Chem.*, 55, 8, 1908.
3. Liebig, J., Kynurenic acid, *Justus Liebys Ann. Chem.*, 86, 125, 1853.
4. Kotake, Y. and Masayama, T., Uber der Mechanismus dert Kynureninbildung aus Tryptophan, *Hoppe-Seyler's Z. Physiol. Chem.*, 243, 237, 1936.
5. Butenandt, A., Weidel, W., Weichert, R., and von Derjugin, W., Kynurenine. Its physiology, constitution and synthesis, *Z. Physiol. Chem.*, 279, 27, 1943.
6. Curzon, G., Hopkins and the discovery of tryptophan, in *Tryptophan Research 1986*, Bender, D. A., Joseph, M. H., Kochen, W., and Steinhart, H., Eds., Walter de Gruyter, Berlin, 1987, xxix-xxxvii.
7. Willcock, E. G. and Hopkins, F. G., The importance of individual amino acids in metabolism. Observations on the effect of adding tryptophane to a diet in which zein is the sole nitrogenous constituent, *J. Physiol.*, 35, 88, 1906.
8. Osborne, T. B. and Mendel, L. B., Amino acids in nutrition and growth, *J. Biol. Chem.*, 17, 325, 1914.
9. Rose, W. C., Lambert, G. F., and Coon, M. J., The amino acid requirement of man. VII. General procedures: The tryptophan requirement, *J. Biol. Chem.*, 211, 815, 1954.
10. Krehl, W. A., Teply, L. J., Sarma, P. S., and Elvehjem, C. A., Growth retarding effect of corn in nicotinic acid low rations and its counteraction by tryptophane, *Science*, 101, 489, 1945.
11. Nishizuka Y. and Hayaishi, O., Studies on the biosynthesis of nicotinamide adenine dinucleotide. I. Enzymatic synthesis of niacin ribonucleotides from 3-hydroxy-anthranilic in mammalian tissues, *J. Biol. Chem.*, 238, 3369, 1963.

12. Nasset, E. S. and Ely, M. T., Nitrogen balance of adult rats fed amino acids low in L-, DL-, and D-tryptophan, *J. Nutr.*, 51, 449, 1953.

13. Bauer, C. D. and Berg, C. P., The amino acids required for growth in mice and the availability of their optical isomer, *J. Nutr.*, 26, 51, 1943.

14. Mertz, E. T., Beeson, W. M., and Jackson, H. D., Classification of essential amino acids for the weanling pig, *Arch. Biochem. Biophys.*, 38, 121, 1952.

15. Rose, W. C. and Rice, E. E., The significance of the amino acids in canine nutrition, *Science*, 90, 186, 1939.

16. Totter, J. R. and Day, P. L., Cataract and other ocular changes resulting from tryptophane deficiency, *J. Nutri.*, 24, 159, 1942.

17. Ferraro, A, and Roizin, L., Ocular involvement in rats on diets deficient in amino acids. I. Tryptophan, *Arch. Ophthalmol.*, 38, 331, 1947.

18. Sydenstricker, V. P., Hall, W. K., Bowles, L. L., and Schmidt, H. L., Jr., The corneal vascularization resulting from deficiencies of amino acids in the rat, *J. Nutr.*, 34, 481, 1947.

19. Von Sallman, L., Reid, M. E., Grimes, P. A., and Collins, E. M., Tryptophan-deficiency cataract in guinea pigs, *Arch. Ophthalmol.*, 62, 662, 1959.

20. Van Heyningen, R., Experimental studies on cataract, *Invest. Ophthalmol.*, 15, 685, 1976.

21. Albanese, A. A., Holt, L. E., Jr., Kajdi, C. N., and Frankston, J. E., Observations on tryptophane deficiency in rats. Chemical and morphological changes in the blood, *J. Biol. Chem.*, 148, 299, 1943.

22. Cole, A. S. and Scott, P. P., Tissue changes in the adult tryptophan-deficient rat, *Br. J. Nutr.*, 8, 125, 1954.

23. Scott, E. B., Histopathology of amino acid deficiencies. IV. Tryptophan, *Am. J. Pathol.*, 31, 1111, 1955.

24. Adamstone, F. B. and Spector, H., Tryptophan deficiency in the rat. Histologic changes induced by forced feeding of an acid hydrolyzed casein diet, *Arch. Pathol.*, 49, 173, 1950.

25. Van Pilsum, J. F., Speyer, J. F., and Samuels, L. T., Essential amino acid deficiency and enzyme activity, *Arch. Biochem.*, 68, 42, 1957.

26. Spector, H. and Adamstone, F. B., Tryptophan deficiency in the rat induced by forced feeding of an acid hydrolyzed casein diet, *J. Nutr.*, 40, 213, 1950.

27. Samuels, L. T., Goldthorpe, H. C., and Dougherty, T. F., Metabolic effects of specific amino acid deficiencies, *Fed. Proc.*, 10, 393, 1951.

28. Kloppel, T. M. and Post, G., Histological alterations in tryptophan-deficient rainbow trout, *J. Nutr.*, 105, 861, 1975.

29. Poston, H. A. and Rumsey, G. L., Factors affecting dietary requirement and deficiency signs of L-tryptophan in rainbow trout, *J. Nutr.*, 113, 2568, 1983.

30. Brown, R. R., A brief history of ISTRY, in *Progress in Tryptophan and Serotonin Research 1986*, Bender, D. H., Joseph, M. H., Kochen, W., and Steinhart, H., Eds., Walter de Gruyter, Berlin, 1987, xix-xx.

31. Brown, R. R., Ed., Tryptophan metabolism, *Am J. Clin. Nutr.*, 24, 653-851, 1971.

32. Allegri, G., De Antoni, A., and Costa, C., Eds., Tryptophan metabolism: Biochemistry, pathology and regulation, *Acta Vitaminol. Enzymol.*, 29, 1–345, 1974.

33. Hayaishi, O., Ishimura, Y., and Kido, O., Eds., Biochemical and medical aspects of tryptophan metabolism, in *Developments in Biochemistry*, Elsevier/North Holland Biochemical Press, 1980, 1–373.

34. Schlossberger, H. G., Kochen, W., Lingen, B., and Steinhart, H., Eds., *Progress in Tryptophan Research*, Walter de Gruyter, Berlin, 1984.

35. Bender, D. A., Joseph, M. H., Kochen, W., and Steinhart, H., Eds., *Progress in Tryptophan and Serotonin Research 1986*, Walter de Gruyter, Berlin, 1987, 1–429.
36. Schwarcz, R., Young, S. N., and Brown, R. R., Eds., Kynurenine and serotonin pathways — progress in tryptophan research, *Adv. Exp. Med. Biol.*, 294, 1–715, 1991.
37. Kochen, W. and Steinhart, H., Eds., *L-tryptophan, Current Prospects in Medicine and Drug Safety*, Walter de Gruyter, Berlin, 1994.
38. Filippini, G. A., Cosla, C. V. L., and Bertazzo, A., Eds., Recent advances in tryptophan research, *Adv. Exp. Med. Biol.*, 398, 1996.
39. Huether, G., Kochen, W., and Steinhart, H., Eds., Tryptophan, serotonin, and melatonin. Basic aspects and applications, *Adv. Exp. Med. Biol.*, 467, 1999.
40. Block, R. J. and Weiss, K. W., The amino acid composition of proteins, in *Amino Acid Handbook*, Charles C Thomas, Springfield, 1956, 288.
41. Harper, A. E., Human amino acid and nitrogen requirements as the basis for evaluation of nutritional quality of protein, in *Food Proteins*, Whitaker, J. R. and Tannenbaum, S. R., Eds., Avi Publishing Co., Inc., Westport, 1977, 363–386.
42. *Recommended Dietary Allowances*, 9th rev. ed., National Academy Press, Washington, D.C., 1980, 43.
43. Schurr, P. E., Thompson, H. T., Henderson, L. M., and Elvehjem, C. A., Determination of free amino acids in rat tissues, *J. Biol. Chem.*, 182, 39, 1950.
44. Mcmenemy, R. M., Lund, C. C., and Oncley, J. L., Unbound amino acid concentrations in human blood plasmas, *J. Clin. Invest.*, 36, 1672, 1957.
45. Fernstrom, J. D. and Wurtman, R. J., Elevation of plasma tryptophan by insulin, *Metabolism*, 21, 337, 1972.
46. Hellmann, H., Die tynthesen des Tryptophans, *Angew. Chem.*, 61, 352, 1949.
47. Gerhartz, W., Ed., *Ullman's Encyclopedia of Industrial Chemistry*, 5th ed., VCH Verlagsgesellschaft mbH, Weinheim, 985, 73–74.
48. Jeschkeit, H. and Griehl, C., Aminosauren, in *Lebensmittel-Biotechnologie*, Ruttloff, H., Ed., Akademie Verlag GmbH, Berlin, 1991, 454-481.
49. Greenstein, J. P. and Winitz, M., *Chemistry of the Amino Acids*, Vol. 3, John Wiley & Sons, New York, 1961, 2316–2347.
50. Meister, A., *Biochemistry of the Amino Acids*, Vols. 1 and 2, 2nd ed., Academic Press, New York, 1965, 841–884.
51. Leahy, M. M. and Warthesen, J. J., The influence of Maillard browning and other factors on the stability of free tryptophan, *J. Food Process. Preserv.*, 7, 25, 1983.
52. Krogull, M. K. and Fennema, O., Oxidation of tryptophan in the presence of oxidizing methyl linoleate, *J. Agric. Food Chem.*, 35, 66, 1987.
53. Kanner, J. D, and Fennema, O., Photo-oxidation of tryptophan in the presence of riboflavin, *J. Agric. Food Chem.*, 35, 71, 1987.
54. Orsi, F. and Dwaechak, E., Study of the Maillard reaction occurring between methionine and tryptophan on the one hand and glucose on the other. Part II. Studies in melts, *Acta Aliment.*, 7, 1, 1978.
55. McLaren, J. A., The reaction of tryptophan and derivatives with some 1,3-dicarbonyl compounds, *Aust. J. Chem.*, 30, 2045, 1977.
56. Kinae, N., Isolation of beta-carboline derivatives from Maillard reaction mixtures that are mutagenic after nitrite treatment, *Dev. Food Sci.*, 13, 343, 1986.
57. Yang, S. F., Destruction of tryptophan during aerobic oxidation of sulfite ions, *Environ. Res.*, 6, 395, 1973.

58. Bercz, J. P. and Bana, R., Oxidation of nutrients in the presence of chlorine based disinfectants used in drinking water treatment, *Toxicol. Lett.*, 34, 141, 1986.
59. Garrison, W. M., Reaction mechanisms in the radiolysis of peptides, polypeptides, and proteins, *Chem. Res.*, 381, 1987.
60. Fontana, A., Advances in chemical modifications of tryptophan in peptides and proteins, in *Progress in Tryptophan and Serotonin Research*, Schlossberger, H. G., Kochen, W., Linzen, B., and Steinhart, H., Eds., de Gruyter, Berlin, 1984, 829.
61. Wolfenden, R., How hydrophilic is tryptophan?, *Trends Biochem. Sci.*, 11, 70, 1986.
62. Sugimura, T., Studies on environmental chemical carcinogenesis in Japan, *Science*, 233, 312, 1986.
63. Friedman, M. and Cua, J.-L., Chemistry, analysis, nutritional value, and toxicity of tryptophan in food. A review, *J. Agric. Food Chem.*, 36, 1079, 1988.

2

Findings in Deficiency States

2.1 Introduction

This chapter is concerned with the biochemical and pathological (morphologic) alterations that occur in cells, tissues, and organs of animals fed a diet deficient in L-tryptophan. Such deficiency disease may be induced in experimental animals by causing a single nutrient to be lacking in the diet. Such conditions are infrequently encountered in naturally occurring nutritional disease of animals and humans. Under most circumstances multiple deficiencies exist, which makes the interpretation complex. Also, the induction of a nutritional deficiency by omission of a single dietary component of an otherwise nutritionally adequate diet in *ad libitum* feeding experiments must be subject to close scrutiny, as will be discussed subsequently. However, this chapter attempts to present experimental results from many studies that were designed and controlled in a variety of ways. It is necessary to keep this in mind as one reviews the findings.

2.2   Pathological Findings

2.2.1   Morphologic Studies

2.2.1.1   Eyes

One of the first pathological changes attributed to tryptophan deficiency was observed in the eyes of experimental animals. Cataracts[1,2] and corneal vascularization[3] were reported in animals subjected to tryptophan deficiency. Ohrloff et al.[4] found that a tryptophan-free diet induced both posterior sub-capsular cataracts and reversible corneal opacities in young rats. Indeed, the only authenticated and reproducible example of experimental cataract caused by dietary deficiencies was that produced in guinea pigs and rats by feeding a diet deficient in or devoid of tryptophan.[5,6] McAvoy et al.[7] conducted a light-microscopic study of the lens of rats fed a tryptophan-deficient diet and reported that the lens was small, and many of the cortical fiber cells had abnormal morphologies (thicker fiber cells and various shapes) as well as changes in number, distribution, and morphology of nuclei in the lens.

2.2.1.2   Blood

Hematological manifestations of anemia[8] and reduction in plasma proteins[9] have been reported with tryptophan deficiency.

2.2.1.3   Liver

Fatty liver has been reported in rats fed tryptophan-deficient diets.[9-14] Adamstone and Specter[11] and Samuels et al.[14] observed a rapid development of fatty liver with a periportal distribution of the lipid in rats after the animals were force-fed a tryptophan-devoid diet.

Bailey et al.[15] reported that omission of tryptophan, as well as of methionine or of threonine, but not of other amino acids, from an otherwise complete diet elevated hepatic nuclear size and the activity of RNA polymerase I.

2.2.1.4   Pancreas

Pancreatic atrophy has been reported in rats force-fed a tryptophan-devoid diet.[14]

2.2.1.5   Spine

Scoliosis has been reported after feeding fish a tryptophan-deficient diet.[16,17] Using tryptophan-deficient and nondeficient synthetic amino acid test diets, Kloppel and Post[16] reported that scoliosis was observed in the tryptophan-deficient rainbow fish after 1 week of feeding. Histological studies of scoliotic fish revealed hyperemia, disorganization of myomere septa and protrusions of the fibrous matrix sheath, which invests the notochord. Conditions returned to normal within 1 week upon replacement of tryptophan in the diet.

2.2.2   Biochemical Studies

2.2.2.1   Liver

Investigations into the biochemical changes in tissues and organs of experimental animals fed tryptophan-deficient diets have been limited. Most of these studies were concerned with changes in the liver. When tryptophan-deficient diets were fed by *ad libitum* or by force-feeding, differences in hepatic metabolism were observed.[12] Also, when animals were fed other single essential amino acid deficient diets, differences in the pathological and biochemical changes in the livers that were dependent upon the route of feeding (*ad libitum* or force-feeding) have been reported.[18] In general, more marked changes were observed after force-feeding than after *ad libitum* feeding of deficient diets.

2.2.2.1.1   Weight or Mass

Increases in liver weight have been reported in rats force-fed a diet devoid of tryptophan.[12,13,19,20] In the livers of such experimental subjects, there was an increase in protein[20] and particularly in lipid[11,13] in comparison with controls.

2.2.2.1.2   Protein

Some insight into the acute effects of L-tryptophan deficiency on hepatic protein synthesis was obtained by early experimental studies by Munro and co-workers[21,22] and Sidransky and co-workers.[23] A number of studies[21,22,24-27] investigated the response of the livers of fasted animals (rats or mice) to one feeding of protein or of a complete amino acid mixture. The livers revealed enhanced protein synthesis with a shift of polyribosomes from lighter to heavier aggregates. Of interest was that a similar response was observed within 1 to 2 h when fasted animals were fed an amino acid mixture devoid of single amino acids: arginine, histidine, isoleucine, leucine, lysine, phenylalanine, threonine, tyrosine, or valine.[23,28] However, this effect was not observed when animals were fed an amino acid mixture devoid only of tryptophan.[21-23] Tryptophan administration alone to fasted animals resulted in enhanced protein synthesis and a shift of hepatic polyribosomes to heavier aggregates.[23,29,30] This important finding suggested that L-tryptophan had a special role in influencing hepatic protein synthesis. Subsequent studies are reviewed in detail in Chapter 4.

In mice fed a tryptophan-deficient diet *ad libitum* for 1 week, Jones et al.[31] reported on tissue serotonin synthesis rates, systemic tryptophan metabolism, and its response to steroid or cycloheximide treatment. In the experimental mice, brain serotonin synthesis was decreased while duodenal serotonin synthesis was increased following a tryptophan load. Liver total protein was depressed in experimental mice but increased following a tryptophan load. Blood tryptophan (total and free) and albumin were decreased in experimental mice, but ratios of albumin-bound tryptophan were increased. Enzyme kinetic studies indicated that, in experimental mice, brain tryptophan-5-hydroxylase had a reduced Vmax but the enzyme response to tryptophan or hydrocortisone injection was increased. However, hepatic tryptophan-2,3-dioxygenase response to tryptophan or hydrocortisone injection was blunted in experimental mice.

2.2.2.1.3   Lipid

Samuels et al.[14] suggested that the fatty livers of rats force-fed a tryptophan-devoid diet were due to increased synthesis of hepatic lipid from carbon chains of amino acids that were not being used normally for protein synthesis. However, other experimental studies did not support this suggestion.[18] Patrich and Bennington[32] reported that the incorporation of labeled amino acids into liver lipids was greater in rats force-fed a tryptophan-devoid diet for 5 days compared with those force-fed a complete diet. Since fatty livers develop after force-feeding other single essential amino acid-devoid diets (other than a tryptophan-devoid diet),[18] the mechanism responsible may be similar regardless of the type of single deficiency. Several studies have suggested that stimulation of hepatic lipid synthesis may be responsible for the genesis of the fatty liver with a single essential amino acid deficiency.[33,34] However, because impairment of lipoprotein release[35,36] was considered to be involved in most cases of experimental fatty liver, further experimentation seems to be necessary to clarify the mechanism with respect to amino acid deficiency. Consequently, impairment of the synthesis of apolipoprotein resulting from a single amino acid deficiency could cause accumulation of triglycerides because of inadequate conversion of triglycerides to lipoprotein.

2.2.2.2   Pancreas

Consistent with the pancreatic atrophy described in rats force-fed a tryptophan-devoid diet,[14] decreases in the activities of pancreatic amylase, lipase, and protease[37] have been reported. Singh[38] fed rats a niacin- and tryptophan-deficient diet and reported decreased pancreatic weight and content of DNA, protein, amylase, lipase, chymotrypsinogen, and trypsinogen but increased secretion of amylase and trypsinogen. These changes differed from those due to feeding a niacin-deficient diet.

2.2.2.3 *Spleen*

A decrease in splenic weight and in protein content has been reported in rats force-fed a tryptophan-devoid diet.[20]

2.2.2.4 *Thyroid*

Using broiler chicks fed a control or tryptophan-deficient diet for 2 to 4 weeks, Carew et al.[39] reported signs of relative hyperthyroidism in chicks fed the tryptophan-deficient diet compared to pair-fed controls (chicks fed the same quantity of diet as consumed by experimental group). Plasma triiodothyronine (T3) was elevated in the experimental group.

2.2.2.5 *Lens of Eye*

In animals with experimental cataracts due to being fed a diet deficient in tryptophan, the soluble lens proteins were proportionally reduced.[4,6] Rats fed a tryptophan-deficient diet had lower lens dry weight and lens water was increased and β-crystallin was decreased compared to that in normal lenses.[40]

2.2.3 Neuropsychiatric Studies

It has been known for many years that diets deficient in tryptophan lead to depletion of brain serotonin and hence to disturbances in serotonin-mediated brain function.[41] Subsequently, in the early 1970s, Fernstrom and Wurtman[42,43] began a systematic investigation of the relationship between tryptophan supply and serotonin synthesis under a variety of circumstances. The role of tryptophan deficiency on neuropsychiatric conditions is reviewed in Chapter 7. In addition, studies of rapid tryptophan depletion have been conducted on a wide variety of neuropsychiatric conditions in humans and in experimental conditions in animals. This approach and the findings are also reviewed in detail in Chapter 7.

2.3 Differences in Methods of Induction of Tryptophan Deficiency

In the older literature, studies dealing with nutritional deficiencies, including tryptophan deficiency, utilized foodstuffs that were fed *ad libitum* to animals. It readily became apparent from such experiments that animals offered diets deficient in one of many essential food constituents consumed progressively less food and, thereby, showed increasing evidence of undernutrition. This was in contrast to the control animals, which consumed much food and gained weight. After weeks or months, the experimental and control animals differed markedly in body weight. Comparisons made under such conditions were difficult to evaluate, since the experimental animals were undernourished owing to inadequate food intake as well as to the effects of the specific dietary deficiency.

In an attempt to overcome the marked variations between the control and experimental groups in *ad libitum* feeding experiments, the technique of pair-feeding was introduced. By pair-feeding, animals on the adequate control diet could be restricted daily to the same total food intake as that of the deficient animals, but such restricted controls tended to consume the limited amount of food quickly and thus starved for the most of the day. Also, the pair-fed controls became undernourished and gained less weight than unrestricted controls. One could compare control undernourished animals fed a controlled limited intake of a good diet with experimental undernourished animals fed a voluntarily restricted intake of a deficient diet. Such studies, of necessity, introduced the undesired variable of undernutrition in both the control and experimental animals.

In an attempt to overcome the problems described above, some investigators resorted to using a force-feeding or tube-feeding technique.[44–47] Purified and synthetic diets could be suspended or dissolved in water, and controlled volumes of complete and deficient diets could be administered via stomach tubes. Animals could be tube-fed several times. A number of control studies with adequate diets[45–49] revealed that the force-fed animals gained weight and manifested no pathological alterations that could be attributed to the force-feeding.

On the basis of studies with amino acid deficiencies, including tryptophan deficiency, it became apparent that the drastic reduction in food intake under *ad libitum* conditions radically altered the morphologic reaction patterns of the tissues to the deficient diets. However, this factor was not usually emphasized in investigations on amino acid deficiencies. In early studies, Spector and Adamstone[13] and Van Pilsum et al.[12] described many pathological tissue changes, including periportal fatty liver, within a short time after the onset of force-feeding diets devoid of tryptophan, phenylalanine, or isoleucine. In contrast, many other investigators1,[9,10,50–53] found far fewer specific tissue changes with diets deficient in single essential amino acids when these were fed *ad libitum* for similar or much longer periods of time. Studies by Sidransky and Farber[54–55] and Sidransky and Baba[56] have likewise reported marked differences in the pathological responses in experimental animals if the same amino acid-deficient diets were fed *ad libitum* or force-fed.

2.4   Concluding Comments

This chapter has reviewed experimental studies designed to determine the effects of feeding animals diets deficient in L-tryptophan. The findings based upon short- and long-term feeding experiments using a variety of deficient diets fed under *ad libitum,* pair-feeding, and force-feeding conditions reveal a number of interesting pathological findings in a number of different organs. The variability in the experimental conditions must be kept in mind when interpreting the significance of the findings. Yet, the results clearly indicate that L-tryptophan is essential for growth and nitrogen balance, and in its absence or in cases of inadequate intake, a number of pathological consequences (morphological, biochemical, and neuropsychiatric) occur. However, since deficiencies of other indispensable amino acids likewise induce a similar variety of pathological changes, it is difficult to attach specific significance to the findings with tryptophan deficiency. Possibly, the finding of cataract formation is special for tryptophan deficiency. Thus, the numerous experimental studies with tryptophan-deficient diets serve to emphasize that specific amino acid deficiencies induce pathological changes that are generally similar to those induced by protein (poor quantity or quality) deficiency. Conceivably, ingestion of a diet deficient or devoid of a single amino acid induces an imbalanced state of amino acids, which leads to pathological changes as occurs with dietary protein deficiency.

References

1. Totter, J. R. and Day, P. L., Cataract and other ocular changes resulting from tryptophane deficiency, *J. Nutr.,* 24, 159, 1942.
2. Ferraro, A. and Roizin, L., Ocular involvement in rats on diets deficient in amino acids. I. Tryptophan, *Arch. Ophthalmol.,* 38, 331, 1947.
3. Sydenstricker, V. P., Hall, W. K., Bowles, L. L., and Schmidt, H. L., Jr., The corneal vascularization resulting from deficiencies of amino acids in the rat, *J. Nutr.,* 34, 481, 1947.
4. Ohrloff, C., Stoffel, C., Koch, H. R., Wefers, U., Bours, J., and Hockwin, O., Experimental cataracts in rats due to tryptophan-free diet, *Albrecht Von Graefes Archiv. Klinisch. Exper. Ophthalmol.,* 205, 73, 1978.
5. Von Sallman, L., Reid, M. E., Grimes, P. A., and Collins, E. M., Tryptophan-deficiency cataract in guinea pigs, *Arch. Ophthalmol.,* 62, 662, 1959.
6. Van Heyningen, R., Experimental studies on cataract, *Invest. Ophthalmol.,* 15, 685, 1976.
7. McAvoy, J. W., Palfrey, L. J., and van Heyningen, R., A light microscope study of the lens of the tryptophan deficient rat, *Exp. Eye Res.,* 28, 533, 1979.
8. Albanese, A. A., Holt, L. E., Jr., Kajdi, C. N., and Frankston, J. E., Observations on tryptophane deficiency in rats. Chemical and morphological changes in the blood, *J. Biol. Chem.,* 148, 299, 1943.
9. Cole, A. S. and Scott, P. P., Tissue changes in the adult tryptophan-deficient rat, *Br. J. Nutr.,* 89, 125, 1954.
10. Scott, E. B., Histopathology of amino acid deficiencies. IV. Tryptophan, *Am. J. Pathol.,* 31, 1111, 1955.
11. Adamstone, F. B. and Spector, H., Tryptophan deficiency in the rat. Histologic changes induced by forced feeding of an acid hydrolyzed casein diet, *Arch. Pathol.,* 49, 173, 1950.

12. Van Pilsum, J. F., Speyer, J. F., and Samuels, L. T., Essential amino acid deficiency and enzyme activity, *Arch. Biochem.*, 68, 42, 1957.

13. Spector, H. and Adamstone, F. B., Tryptophan deficiency in the rat induced by forced feeding of an acid hydrolyzed casein diet, *J. Nutr.*, 40, 213, 1950.

14. Samuels, L. T., Goldthorpe, H. C., and Dougherty, T. F., Metabolic effects of specific amino acid deficiencies, *Fed. Proc.*, 10, 393, 1951.

15. Bailey, R. P., Vrooman, M. J., Sawai, Y., Tsukada, K., Short, K., and Lieberman, I., Amino acids and control of nucleolar size, the activity of RNA polymerase I, and DNA synthesis in liver, *Proc. Nat. Acad. Sci.*, 73, 3201, 1976.

16. Kloppel, T. M. and Post, G., Histological alterations in tryptophan-deficient rainbow trout, *J. Nutr.*, 105, 861, 1975.

17. Poston, H. A. and Rumsey, G. L., Factors affecting dietary requirement and deficiency signs of L-tryptophan in rainbow trout, *J. Nutr.*, 113, 2568, 1983.

18. Sidransky, H., Chemical and cellular pathology of experimental acute amino acid deficiency, *Meth. Achie. Exp. Pathol.*, 6,1, 1972.

19. Deo, M. G. and Ramalingaswami, V., Production of periportal fatty infiltration of liver in rhesus monkey by protein-deficient diet, *Lab. Invest.*, 9, 319, 1960.

20. Sidransky, H. and Verney, E., Enhanced hepatic protein synthesis in rats force-fed a tryptophan-devoid diet, *Proc. Soc. Exp. Biol. Med.*, 135, 618, 1970.

21. Fleck, A., Shepherd, J., and Munro, H. N., Protein synthesis in rat liver. Influence of amino acids in diet on microsomes and polysomes, *Science*, 150, 628, 1965.

22. Wunner, W. H., Bell, J., and Munro, H. N., The effect of feeding with a tryptophan-free amino acid mixture on rat liver polysomes and ribosomal ribonucleic acid, *Biochem. J.*, 101, 417, 1966.

23. Sidransky, H., Sarma, D. S. R., Bongiorno, M., and Verney, E., Effect of dietary tryptophan on hepatic polyribosomes and protein synthesis in fasted mice, *J. Biol. Chem.*, 24, 1123, 1968.

24. Sox, H. C., Jr. and Hoagland, M. B., Functional alterations in rat liver polysomes associated with starvation and refeeding, *J. Mol. Biol.*, 20, 113, 1966.

25. Staehelin, T., Verney, E., and Sidransky, H., The influence of nutritional change on polyribosomes of the liver, *Biochim. Biophys. Acta*, 145, 105, 1967.

26. Webb, T. E., Blobel, G., and Potter, V. R., Polyribosomes in rat tissues. III. The response of the polyribosome pattern of rat liver to physiologic stress, *Cancer Res.*, 26, 253, 1966.

27. Wilson, S. H. and Hoagland, M. B., Physiology of rat-liver polysomes. The stability of messenger ribonucleic acid and ribosomes, *Biochem. J.*, 102, 556, 1967.

28. Pronezuk, A. W., Baliga, B. S., Triant, J. W., and Munro, H. N., Comparison of the effect of amino acid supply on hepatic polysome profiles *in vivo* and *in vitro*, *Biochim. Biophys. Acta*, 157, 204, 1968.

29. Cammarano, P., Chinali, G., Gaeteni, S., and Spandoni, M. A., Involvement of adrenal steroids in the changes of polysome organization during feeding of imbalanced amino acid diets, *Biochim. Biophys. Acta*, 155, 302, 1968.

30. Rothschild, M. A., Oratz, M., Mongelli, J., Fishman, L., and Schreiber, S. S., Amino acid regulation of albumin synthesis, *J. Nutr.*, 98, 395, 1969.

31. Jones, M. L., Kimbrough, T. D., and Weekley, L. B., Disturbances of tryptophan metabolism in mice acutely deprived of tryptophan, *Ann. Nutr. Metab.*, 29, 209, 1985.

32. Patrich, H. and Bennington, L. K., Biochemical changes in the rat produced by feeding a tryptophan deficient ration, *Proc. West. VA Acad. Sci.*, 41, 161, 1969.
33. Wilfred, G. and Sekhara Varma, T. N., The mechanism of hepatic fatty infiltration in acute threonine deficiency, *Biochim. Biophys. Acta*, 187, 442, 1969.
34. Sidransky, H., Wagle, D. S., Bongiorno, M., and Verney, E., Chemical pathology of acute amino acid deficiencies. Studies on hepatic enzymes in rats force-fed a threonine-devoid diet, *J. Nutr.*, 100, 678, 1970.
35. Lombardi, B., Considerations on the pathogenesis of fatty liver, *Lab. Invest.*, 15, 1, 1966.
36. Dianzani, M. U., Biochemical aspects of fatty liver, *Biochem. Soc. Trans.*, 1, 903, 1973.
37. Lyman, R. L., and Wilcox, S. S., Effect of acute amino acid deficiencies on carcass composition and pancreatic function in the force-fed rat. I. Efficiencies of valine, lysine, tryptophan, leucine, and isoleucine, *J. Nutr.*, 79, 37, 1963.
38. Singh, M., Effect of niacin and niacin-tryptophan deficiency on pancreatic acinar cell function in rats *in vitro*, *Am. J. Clin. Nutr.*, 44, 512, 1986.
39. Carew, L. B., Jr., Alster, F. A., Foss, D. C., and Scanes, C. G., Effect of a tryptophan deficiency on thyroid gland, growth hormone and testicular functions in children, *J. Nutr.*, 113, 1756, 1983.
40. Koch, H. R., Ohrloff, C., Bours, J., Riemann, C., Dragomirescu, V., and Hockwin, O., Separation of lens proteins in rats with tryptophan deficiency cataracts, *Exp. Eye Res.*, 34, 479, 1982.
41. GáL, E. M. and Dreves, P. A., Studies on the metabolism of 5-hydroxy-tryptamin (serotonin). II. Effect of tryptophan deficiency in rats, *Proc. Soc. Exptl. Biol. Med.*, 110, 368, 1962.
42. Fernstrom, J. D. and Wurtman, R. J., Brain serotonin content: Physiological dependence on plasma tryptophan levels, *Science*, 173, 149, 1971.
43. Fernstrom, J. D. and Wurtman, R. J., Brain serotonin content: Physiological regulation of plasma neutral amino acids, *Science*, 178, 414, 1972.
44. Shay, H. and Gruenstein, M., A simple and safe method for the gastric instillation of fluids in the rat, *J. Lab. Clin. Med.*, 31, 1384, 1946.
45. Denton, A. E., Williams, J. N., Jr., and Elvehjem, C. A., Methionine deficiency under *ad libitum* and force-feeding conditions, *J. Nutr.*, 42, 423, 1950.
46. Bothwell, J. W. and Williams, J. N., Jr., A study of histidine deficiency and nitrogen balance under *ad libitum* and force-feeding conditions, *J. Nutr.*, 45, 245, 1951.
47. Bothwell, J. W. and Williams, J. N., Jr., A study of lysine deficiency and nitrogen balance under *ad libitum* and force-feeding conditions, *J. Nutr.*, 47, 375, 1952.
48. Forbes, R. M. and Vaughan, L., Nitrogen balance of young albino rats force-fed methionine- or histidine-deficient diet, *J. Nutr.*, 52, 25, 1954.
49. Greenstein, J. P., Birnbaum, S. M., Winitz, M., and Otey, M. C., Quantitative nutritional studies with water-soluble, chemically defined diets. I. Growth, reproduction and lactation in rats, *Arch. Biochem.*, 72, 396, 1957.
50. Cannon, P. R., *Some Pathologic Consequences of Protein and Amino Acid Deficiencies*, Charles C Thomas, Springfield, IL, 1948.
51. Follis, R. H., Jr., *Deficiency Disease*, Charles C Thomas, Springfield, IL, 1958.
52. David, H., *Die Leber bei Nahrungsmangel und Mangelernährung*, Akademie Verlag, Berlin, 1961.
53. Sós, J., *Die Pathologie der Eiweissernährung*, Verlag der Ungarischen Akademie der Wissenschaften, Budapest, 1964.

54. Sidransky, H. and Farber, E., Chemical pathology of acute amino acid deficiencies. I. Morphologic changes in immature rats fed threonine-methionine-, or histidine-devoid diets, *Arch. Path.*, 66, 119, 1958.
55. Sidransky, H. and Farber, E., Chemical pathology of acute amino acid deficiencies. II. Biochemical changes in rats fed threonine- or methionine-devoid diets, *Arch. Path.*, 66, 135, 1958.
56. Sidransky, H. and Baba, T., Chemical pathology of acute amino acid deficiencies. III. Morphologic and biochemical changes in young rats fed valine- or lysine-devoid diets, *J. Nutr.*, 70, 463, 1960.

3

Genetics

CONTENTS

3.1 Biochemical Genetics of Tryptophan Synthesis

Genetic and biochemical techniques have been utilized in studying the regulation of tryptophan biosynthesis in prokaryotes, specifically in *Escherichia coli*. The emerging picture is that the *trp* aporepressor is the product of the *trpR* gene located at 0 min on the *E. coli* genetic map.[1] On binding with L-tryptophan, the *trp* aporepressor forms the active complex or *trp* repressor, which in turn is able to bind with high affinity at the DNA operator sites of the three operons it regulates. Besides the two operons, *trp* EDCBA and *aro* H, which encode six enzymes essential for the biosynthesis of L-tryptophan itself, the third operon, namely, *trpR*, encodes the *trp* aporepressor protein.[2-4] The *trp* aporepressor is composed of a single polypeptide of 108 residues with a molecular weight of about 12,356, as is apparent from the DNA sequence of the gene.[5]

In studying the biochemical genetics of tryptophan synthesis in *Pseudomonas acidovorans*, Buvinger et al.[6] isolated 60 independent tryptophan auxotrophs of *Pseudomonas acidovorans* and characterized them for nutritional response to intermediates of the pathway, accumulation of intermediates, and levels of tryptophan-synthetic enzymes. Mutants for each of the seven proteins catalyzing the five steps of tryptophan synthesis were obtained. Transductional analysis established three unlinked chromosomal regions: *trp*E, *trp*GDC, and *trp*FBA. The levels and enzymatic activities of wild-type and mutant strains indicated that *trp*E and *trp*GDC were repressed by tryptophan. In contrast, *trp*FBA was not derepressed significantly by starvation for tryptophan. The *trp*G mutants had an additional requirement for p-aminobenzoate, which suggested that anthranilate synthase subunit II also served as glutamine-binding protein in the analogous reaction catalyzed by p-aminobenzoate synthase. In addition, *trp*D mutants revealed the ability of *P. acidovorans* to degrade anthranilate via the beta-ketoadipate pathway.

Two DNA fragments (3941 and 7152 base pairs) from the prokaryotic endosymbiont (*Buchnera*) of the aphid *Schlechtendalia chinensis* were cloned and sequenced.[7] The smaller fragment contained trpEG, and the larger fragment contained trpDC(F)BA, genes coding for enzymes of the tryptophan biosynthetic pathway which convert chorismate to tryptophan. Both of these gene clusters were present as one copy of the endosymbiont chromosome and probably constitute two transcription units. The deduced amino acid sequences of the proteins was 51 to 61%, identical to the corresponding proteins previously studied in *Buchnera* of the aphid *Schizaphis graminum*. In this endosymbiont, *trp*EG is amplified and located on a plasmid, whereas, in the endosymbiont of *S. chinensis*, as in other eubacteria, *trp*EG occurs as a single copy on the bacterial chromosome.

In contrast to prokaryotes, in mammals, tryptophan is not synthesized in the body and, therefore, must be provided through a dietary source. The essential amino acid is not only a building block of proteins but also a precursor of serotonin and of the nicotinamide ring of NAD^+.

3.2   Biochemical Genetics of Tryptophan 2,3-Dioxygenase

In considering genetic aspects of L-tryptophan, it probably is best to consider the molecular genetics of L-tryptophan 2,3-dioxygenase (EC 1.13.1.12), the enzyme which catalyzes the first reaction in the major catabolic route of L-tryptophan. In another section the action and control of this enzyme are discussed.

Schmid et al.[8] isolated the tryptophan oxygenase gene from rats. Identification of a DNA clone from a rat liver cDNA library was achieved by hybridizing rat liver mRNA to pools of clones, and subsequently identifying specifically bound tryptophan oxygenase mRNA by precipitation of *in vitro* translated tryptophan oxygenase enzyme with a specific antibody against the enzyme. With such a cDNA, genomic DNA clones could be identified and isolated. Progress in the molecular genetics of tryptophan oxygenase in rat liver up to 1986 was reviewed by Renkawitz.[9]

Subsequently, reports have characterized the tryptophan oxygenase gene of *Anopheles gambiae.*[10,11] In the rat, nucleotide sequence (3.2 kb) of a DNA region located approximately between introns 4 and 7 of the rat tryptophan oxygenase gene was determined.[12] Using filter binding studies and monoclonal antibodies against the glucocorticoid receptor, a high affinity binding of this region to the glucocorticoid receptor was demonstrated. Also, in rat liver, expression of the gene coding for tryptophan oxygenase (TO) is switched on at about 2 weeks after birth.[13] Two clusters of DNAse I hypersensitive (HS) sites in the TO gene upstream region, one near the promoter and the other at a distant upstream location (-8.5 kb), were described. Hypersensitivity of upstream sites was present in adult and in 7-day-old rat liver but absent in kidney. To investigate the role of these sites in transcriptional regulation, a reporter gene controlled by both HS site regions was used to generate transgenic mice. In these animals the transgene followed the cell-specific and developmental regulation of the endogenous gene, inactive after birth and active in adult liver. Transgenes containing only the promoter proximal HS site were nonfunctional.

Nuclear proteins that specifically bind to the regulatory region of rat liver tryptophan oxygenase have been reported.[14] Using electrophoretic mobility shift assay, the binding of rat liver nuclear proteins to the fragments from −466 to −292 and from −292 to −178 relative to the transcriptional start site of the rat tryptophan oxygenase gene were observed. Studies of the competition with a synthetic consensus sequence for the NF 1 recognition site have shown that the liver nuclear proteins responsible for the formation of specific complexes with these fragments belong to the family of the nuclear factor 1 (NF 1). The *trans*-acting factors of the NF 1 family form several complexes with each of the two tested fragments of the tryptophan oxygenase gene. Investigation of transcription factors that bind to DNA from the −292nd to the −178th nucleotide of gene *in vitro* indicate that this DNA region contains a site corresponding to the constitutive DNAse I hypersensitive site *in vivo*.[15] Using electrophoretic mobility shift assay, binding of rat liver proteins to this DNA region was analyzed. NF 1-rich nuclear protein fraction was purified from the rat liver nuclear extract by DEAE-cellulose and heparin-sepharose chromatography. Studies of the competition with a consensus sequence site for NF 1 recognition sites have shown that it is the NF 1 family transcription factors that are responsible for the formation of these specific complexes.

A human tryptophan oxygenase clone was isolated by screening a liver cDNA library with a rat tryptophan oxygenase cDNA clone.[16] Analysis showed extensive homology between the rat and the human DNA and protein sequences. The combined use of cell hybrids and *in situ* hybridization indicated that human tryptophan oxygenase was localized to chromosome band 4q31. The tryptophan oxygenase gene has been considered to be important in some human behavior disorders, especially those associated with abnormalities of serotonin metabolism.

3.3   Species and Strain Differences in Tryptophan Metabolism and in Responses to Tryptophan Administration

3.3.1   Species Differences

Fujigaki et al.[17] reported on species differences in tryptophan-kynurenine pathway metabolism by quantitative studies of anthranilic acid (AA) and its related enzymes. Serum and cerebrospinal fluid (CSF) AA concentrations in different animal species were measured using reversed-phase high-performance liquid chromatography with electrochemical detection. CF AA concentrations in rabbits were 5.7 to 33.0 times lower than those in other species studied, including rat, mice, and gerbils. However, serum AA concentrations were slightly higher in rabbits than in the other species. In contrast, the concentrations of L-kynurenine in both serum and CSF were substantially higher in rabbits than in the other species. Tissue kynurenine pathway enzymes, indolamine 2,3-dioxygenase (IDO), tryptophan 2,3-dioxygenase, kynurenine 3-hydroxylase, and kynureninase were determined in rabbits, rats, gerbils, and mice, and these enzymes varied among species. Lung IDO activities in rabbits were 146 to 516 times higher than those found in the other species, but rabbit liver kynurenine 3-hydroxylase activities were lower by one order of magnitude than those of the other species tested. Furthermore, brain kynurenine 3-hydroxylasae activities were 12.3 to 23.2 times higher in gerbils than in the other species tested.

Pranzatelli et al.[18] measured seven serotonin (5-HT) receptor binding sites and the 5-HT uptake site in guinea pig brainstem and compared them to the rat. In guinea pig brainstem, the rank order of binding site density was 5-HT transporter site > 5-HT1D > antagonist-labeled 5-HT2 > 5-HT1A, 5-HT1C > 5-HT1E > agonist-labeled 5-HT2 binding site. There were fewer 5-HT1A and 5-HT1C binding sites and 5-HT uptake sites in guinea pig than rat brainstem, and there were more 5-HT1D and antagonist-labeled 5-HT2 sites, but the differences were two-fold or less. The major species difference was that 5-HT1B sites were virtually undetectable in guinea pig brainstem. Limited competition experiments with related 5-HT receptor subtype-selective agonists and antagonists suggested that the sites in guinea pig brainstem conformed to those described in the rat.

Sidransky and Verney[19] reported that the *in vitro* nuclear binding affinity for L-tryptophan of livers of hamsters was significantly less than that of livers of guinea pigs or mice (Swiss). In general, the basal nuclear-specific binding affinity to L-tryptophan of the species of animals used correlated with the degree of stimulatory effect on hepatic protein synthesis (high in mice and low in hamsters) by tube-feeding L-tryptophan 1 h before killing compared to that of animals tube-fed water.

3.3.2 Strain Differences

Costa et al.[20] reported on strain differences of rats in the urinary excretion of the tryptophan metabolites along the kynurenine pathway and the variations of enzyme activities metabolizing the tryptophan in different strains of rats. While there was a good correlation between urinary excretory values of the metabolites and enzyme activities in the same strain of rats, some differences appeared when the data were compared among different strains. Wistar, heterozygous Gunn, and Sprague-Dawley rats showed similar total urinary excretion of tryptophan metabolites, while the Long Evans rats had significantly lower values, in accordance with the lower activity of tryptophan oxygenase. Kynureninase activity was slightly but not significantly higher in Sprague-Dawley rats, in agreement with the high levels of anthranilic acid excreted. Regarding kynurenine aminotransferase, Sprague-Dawley rats showed lower activity in the liver, but higher activity in the kidneys in comparison to other strains of Wistar, Long Evans, and heterozygous Gunn rats.

Knapp et al.[21] reported that the levels of forebrain tryptophan, serotonin (5-HT), 5-hydroxyindoleacetic acid (5-HIAA), and hydroxylase cofactor (BH4) were comparable in two experimental mouse strains (A/J and C57B1/6J), despite two- to three-fold differences *in vitro* in the relative activities of forebrain and midbrain tryptophan-5-monoxygenase. The enzyme activities did not differ with respect to Km for cofactor at saturating levels, but manifested different degrees of cooperativity with respect to cofactor when examined with BH4 concentrations within a physiological range.

Strain differences in the activity of tryptophan hydroxylase, the rate-limiting enzyme in serotonin biosynthesis, have been reported in rats[22,23] and in mice.[24] Chaouloff et al.[22] reported that the activity of tryptophan hydroxylase was decreased in Lewis rats compared with Fisher 344 rats. Kulikov et al.[23] reported that *in vitro* central tryptophan hydroxylase activity was higher in the Lewis strain of rats than in spontaneously hypertensive rats. In mice, Knapp and Mandell[24] reported that midbrain tryptophan hydroxylase from two behaviorally different mouse strains, C57B1/6J and A/J, had different stabilities and regulatory properties.

It has been reported that $NZBWF_1$ mice, routinely used as a model of systemic lupus erythematous,[25,26] have less affinity for L-tryptophan binding to hepatic nuclei than do other mice strains (Swiss, DBA, SJL, and BALB/c).[27] This decreased binding affinity of $NZBWF_1$ mice appears to correlate with the decreased effect of L-tryptophan administration on hepatic protein synthesis as compared to Swiss mice.[27] Also, hepatic nuclei of $NZBWF_1$ mice revealed a significantly decreased binding response of ^3H-tryptophan in comparison to those of Swiss mice when nuclei of both groups were affected by Showa Denko L-tryptophan (implicated in eosinophilia-myalgia syndrome) or to its contaminants, 1,1'-ethylidenebis-(tryptophan) and 3-phenylamino-L-alanine, in contrast to that of control nonimplicated L-tryptophan.[28]

In rats, a decrease in the affinity of *in vitro* L-tryptophan binding to hepatic nuclei and nuclear envelopes has been reported in Lewis rats compared with Sprague-Dawley rats.[29] While the K_D values were similar in both rat strains, the B_{max} values were significantly less in Lewis rats compared with Sprague-Dawley rats. Lewis rats are known to be quite susceptible to many inflammatory diseases in response to a wide range of stimuli.[30]

3.3.3   Concluding Remarks

It is apparent from the above reports that differences in tryptophan metabolism and in biological responses to tryptophan exist in certain species and strains of animals. These findings suggest the importance of considering species and strains when evaluating experimental results dealing with tryptophan. These variations need to be considered in various alterations that may occur in humans under normal and pathological conditions. Also, these variations in experimental animals may serve as models offering valuable clues to the pathogenesis of disease states relating to or involving L-tryptophan.

3.4   General Comments

In considering nutrients and gene expression, many investigators have used a molecular approach to establish that certain micro- and macronutrients affect cell function through changes in gene expression. Such effects can alter cell metabolism, growth, or differentiation. Among the micronutrients, vitamins A and D have been reported to have important effects on metabolism/growth and whole body calcium homeostasis, respectively. Derivatives of these micronutrients alter cell function by binding to intracellular receptors that interact with promoters of specific genes. Such interaction leads to changes in gene expression and subsequent changes in cell function. Among the macronutrients, cholesterol can best be cited as an example of macronutrient control of gene expression (dietary cholesterol and fat regulation of cholesterol and lipid homeostasis). Based upon existing background information about L-tryptophan, there is great need for in-depth investigation into how this indispensable amino acid may affect gene expression in health and disease. Such research will be rewarding.

References

1. Bachmann, B. J. and Low, K. B., Linkage map of *Escherichia coli* K-12, edition 6, *Microbiol. Rev.*, 44, 1, 1980.

2. Platt, T., Regulation of gene expression in the tryptophan operon of *Escherichia coli*, in *The Operon*, Miller, J. H. and Reznikoff, W. S., Eds., Cold Spring Harbor Laboratory, Cold Spring Harbor, NY, 1980, 2, 263–302.

3. Crawford, I. P. and Stauffer, G. V., Regulation of tryptophan biosynthesis, *Annu. Rev. Biochem.*, 49, 163, 1980.

4. Somerville, R. L., Tryptophan: Biosynthesis, regulation, and large-scale production, in *Amino Acid Biosynthesis and Genetic Regulation*, Herrmann, K. M. and Somerville, R. L., Eds., Addison-Wesley, Reading, MA, 1983, 351–378.

5. Gunsalus, R. P. and Yanofsky, C., Nucleotide sequence and expression of *Escherichia coli TrpR*, the structural gene for the trp aporepressor, *Proc. Natl. Acad. Sci., USA*, 77, 7117, 1980.

6. Buvinger, W. E., Stone, L. C., and Heath, H. E., Biochemical genetics of tryptophan synthesis in *Pseudomonas acidovorans*, *J. Bact.*, 147, 62, 1981.

7. Lai, C. Y., Baumann, P., and Moran, N. A., Genetics of the tryptophan biosynthetic pathway of the prokaryotic endosymbiont (Buchnera) of the aphid *Schlechtendalia chinensis*, *Insect Mol. Biol.*, 4, 47, 1995.

8. Schmid, W., Scherer, G., Danesch, U., Zentgraf, H., Matthias, P., Strange, C. M., Rowekamp, W., and Schutz, G., Isolation and characterization of the rat tryptophan oxygenase gene, *EMBO J.*, 1, 1287, 1982.

9. Renkawitz, R., Molecular genetics of L-tryptophan 2,3-dioxygenase in rat liver, in *Progress in Tryptophan and Serotonin Research 1986*, Bender, D. A., Joseph, M. H., Kochen, W., and Steinhart, H., Eds., Walter de Gruyter, Berlin, 1987, 1–6.

10. Mukabayire, O., Cornel, A. J., Dotson, E. M., Collins, F. H., and Besansky, N. J., The tryptophan oxygenase gene of *Anopheles gambiae*, *Insect Biochem. Mol. Biol.*, 26, 525, 1996.

11. Besansky, N. J., Mukabayire, O., Benedict, M. Q., Rafferty, C. S., Hamm, D. M., and McNitt, L., The *Anopheles gambiae* tryptophan oxygenase gene expressed from a baculovirus promoter complements *Drosophilia melanogaster vermilion*, *Insect Biochem. Mol. Biol.*, 27, 803, 1997.

12. Merkulov, V. M. and Merkulova, T. I., Nucleotide sequence of a fragment of the rat tryptophan oxygenase gene showing high affinity to glucocorticoid receptor *in vitro*, *Biochim. Biophys. Acta*, 1132, 100, 1992.

13. Kaltschmidt, C., Muller, M., Brem, G., and Renkawitz, R., DNAse I hypersensitive sites far upstream of the rat tryptophan oxygenase gene direct developmentally regulated transcription in livers of transgenic mice, *Mech. Dev.*, 45, 203, 1994.

14. Chikhirzhina, G. I., Fedorova, S. A., Chespokov, I. N., and Romanovskaia, E. V., Nuclear proteins, specifically binding the regulatory region of rat tryptophan oxygenase, *Biokhimiia*, 58, 392, 1993.

15. Chikhirzhina, G. I., Romanovskaia, E. V., Nazarova, N. Iu., and Fedorova, S. A., Interaction of the regulatory region of the tryptophan oxygenase gene with transcription factors of the nuclear factor 1 (NF 1) family, *Tsitologiia*, 41, 939, 1999.

16. Comings, D. E., Muhleman, D., Dietz, G. W., Jr., and Donlon, T., Human tryptophan oxygenase localized to 4q31: Possible implications for alcoholism and other behavioral disorders, *Genomics*, 9, 301, 1991.

17. Fujigaki, S., Saito, K., Takemura, M., Fujii, H., Wada, H., Noma, A., and Seishima, M., Species differences in L-tryptophan-kynurenine pathway metabolism: Quantification of anthranilic acid and its related enzymes, *Arch. Biochem. Biophys.*, 358, 329, 1998.

18. Pranzatelli, M. R., Tailor, P. T., and Razi, P., Brainstem serotonin receptors in the guinea pig: Implications for myoclonus, *Neuropharmacology,* 32, 209, 1993.
19. Sidransky, H. and Verney, E., L-tryptophan binding to hepatic nuclei: Age and species differences, *Amino Acids,* 12, 77, 1997.
20. Costa, C., De Antoni, A., Baccichetti, F., Vanzan, S., Appodia, M., and Allegri, G., Strain differences in the tryptophan metabolite excretion and enzyme activities along the kynurenine pathway in rats, *Ital. J. Biochem.,* 31, 412, 1982.
21. Knapp, S., Mandell, A. J., Russo, P. V., Vitto, A., and Stewart, K. D., Strain differences in kinetic and thermal stability of two mouse brain tryptophan hydroxylase activities, *Brain Res.,* 230, 317, 1981.
22. Chaouloff, F., Kulikov, A., Sarrieau, A., Castanon, N., and Mormede, P., Male Fischer 344 and Lewis rats display differences in locomotor reactivity, but not in anxiety-related behaviours: Relationship with the hippocampal serotonergic system, *Brain Res.,* 693, 169, 1995.
23. Kulikov, A., Aguerre, S., Berton, O., Ramos, A., Mormede, P., and Chaouloff, E., Central serotonergic systems in the spontaneously hypertensive and Lewis rat strains that differ in the elevated plus-maze test of anxiety, *J. Pharmacol. Exp. Ther.,* 281, 775, 1997.
24. Knapp, S. and Mandell, A. J., Mouse midbrain tryptophan hydroxylase: Strain differences in variational properties, *J. Physiol.,* 77, 281, 1981.
25. Hirose, S., Nakanishi, K., Yoshimoto, T., Kashiwamura, S., Hiroishi, K., Matsumoto, H., Hamaoka, T., Shenka, S., and Higoshino, K., Identification and characterization of 1L-2-hyper-responsive NZB/WF_1 CD5-B cells, *J. Immunol.,* 15, 1847, 1994.
26. Wantanabe, Y., Yoshida, S. H., Ansari, A. A., and Gershwin, M. E., The contribution of H-2bm12 and non-H-2 background genes on murine lupus in NZB. H-2bm12b mice, *J. Autoimmun.,* 7, 153, 1994.
27. Sidransky, H. and Verney, E., Differences in tryptophan binding to hepatic nuclei of $NZBWF_1$ and Swiss mice: Insight into mechanism of tryptophan's effects, *J. Nutr.,* 127, 270, 1997.
28. Sidransky, H. and Verney, E., Mouse strain and source of L-tryptophan affects hepatic nuclear tryptophan binding, *Toxicology,* 118, 37, 1997.
29. Sidransky, H. and Verney, E., Comparative studies on tryptophan binding to hepatic nuclear envelopes in Sprague-Dawley and Lewis rats, *Am. J. Physiol.,* 267(36), R502, 1994.
30. Sternberg, E. M., Hill, J. M., Chrousos, G. P., Kamilaris, T., Listnvak, S. J., Gold, P. W., and Wilder, R. L., Inflammatory mediator-induced hypothalamic-pituitary-adrenal axis activation in defective streptococcal cell wall arthritis-susceptible Lewis rats, *Proc. Natl. Acad. Sci. USA,* 86, 2374, 1989.

4

Chemical Pathways, Protein Metabolism, and Interrelationships

CONTENTS

4.1   Introduction

This chapter discusses the pathways by which L-tryptophan is metabolized into a variety of metabolites, many of which have important physiological functions. A few metabolites are cited here briefly. Quinolinic acid is involved in the regulation of gluconeogenesis. Picolinic acid is involved in normal intestinal absorption of zinc. The body's pool of nicotinamide adenine dinucleotide (NAD) is influenced by L-tryptophan's metabolic conversion to niacin. Finally, L-tryptophan is the precursor of several neuroactive compounds, the most important of which is serotonin (5-HT), which participates as a neurochemical substrate for a variety of normal behavioral and neuroendocrine functions. Serotonin derived from L-tryptophan allows it to become involved in behavioral effects, reflecting altered central nervous system function under conditions that alter tryptophan nutrition and metabolism.

Since L-tryptophan is an indispensable amino acid, its role as a substrate for protein synthesis is necessarily of much importance. However, L-tryptophan has other roles that are vital in maintaining normal physiological functions. For example, L-tryptophan has been reported to play a unique role in regulating protein synthesis, particularly in the liver, but also in other organs in a manner unrelated to its function as a precursor amino acid. This action of L-tryptophan is reviewed in this chapter.

Also, L-tryptophan has important interrelationships with a number of components: blood albumin, other amino acids, and vitamins. These interrelationships are also reviewed in this chapter.

4.2   Chemical Pathways

Tryptophan appears to be converted to a larger number of metabolites than any of the other amino acids. The degradation of tryptophan in animals occurs mainly in two pathways, I and II (Figure 4.1). The first major pathway (I), initiated by the action of tryptophan dioxygenase, involves oxidation of tryptophan to N-formylkynurenine and the formation of a series of intermediates and byproducts, most of which appear in varying amounts in the urine, the sum of which accounts for the total metabolism of tryptophan, approximately. The second pathway (II) involves hydroxylation of tryptophan to 5-hydroxytryptophan and decarboxylation of this compound to 5-hydroxytryptamine (serotonin), a potent vasoconstrictor found particularly in the brain, intestinal tissues, blood platelets, and mast cells. A small percentage (3%) of dietary tryptophan is metabolized via the pathway (III) to indoleacetic acid. Other minor pathways also exist in animal tissues.

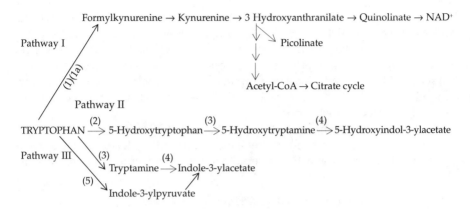

FIGURE 4.1

Pathways of tryptophan metabolism in the rat. Enzymes include (1) tryptophan dioxygenase (EC 1.13.11.11), (1a) indoleamine dioxygenase, (2) tryptophan 5-monooxygenase (EC 1.14.16.1), (3) aromatic L-amino acid decarboxylase (EC 4.1.1.28), (4) monoamine oxidase (EC 1.4.3.4), (5) tryptophan aminotransferase (EC 2.6.1.27).

Among its physiological and biochemical functions, tryptophan is a precursor of NAD (Figure 4.1).[1] Tryptophan, ingested via the portal vein, affects many processes in the liver, RNA synthesis, gluconeogenesis, and the induction of many enzymes. These aspects of tryptophan's action are covered in other sections.

4.2.1   Importance of enzymes

4.2.1.1   Degradative Enzymes

Figure 4.1 reveals a number of enzymes that are directly involved at different steps in the catabolism of tryptophan.

For many years tryptophan dioxygenase was considered a very important enzyme in the kynurenine-niacin pathway. The induction of liver tryptophan dioxygenase by glucocorticoids and stabilization by elevated tryptophan levels were utilized in explaining elevated metabolite levels in a variety of conditions. This enzyme will be discussed in greater detail in another section.

From 1978 to 1985 renewed interest in tryptophan metabolism via the kynurenine-niacin pathway was generated by the findings of Hayaishi et al. and others of a second enzyme, namely, indoleamine-2,3-dioxygenase (IDO).[2,3] This enzyme was found to be present in several nonhepatic tissues (lung, intestine, brain, and epididymis) and cells (blood monocytes, macrophages, and eosinophils). The enzyme normally has very low activity but is induced to very high activity by stimulation of immune systems with interferon-γ[4–8] or interleukin-2 (cytokines).[9] Thus, inflammatory processes, infections, and immune stimulation that induce interferon-γ could lead to the induction of IDO and enhanced catabolism of tryptophan via the kynurenine pathway.[10,11] IDO has a low K_m and, once induced, can cause very low levels of tryptophan in blood or tissue or cultures. For example, cancer patients treated with interferon-γ or interleukin-2 (which induces interferon-γ) within 24 h showed a marked drop in blood tryptophan levels, while other blood amino acids were unchanged.[9,10,12] At the same time, kynurenine (blood and urine) was elevated.

Liver dioxygenase has a high K_m and is probably active only when levels of tryptophan are high, such as after a meal or a loading dose, but this enzyme is probably not very effective when blood levels of tryptophan are normal.

4.2.1.2 Induction of Enzymes (Primarily in Liver)

Many studies have demonstrated that the administration of tryptophan causes an enhancement in the activity of a variety of liver enzymes. Table 4.1 summarizes a number of hepatic enzymes that have reportedly increased in activity due to tryptophan. Tryptophan has been demonstrated to have specific effects on the activities of hormonally and nutritionally sensitive enzymes, many of which are not necessarily related to tryptophan metabolism itself.[13-17] The mechanisms by which tryptophan acts to affect these enzyme levels are not clear. In some instances, there is evidence that the specific regulation by tryptophan involves enzyme degradation rather than synthesis.[15] Deguchi and Barchas[18] suggested that a metabolite, rather than tryptophan itself, may be the actual active component. Such is indeed the case for tryptophan-induced hypoglycemia *in vivo*.[19] In searching for a unifying mechanism, Smith et al.[20] conducted a systematic study involving the activities of a number of tryptophan-sensitive enzymes: tyrosine and tryptophan transaminases, tryptophan dioxygenase, histidase, serine dehydratase, and phosphoenopyruvate carboxykinase. Their conclusion did not support the concept that a single, simple mechanism was responsible for explaining how tryptophan affects enzyme activities. They concluded that a variety of mechanisms must be involved.

In considering the mechanisms by which tryptophan causes an increase in certain hepatic enzymes, Kenney[21] suggested that tryptophan may increase the rates of synthesis of tyrosine aminotransferase, phosphopyruvate carboxylase, and other enzymes indirectly via cyclic AMP (cAMP). Indeed, cAMP will induce these enzymes. Also, Kato[22] indicated that the mechanism of tryptophan-mediated induction of tyrosine aminotransferase includes a cAMP-accumulating process that is sensitive to phentolamine, an adrenergic-blocking agent. Also, Schumm and Webb[23] reported that the addition of physiological concentrations of cAMP stimulated the release of RNA from isolated prelabeled rat liver nuclei to a fortified cytosol in a cell-free system.

TABLE 4.1

Tryptophan-Induced Hepatic Enzymes

Enzyme	Ref.
Alanine aminotransferase	16
Aniline hydroxylase	204
Aspartate aminotransferase	16
Cytochrome b_5	205
Cytochrome P450	204–206
DNA-dependent RNA polymerase (I and II)	16, 79–82
Histidase	13, 20
Indoleamine-2,3-dioxygenase	10, 11
Nitrosodimethylamine demethylase	207
Ornithine σ-transaminase	13, 16, 17
Ornithine decarboxylase	208
Nucleoside triphosphatase	112
Phosphoenolpyruvate carboxykinase	13, 15, 16, 20
Phosphoprotein phosphohydrolase	103
Protein phosphokinase	103
Serine (threonine) dehydratase	13, 16, 20
Tryptophan dioxygenase	14, 16, 20
Tyrosine α-ketoglutarate transaminase	16, 20, 22

4.3   Protein Metabolism

4.3.1   Significance of Tryptophan in Proteins

It is known that tryptophan is a structural amino acid in proteins. However, a number of studies have indicated that specific locations of tryptophan within certain proteins play an essential role in the function of these proteins (or enzymes). An extensive review of some reported functions of tryptophan in proteins was conducted by Brown.[24] Such roles include receptor binding of protein hormones such as insulin-like growth factor-1,[25] human growth hormone,[26] binding of the 2-acyl fatty acid of phospholipids to Annexin V,[27] and receptor binding of 25-hydroxy-vitamin D3.[28] Tryptophan-50 in diphtheria toxin is a major determinant of NAD affinity to this toxin, and replacement of this tryptophan with another amino acid inactivates the toxin.[29] Such nontoxic forms of toxins, as in vaccines, may be of great importance. The importance of Tryptophan-62 in egg white lysozyme for protein-carbohydrate interaction has been reported.[30] A tryptophan residue, Tryptophan-221, is involved with GTP/GDP binding in elongation factor eEF-2 and is important for its function on the ribosome.[31,32] Similarly, Tryptophan-207 in transducin-t*a* is involved in binding of the G-protein activation switch.[33] Binding of the immunosuppressant cyclosporin A to its receptor cyclophylins depends upon a specific tryptophan residue in the receptor.[34] Mouse

P-glycoprotein, involved in multidrug resistance of cancer cells, contains five tryptophan residues, one of which is involved in the function of this protein.[35]

These data indicate that specific tryptophan residues in various proteins may be involved in binding to (1) guanine or adenine nucleotide cofactors, (2) phospholipids, (3) certain glycosides, (4) cyclosporin A, and possibly other xenobiotics, (5) growth hormone, (6) insulin-like growth factor, and (7) vitamin D.

There are numerous reports of binding of the indole ring of tryptophan with adenine or guanine nucleotides and with nucleic acids[36–40] by sharing of π electrons (stacking, charge-transfer complexing). The energy of such associations may be as high as 7 Kcal/mol, i.e., stronger than hydrogen bonds. Thus, it seems likely that exposed tryptophans in certain proteins may function to orient and bind various purine-containing cofactors (e.g., NAD, NADP, FAD, ATP, GTP, etc.) and to bind DNA or RNA. It is also of interest to note that certain proteins have their tryptophan residues concentrated at one end of the protein chain, and that the tryptophan residues are often in a regular, repeating configuration.

In view of the relatively strong binding between tryptophan sidechains and purine bases, it is tempting to speculate that the tryptophan residues in such proteins may be important in orienting and attaching such proteins to nucleic acids of virus nucleic acid cores. Similarly, binding of tryptophan residues to phospholipids[27] may be important in orienting certain receptor proteins in phospholipid membranes of cells. The repeated tryptophan-containing sequences found in prion proteins suggest that these proteins may bind strongly to nucleic acids and that such binding may be important in the as yet unclear mechanism of prion pathogenesis.[41]

Yau et al.[42] reported that one of the ubiquitous features of membrane proteins is the preference of tryptophan and tyrosine residues for membrane surfaces that presumably arise from enhanced stability due to distinct interfacial interactions. Indeed, the presence of tryptophan and tyrosine residues for regions corresponding to membrane surfaces is a remarkable feature shared by 10 or so membrane proteins with known three-dimensional structures.[43]

4.3.2 Protein Synthesis

Tryptophan is one of 20 to 22 amino acids that are required for the synthesis of protein within tissues. Tryptophan is assumed to consist of 1.5% of the total amino acids in tissue protein. Assuming that the adult male at nitrogen equilibrium synthesizes approximately 225 to 250 g of protein daily (approximately 3 g/kg/d), then approximately 3.5 g of tryptophan is utilized daily for protein synthesis. This is of special interest because there is no net accretion of body protein at nitrogen balance. Thus, a large flux of amino acids, including tryptophan, participates in this pathway daily. Actually, the tryptophan involved is much greater than the daily dietary intake of tryptophan and, therefore, must involve protein catabolism, liberating tryptophan. This is probably the most significant pathway in the utilization of tryptophan.

4.3.2.1 Regulatory Role of Tryptophan

Protein synthesis in the whole organism (animal) has been recognized as being sensitive to a variety of nutritional factors, including the pattern and amount of amino acids provided in relation to amino acid requirement (nutritional amino acid balance or imbalance) and the supply and source of energy. During the past 30 to 35 years, many experimental studies have provided information and data that suggest that L-tryptophan has a unique role in the regulation of protein synthesis in a number of organs, such as the liver,[44,45] lung,[46] kidney,[47] gastric mucosa,[48] muscle,[49] and brain.[47,50] Most of these experimental studies have dealt with protein synthesis in liver and have provided information on the vital role of L-tryptophan. It is appropriate that the developments be reviewed chronologically.

From 1965 to 1968, a number of reports described how the livers of fasted animals responded rapidly to a single feeding of good quality protein or of complete amino acids, with enhanced protein synthesis and a shift in poly-ribosomes toward heavier aggregation.[51–58] In general, a good correlation was demonstrated between the protein synthetic ability of cells and tissues and the state of polyribosomal aggregation.[59] Next, investigators determined how animals responded to a single feeding of an incomplete amino acid mixture (a complete amino acid mixture free of single essential amino acids). Such early studies[53,60] revealed that when fasted animals were tube-fed a complete amino acid mixture devoid of single essential amino acids (argin-ine, histidine, isoleucine, leucine, lysine, methionine, phenylalanine, threo-nine, or valine), the overall response was the same as that found after feeding the complete amino acid mixture. One notable exception was observed, that of the deletion of tryptophan, where the hepatic polyribosomes did not respond but remained as those of the fasted animals.[52–53,60–61] These findings led to studies that examined the role that L-tryptophan alone may have on hepatic polyribosomes and protein synthesis.

The laboratory of Sidransky et al.[52,53,62] in 1967–1968 demonstrated that L-tryptophan alone elicited a response of hepatic polyribosomes toward heavier aggregation as well as an enhancement of protein synthesis as meas-ured *in vivo* or *in vitro*. The single administration of tryptophan alone, but not of one of three other essential amino acids (threonine, methionine, or isoleucine), elicited a stimulatory hepatic response that was similar to that obtained with a complete amino acid mixture.[53] Earlier, Feigelson et al.[63] in 1959 had reported that the parenteral administration of tryptophan in the rat produced a transient elevation in hepatic protein synthesis as determined by measuring 2[^{14}C]glycine incorporation into hepatic protein. Subsequent studies from other laboratories[60,64–69] confirmed the stimulatory effect of tryp-tophan on hepatic protein synthesis.

After establishing that L-tryptophan alone stimulated overall hepatic protein synthesis, it became important to determine which proteins were
involved. Increased synthesis of albumin due to L-tryptophan was reported
by Rothschild et al.[65] and by Jorgensen and Majumdar.[47,68] The latter investigators also reported that tryptophan increased the synthesis of transferrin,
fibrinogen, and ferritin. Thus, extracellular as well as intracellular proteins
that are synthesized by the liver were affected by L-tryptophan. Furthermore,
it was demonstrated that after L-tryptophan administration, both free and
membrane-bound polyribosomes of the liver showed a shift toward heavier
aggregation, more marked for free polyribosomes than for membrane-bound
polyribosomes.[62] Also, *in vitro* protein synthesis revealed a greater increase
with free polyribosomes than with membrane-bound polyribosomes of the
livers of tryptophan-treated animals in comparison with similar fractions of
livers of control animals.

The preceding findings regarding the role of L-tryptophan on hepatic protein synthesis should not be interpreted to mean that other single amino acids
could not under certain conditions stimulate hepatic protein synthesis. For
example, Pronczuk et al.[70] reported that when animals were fed threonine-
or isoleucine-imbalanced diets, which depleted tissue pools of these amino
acids, hepatic polyribosomes were disaggregated and stimulated by the
addition of the limiting amino acid to the meal. Ip and Harper[71] extended
these findings in studies of rats fed a threonine-imbalanced diet. Feeding
animals a threonine-imbalanced diet for 7 days resulted in hepatic ribosomes
that were largely disaggregated. Oral administration of threonine caused the
ribosomes to reaggregate and stimulated the incorporation of ^{14}C-leucine
into tissue proteins. Under these experimental conditions, administration of
tryptophan to threonine-depleted animals did not improve protein synthesis,
suggesting that liver protein synthesis in such cases was most sensitive to
the inadequate supply of the amino acid (threonine) most limiting in the
tissue. However, the role of L-tryptophan described in the previous reports
dealt with normal animals that were fasted overnight, as well as with nor-
mal-fed animals.[72]

4.3.2.2   Considerations of Mechanisms Involved

Since the free tryptophan content of serum and tissues was the lowest of
any indispensable amino acid,[73] it was understandable that this raised the
possibility that tryptophan might be the limiting amino acid for protein
synthesis in fasted animals. Studies by Hori et al.[74] and by Hunt et al.[75] using
reticulocytes suggested that tryptophan tRNA may become limiting. Similarly, it was considered that tryptophan tRNA could become limiting in the
livers of fasted animals because of no dietary tryptophan intake and, therefore, would restrict the rate of hepatic protein synthesis. Also, the finding
that the tryptophan-tRNA content of liver falls more rapidly during food
deprivation than do the t-RNAs of other indispensable amino acids[76] suggested that tryptophan may be an important effector of hepatic protein

synthesis under many physiological circumstances. However, data from a variety of other studies[72,77] suggested that the effect of tryptophan on hepatic polyribosomes and protein synthesis involved a more complex process than one consisting only of raising the low levels of tryptophan in the blood or liver. When L-tryptophan was administered to fed mice in which the blood and hepatic levels of tryptophan were much higher than in fasted mice, the hepatic polyribosomes shifted toward heavier aggregation, and hepatic protein synthesis (*in vitro*) was enhanced, similar to that which occurred in fasted animals.[72] Also, it is of interest that Allen et al.[78] reported no differences in the levels of tryptophan-tRNA in fasted and fed rats, suggesting that this may not be rate-limiting in fasted animals. In addition, L-tryptophan has been effective in enhancing hepatic protein synthesis in animals treated with selected hepatotoxic agents where the tryptophan levels in the blood and liver were not changed but were similar to those in control animals.[77]

A number of studies investigated whether L-tryptophan may act at the translational level of control of hepatic protein synthesis. In these studies, actinomycin D was administered to inhibit RNA synthesis and then L-tryptophan was administered. In such studies, L-tryptophan was still found to be able to stimulate the effect on hepatic polyribosomes and on protein synthesis in fasted mice.[53] Also, Jorgensen and Majumdar[47] reported that the administration of tryptophan to well-fed adrenalectomized rats pretreated with actinomycin D caused an increase in ^{3}H-leucine incorporation into ferritin, transferrin, albumin, and fibrinogen, compared to that in water-fed controls. Tryptophan without pretreatment with actinomycin D caused a larger increase in ^{3}H-leucine incorporation into the same components. A number of studies suggested that L-tryptophan administration may act at the transcriptional level of control of hepatic protein synthesis. L-tryptophan administration has been reported to cause an increase of DNA-dependent RNA polymerase activity,[79–81] nuclear RNA synthesis,[79,80,82] polyribosomal RNA synthesis,[79,83] and cytoplasmic mRNA[84,85] in the liver. It has been reported that the nuclei of rat liver contain at least three forms of DNA-dependent RNA polymerase that play specific roles in genetic transcription.[86,87] Polymerase I is presumed to transcribe ribosomal genes and is Mg^{2+} dependent and amanitin resistant. Polymerase II and III are considered to synthesize, respectively, heterogeneous and smaller molecular weight RNAs. Polymerase II is $Mn^{2+}/(NH_4)_2SO_4$ dependent and amanitin sensitive. Vesley and Cihak,[80] Majumdar and Jorgensen,[88] and Majumdar[89] reported that following tryptophan administration, the activities of both polymerase I and II were rapidly elevated, and this was unrelated to adrenal secretion. Also, Majumdar[81] studied the activities of the engaged (chromatin-bound) and free states of nuclear RNA polymerases in young and adult rats tube-fed tryptophan and observed marked increases in the activities of both engaged and free polymerase in 2-week-old rats but an increase only in the engaged polymerase of the adult rats.

A number of reports have demonstrated that L-tryptophan has a regulatory effect at the posttranscriptional level of hepatic protein synthesis. Details of such experiments follow. After first observing that there was an elevation in hepatic cytoplasmic mRNA following L-tryptophan administration,[84,85] whether this effect could be due, in part or totally, to increased nucleocytoplasmic transport of mRNA was explored. In experiments using fasted mice, hepatic RNA was prelabeled with [6-^{14}C]orotic acid, and then the animals were treated with actinomycin D to inhibit further RNA synthesis. Next, the animals were tube-fed either tryptophan or water. The livers showed elevated levels of cytoplasmic mRNA and a shift in polyribosomes toward heavier aggregates caused by tryptophan.[84] This suggested that, even in the absence of RNA synthesis, tryptophan acted to stimulate the transfer of mRNA from the nucleus into the cytoplasm of hepatic cells. In further studies, the administration of tryptophan to fasted animals resulted in significant increases in the amounts of hepatic polyadenylic acid [poly(A)] and poly(A)-mRNA in the cytoplasm, and this stimulation occurred even following the administration of cordycepin (an inhibitor of poly(A) synthesis) and/or actinomycin D (an inhibitor of RNA synthesis).[85] Administration of L-tryptophan to fasted rats pretreated with cordycepin or actinomycin D, or both, induced a shift in hepatic polyribosomes toward heavier aggregates and an increase in *in vitro* protein synthesis. Also, fasted rats that received [U-^{14}C]adenosine to prelabeled hepatic poly(A) and then were treated with cordycepin or actinomycin D or both before tube-feeding L-tryptophan revealed increased hepatic levels of labeled polyribosomal poly(A) in comparison with controls.[85] The administration of tryptophan to fasted rats pretreated with cordycepin and actinomycin D led to decreased levels of nuclear poly(A)-mRNA and a concomitant increase in the levels of polyribosomal poly(A)-mRNA in the cytoplasm.[90] These findings indicted that L-tryptophan played a role in stimulating the rate of translocation of poly(A)-mRNA from the nucleus into the cytoplasm of the livers of normal animals[84,85] and in those treated with selected inhibitors.[77,91,92]

The possible role that informosomal mRNA may play in the stimulation of hepatic protein synthesis induced by L-tryptophan was investigated.[93] While L-tryptophan induced an increase (20%) in the amount of polyribosome-associated poly(A)-mRNA in the liver within 1 h, the amount of the informosomal poly(A)-mRNA revealed no significant increase or decrease. Since the size of the increase in the polyribosome-associated poly(A)-mRNA was equal to the entire amount of informosomal poly(A)-mRNA present in the hepatic cells, it was concluded that the failure to detect a significant decrease in the size of the informosomal mRNA pool indicated that the increase in the polyribosome-associated poly(A)-mRNA must be due to a different mechanism, such as enhanced nucleocytoplasmic translocation of poly(A)-mRNA, which has been reported earlier and will be further discussed. Hybridization studies with DNA-RNA were also conducted using hepatic polyribosome-associated poly(A)-mRNA from L-tryptophan-treated and control rats to determine if qualitative or quantitative changes occurred in the RNA sequences along with the increase in poly(A)-mRNA following tryptophan administration.[93] Although qualitatively no new species of mRNA were detected in the mRNA from the tryptophan-treated rats, kinetic analysis of the hybridization curves indicated that there was a shift or accumulation of hepatic poly(A)-mRNA belonging to the intermediate- and possibly the high-frequency classes of polyribosome-associated poly(A)-mRNA in the livers of the tryptophan-treated rats.

Since posttranscriptional controls can operate within the nucleus, at the nuclear membrane, and/or in the cytoplasm to regulate the rate of nucleocytoplasmic translocation of ribo-nucleoprotein particles both qualitatively and quantitatively,[94,95] this aspect was investigated in regard to L-tryptophan. Evidence for modification of nucleocytoplasmic transport of RNA owing to chemical carcinogens,[96,97] in transformed cells,[98,99] and during aging[100] has been demonstrated. In view of this information, studies were undertaken relating to the enhanced hepatic nucleocytoplasmic translocation of mRNA occurring following L-tryptophan administration. Experiments were conducted using a cell-free system, modeled after that used by Schumm and Webb,[101] in which the release of RNA from isolated nuclei into a defined medium could be studied. These researchers observed that the release of RNA from isolated hepatic nuclei was influenced by dialyzed cell sap (cytosol) and suggested that the cell sap contained nondialyzable components that act posttranscriptionally to regulate the nuclear processing and/or transport of mRNA to the cytoplasm. Using this assay system, evidence that L-tryptophan affected both the nucleus and the cytoplasm in the process of enhancing intracellular transport of RNA was observed. First, using control liver cell sap, there was greater release of labeled poly(A)-mRNA (prelabeled *in vivo*, with [^{14}C]orotic acid) in the medium from isolated hepatic nuclei of L-tryptophan-treated (10 min) rats than from nuclei of control animals.[90] This effect was detected as early as 3 or 6 min after the administration of L-tryptophan.[102] Tryptophan concentrations became elevated in the plasma and in the liver (including hepatic nuclei) within 5 min,[102] and increased hepatic protein synthesis was evident within 10 min.[53] To determine whether the increased hepatic protein synthesis was involved in the nuclear effect of the L-tryptophan-treated animals, rats received puromycin treatment 10 min before L-tryptophan administration. Using the *in vitro* assay system, hepatic nuclei of rats that received L-tryptophan following puromycin exhibited greater release of labeled RNA (poly(A)-mRNA) into the medium in comparison with control nuclei of puromycin-treated rats.[102] Next, liver cell sap of the tryptophan-treated animals was evaluated. Since *in vivo* hepatic protein synthesis was already stimulated within 10 min after tryptophan administration,[53] it was conceivable that some regulatory protein(s) in the cytosol might play a role in the transport activity. To test for this possibility, cell saps were prepared from livers of rats tube-fed water or L-tryptophan 10 min before killing, and their effects on *in vitro* release of labeled poly(A)-mRNA from control hepatic nuclei in the presence of added L-tryptophan in the medium were investigated. There was more release of total RNA and poly(A)-mRNA from control hepatic nuclei incubated with liver cell sap of L-tryptophan-treated rats compared with release using liver cell sap of control rats.[102] The addition of L-tryptophan to the incubation medium was essential for the increased release of labeled RNA by the experimental liver cell sap. Since the dialyzed cell saps used in the incubation medium lacked L-tryptophan, its addition was important.

To determine whether the rapidly stimulated hepatic protein synthesis following L-tryptophan administration was involved in this process, pre-treatment of the animals with inhibitors of protein synthesis was followed for their influence on the increased transporting effect of the liver cell sap of L-tryptophan-treated rats. Animals were pretreated with cycloheximide for 2.5 h or with puromycin for 20 min before the L-tryptophan or water administration, which was given 10 min before killing. The effects of liver saps prepared from the control and experimental groups on *in vitro* release of labeled RNA from hepatic nuclei were investigated. Liver cell saps from rats treated with cycloheximide or puromycin before L-tryptophan administration were not able to stimulate the release of labeled RNA, as could liver cell saps of L-tryptophan-treated rats.[102]

A dichotomy existed between the effect of inhibition of hepatic protein synthesis, as induced by puromycin or cycloheximide, and the action of L-tryptophan on the nuclear cytosol involvement in the enhanced RNA transport activity as measured *in vitro*. While inhibition of protein synthesis did not affect the stimulatory effect of nuclei, it inhibited the stimulatory effect of liver cytosol of L-tryptophan-treated rats. To explain these differences, one may speculate that in animals treated with inhibitors of protein synthesis, L-tryptophan may be able to act in one of two ways: (1) to stimulate the synthesis of regulatory proteins in the nucleus, or (2) to enhance the transfer of the existing amounts of regulatory factors in the cytosol to the nuclear membrane. The question of whether protein synthesis occurs in the nucleus is not yet resolved definitively. Some investigators have implicated the nucleus and nuclear envelope as sites of protein synthesis and have reported that nuclear protein synthesis is inhibited to a lesser extent by puromycin and cycloheximide than is cytoplasmic protein synthesis.[103,104] Evidence suggesting that pre-existing proteins of the cytosol may act on the nuclear envelopes has been obtained in other experiments.[105] It is quite difficult to unravel the complex mechanisms that come into play following the use of L-tryptophan alone in normal animals and possibly even more so when L-tryptophan is used in combination with a variety of inhibitors. Indeed, inhibitors that are considered to have one primary action often cause a variety of secondary effects *in vivo* in animals. Although inhibitors of RNA and protein synthesis have been of great value in experiments attempting to unravel mechanisms, caution must be exercised in interpreting data based upon their use in normal animals.

Summarizing the above findings, it appears that the enhanced nucleocytoplasmic translocation of mRNA in the livers of L-tryptophan-treated animals affects both the nucleus and the cytosol. The nuclear effect appears to be independent of changes in hepatic protein synthesis, while the cytosol effect is dependent on hepatic protein synthesis. Thus, while both (nuclear and cytosol) effects are probably operative in normal animals treated with L-tryptophan, only one effect, that on the nucleus, is probably operative in animals treated with hepatotoxic agents that act to inhibit hepatic protein synthesis. The latter mechanism could be invoked in explaining the stimulatory effect of L-tryptophan on hepatic polyribosomal aggregation and protein synthesis of rats treated with inhibitors of protein synthesis, such as ethionine, puromycin, or hypertonic NaC1.[91,106,107] Also, experimental studies with ethionine, puromycin, and hypertonic NaC1 support this conclusion.[77]

In probing further into the mechanism by which L-tryptophan stimulates hepatic nucleocytoplasmic translocation of mRNA, it became necessary to investigate special components of the nucleus — the nuclear envelope and the nuclear pore complex — that are considered to play a key role in the regulation of nucleocytoplasmic RNA translocation.[108] A nucleoside triphosphatase (NTPase) has been identified in the mammalian liver nuclear envelope, and this enzyme appears to be involved in the nucleocytoplasmic translocation of RNA.[109–111] Furthermore, following treatment of rats with thioacetamide or CC1$_4$, a parallelism between alterations in nuclear RNA transport and nuclear envelope NTPase activity in the liver has been demonstrated.[109] Therefore, the question of whether the enhanced nucleocytoplasmic translocation of mRNA caused by tryptophan was related to an alteration in the activity of nuclear envelope NTPase was investigated. The levels of nuclear envelope NTPase activity were significantly elevated in the livers of rats tube-fed L-tryptophan at 10, 30, or 60 min before killing.[112] As described earlier, concomitant with this rapid (10 min) increase in the NTPase activity, there was a greater release of labeled RNA from isolated hepatic nuclei of livers of L-tryptophan-treated rats than from those of control rats. The parallel increases in both NTPase activity of nuclear envelopes and the translocation of RNA suggested that these two processes may be associated with or related to one another. In further experiments, the administration of L-tryptophan was found to stimulate the levels of hepatic nuclear envelope NTPase activity in rats pretreated with puromycin, similar to the increases in the control rats that received tryptophan alone.[112] This finding added further support to the view that the increased activity of nuclear envelope NTPase was related to or probably responsible for the enhanced RNA transport activity of hepatic nuclei of puromycin-treated plus L-tryptophan-treated rats compared with that of the hepatic nuclei of control rats.

Activities of two other enzymes, protein phosphokinease and phosphoprotein phosphohydrolase, have also been identified on the mammalian nuclear envelope.[113–115] It has been suggested that the levels of phosphorylation and dephosphorylation of the nuclear envelope protein by these two enzymes may regulate nucleocytoplasmic RNA translocation.[116] Because these nuclear envelope-associated enzymes may play a key role in the regulation of nuclear RNA transport, a study was conducted to investigate whether the administration of tryptophan would influence the phosphorylation and dephosphorylation process in the hepatic nuclear envelopes, which may then modulate nucleocytoplasmic transport of RNA. The activities of protein phosphokinase (PK) and phosphoprotein phosphohydrolase (PH) were investigated in the livers of rats that received a single tube-feeding of L-tryptophan 10 min before killing, and the hepatic nuclear envelope activities of both enzymes were found to be increased.[155] Furthermore, L-tryptophan administration increased the *in vivo* incorporation of [³H]leucine into proteins of the nuclear envelopes (+83%) and also into proteins of the other subcellular fractions (+34 to +43%) of the liver compared with incorporation into proteins of the corresponding fractions of the control rats. Rats that received [³H]leucine to prelabel hepatic proteins and then were treated with puromycin to inhibit further protein synthesis followed by tube-feeding of L-tryptophan revealed greater radioactivity associated with nuclear envelope proteins than did controls. The latter findings suggested that L-tryptophan may act to stimulate the movement or availability of proteins to the vicinity of the nuclear envelope, possibly specific regulatory proteins, such as NTPase, PIK, and PH, which show increased activities and may be responsible for the increase in the rate of nucleocytoplasmic translocation of mRNA.

In view of the involvement of the nuclear envelope in controlling active nucleocytoplasmic transfer of RNP particles, several studies have examined the ultrastructure of the nuclear envelope. The intact nuclear envelope is composed of inner and outer nuclear membranes and nuclear pore complexes.[117] Treatment of nuclei with nonionic detergents, such as Triton X-100, completely removes the outer nuclear membrane, leaving intact nuclei with preservation of nuclear pore complexes. The nuclear pores are considered to be the major sites of nucleocytoplasmic transfer of macromolecules.[118,119] Therefore, studies were conducted on the effect of removing the outer nuclear membranes (by Triton X-100 treatment of isolated hepatic nuclei) on the capacity of the nuclei of control or L-tryptophan-treated rats to transport RNA *in vitro* and on the activity of nuclear envelope NTPase. Following treatment with Triton X-100, there was greater release of labeled RNA from the isolated hepatic nuclei of L-tryptophan-treated rats compared with that from control hepatic nuclei.[112] These findings were similar to those observed with untreated nuclei (not treated with Triton X-100). Similar increases in the activity of nuclear envelope NTPase were found with the experimental compared with the control samples.[112] The findings that the increased translocation of mRNA occurred along with the increased activity of nuclear envelope NTPase in the livers of the experimental rats were in general agreement with data of others which demonstrated that (1) detergent treatment was not deleterious to the ability of nuclei to transport RNA, (2) the transported RNA was of intranuclear origin, and (3) nuclear pore complexes and NTPase activity were probably responsible for the nucleocytoplasmic translocation of mRNA.[110,119,120]

Since L-tryptophan administration rapidly enhanced nucleocytoplasmic translocation of RNA in the liver, it was of interest to learn whether tryptophan deprivation would be inhibitory to this process. A few experimental studies suggested that indeed this was the case. Bocker et al.,[121] using rats fed *ad libitum* a tryptophan-free or complete diet (pair-fed controls) for 15 days, studied the incorporation of [^{3}H]orotic acid into RNA fractions separated from the hepatic nucleus and cytoplasm. The incorporation of orotic acid into the high-weight components of the RNA of the nucleus was increased, but no increase was found in the cytoplasmic RNA. These findings were interpreted as indicating that RNA in the nuclei in the livers of the experimental rats was synthesized but not delivered to the cytoplasm. Similarly, Wannemacher et al.[122] reported that in rats fed an amino acid-deficient diet (6% casein) nuclear RNA was synthesized but was not properly processed and therefore not transported to the cytoplasm. Further studies are needed to elucidate if indeed long-term feeding of tryptophan-devoid diets impairs hepatic nucleocytoplasmic translocation of mRNA.

Schumm and Webb[23] suggested that cyclic nucleotides can exert an influence on the posttranscriptional events of RNA processing and transport since they found that the addition of cyclic AMP or GMP stimulated the release of RNA from isolated hepatic nuclei. Subsequently, in preliminary experiments, the addition of cAMP to the cell-free system composed of cell saps of livers of control rats, but not composed of cell saps of livers of tryptophan-treated rats, caused increases in the release of labeled RNA from the liver nuclei of control rats. This response in the cell-free system to added cAMP probably reflects the *in vivo* concentrations of cAMP in the tissues from which the cytosol was prepared. Thus, these preliminary findings suggest that tryptophan may elevate *in vivo* the cAMP levels in liver cytosol, and this may be of importance in the enhanced nucleocytoplasmic translocation of mRNA in liver owing to tryptophan. However, preliminary assays of cAMP activities in the livers of control and tryptophan-treated rats have failed to reveal significant differences.

Based upon many of the described studies regarding the actions and effects of L-tryptophan, it was appropriate to consider that the actions of L-tryptophan on hepatic cells may be similar to those of a hormone, such as insulin, steroid hormones, or triiodothyronine. Analogous to insulin, its first step may be the binding of L-tryptophan to a specific receptor protein on the surface of the target cells. As described for insulin,[123,124] L-tryptophan may bind at specific receptors on the plasma membranes of target cells such as liver. After binding, the tryptophan-receptor complex may lead to many of the subsequent actions of L-tryptophan. On the other hand, based upon other findings with insulin, there is evidence that insulin has a direct effect upon nuclei. Goldfine and Smith[125] and Goldfine et al.[126] have reported that purified nuclei from both rat liver and cultured lymphocytes contain specific binding sites for insulin. Also, Vigneri et al.[127] have reported that the nuclear envelope is the major site of insulin binding to the cell nucleus. Goldfine et al.[128,129] have reviewed the evidence that nuclear envelopes contain specific high-affinity binding sites for insulin, that insulin stimulates nuclear envelope NTPase activity, and that the insulin directly stimulates the release of mRNA from isolated nuclei. Roth and Cassell[130] have reported, in studies using a highly purified preparation of insulin receptor, that the insulin receptor itself may be a protein kinase. In considering that L-tryptophan may be acting directly on the nuclei (nuclear membranes) of liver cells, studies were undertaken to explore whether or not L-tryptophan may have some effects on hepatic nuclei similar to those of insulin.

Steroid hormones act on target cells essentially through a sequence of early events involving (1) the penetration of the hormone into the target cell, (2) its binding to specific receptor proteins, and (3) the temperature-dependent activation of the steroid-receptor complex, activation necessary to the migration of the complexes to the nucleus. Finally, the attachment of the activated complexes to chromatin is probably responsible for the alteration of transcription of specific genes.[131,132] The finding of specific reports for glucocorticoids in the cytosol of most of the target organs including liver is considered one of the strongest pieces of evidence in support of this model.[133,134]

Markovic and Petrovic[135] have reported that the radioactive profiles on sucrose density-gradient analysis of the macromolecular liver cytosol fraction incubated with tritiated hydrocortisone and tryptophan were similar. This resemblance suggested to them that both compounds bind to rat liver proteins of similar size and that a competition may exist between hydrocortisone and tryptophan for receptor proteins of rat liver cytosol. Baker et al.[136] have reported that tryptophan methyl ester, a competitive inhibitor of chymotrypsin, is also a competitive inhibitor of dexamethasone binding to the glucocorticoid receptor in HTC cells, which suggests that the binding sites of tryptophan methyl ester and dexamethasone are partially contiguous. The findings by Markovic and Petrovic[135] pointed to the possibility that the maximal biological activity of one compound might be impaired by the presence of the other. Majumdar and Jorgensen[137] observed, using well-fed adrenalectomized rats, that while the stimulatory effect on hepatic protein synthesis of tryptophan was not fully expressed in the presence of cortisol, the reverse is true for cortisol, in that the amino acid blocks the cortisol-mediated stimulation of hepatic protein synthesis to a great extent, as measured by [³H]leucine incorporation into plasma albumin, fibrinogen, and liver ferritin *in vivo*. However, using normal rats, tryptophan administration to rats that had hepatic protein synthesis enhanced by previous treatment with cortisone acetate revealed further stimulation of hepatic polyribosomes toward heavier aggregation and hepatic protein synthesis *in vivo*.[138]

The nuclear receptor for T_3 belongs to the same superfamily as steroid hormone receptors, especially in their DNA-binding domains and in the organization of their functional domains, which appear to correlate with similarities in their mechanism of action.[139–141]

Interactions and interrelationships among receptors, their ligands, and transcriptional actions have been described. A few selected examples can be cited. The functional interaction of the glucocorticoid receptor with liver-specific transcription factors and the functional synergy of the glucocorticoid receptor with the thyroid hormone receptor have been reported.[142] Both thyroid hormones and glucocorticoids are required for optimal induction of several genes, for example, rat phosphoenolypyruvate carboxykinase gene.[143] The growth hormone gene requires either T_3 or retinoic acid for induction by glucocorticoids.[144,145] T_3, but not retinoic acid, increases estrogen receptor levels in pituitary cells by a process requiring protein synthesis and which is accompanied by an increase in the mRNA.[146] The biologic effects of T_3, estrogen, and retinoic acid indicate that their cognate receptors can act to regulate distinct but overlapping sets of genes.[147] Recent findings suggest a probable interrelationship between nuclear receptors for T_3 and tryptophan. Both ligands, T_3 and tryptophan, affect the binding affinity of the nuclear receptor for tryptophan, and this competitive binding effect appears to diminish a biological response induced by tryptophan alone (enhanced hepatic protein synthesis and increased hepatic nuclear PAP enzyme activity).[148]

A possible consideration in the *in vivo* experiments where T_3 and tryptophan were administered to rats was that T_3 may inhibit tryptophan transport to the liver. A mutual competitive inhibition between the transport of tryptophan (mediated by the aromatic amino acid transport system T) and T_3 has been reported.[149,150] Though system T transport activity has been studied mainly in erythrocytes, it is also expressed in hepatocytes.[151] Interactions between thyroid hormone and tryptophan transport in rat liver have been reported to be modulated by thyroid status.[152] For this reason, whether the administration of T_3 and tryptophan under selected experimental conditions would affect free tryptophan levels in liver was investigated. The results revealed that rats tube-fed tryptophan and given T_3 intraperitoneally at 0 time and killed after 1 h[148] had the same increase (10%) in free tryptophan levels in liver as that of rats tube-fed tryptophan alone.

Many hormones have been demonstrated to bind to proteins (receptors) of cellular components, and this enables them to exert regulatory controls and actions. Therefore, experiments were undertaken to determine whether L-tryptophan may bind to cellular proteins (receptors), as occurs with certain hormones.

4.3.3 Tryptophan Binding to Serum Protein

For many years, it has been known that L-tryptophan in blood binds to serum albumin, which is then transported in this manner throughout the circulatory system. McMenamy[153] described this binding, and it is also reviewed in Chapter 5. Normally, L-tryptophan in the blood is approximately 85% bound to albumin and 15% free.

It became of interest to determine whether L-tryptophan that enters cells may bind to cytosolic proteins. This was tested by orally administering L-tryptophan or nothing to fasted rats, followed by killing the rats after 15 min or 2 h. Following the tube-feeding of tryptophan (30 mg per 100 g body weight) to fasted rats, total tryptophan concentrations after 15 min became markedly elevated in serum (+727%) and in liver (+797%), and after 2 h the levels were still elevated in serum (+458%) and in liver (+95%). Similar changes were reported earlier.[102] In several experiments, the free- and bound-tryptophan levels of serum and of liver homogenates or postmitochondrial supernatants of rats treated with water or tryptophan 15 min or 2 h before killing were determined. The methodology employed was that of Badawy and Smith[154] using supernatants after trichloroacetic acid (TCA) precipitation to determine total tryptophan levels and using ultrafiltrates prepared by centrifuging liver homogenates through Amicon Centriflo membrane cones and measuring free-tryptophan levels on pass throughs. Protein-bound tryptophan was determined by differences. While in the control rats the serum contained 10% free and 90% bound tryptophan and the liver contained 76% free and 24% bound tryptophan, after tryptophan tube-feeding (15 min or 2 h) the serum changed to 36% free and 62% bound and the liver changed to 38% free and 62% bound. Combining the data of the increases in total tryptophan levels with the free and bound percentages, it appears that the serum shows greater increases in the amounts of free than of bound tryptophan, while in the liver there are greater increases in bound than in free tryptophan.

Next, in the absence of protein synthesis, the *in vitro* binding of [³H]tryptophan into proteins of dialyzed liver cell saps of control and tryptophan-treated (10 min) rats was studied. A similar percentage of binding in the free and bound fractions of control and experimental groups was found.[44] Only in the TCA-precipitable fractions of dialyzed cell saps (where only 5% of the total counts resided) was there a significant increase in the experimental over the control groups. When [³H]leucine binding *in vitro* was measured instead of [³H]tryptophan binding under the same experimental conditions, there were no differences in the binding to TCA-precipitable proteins of the dialyzed liver cell saps of control and experimental (tryptophan-treated, 10 min) groups. Thus, the [³H]tryptophan binding to TCA-precipitable proteins under the experimental conditions did not appear to be related to the normal binding of tryptophan to serum albumin or to general hepatic proteins. Other types of bindings are possible. In considering that L-tryptophan may rapidly bind to or become absorbed by certain proteins of the cytosol or nuclei of livers, a number of experiments were designed to determine whether or not this reaction occurs. Initially, these experiments were designed to determine whether such an effect could be demonstrated. Second, if an effect was found, it was necessary to determine which proteins were involved.

4.3.4 Tryptophan Binding to Cellular Organelles of Liver

Tryptophan rapidly becomes incorporated into proteins, and it also binds to proteins of liver cells, particularly to proteins of the nuclear envelopes.[44] Increased *in vitro* bindings of [³H]tryptophan to proteins (TCA-precipitable) of nuclei and cytosols of livers of tryptophan-treated (10 min) rats were observed, and this reaction appears to correlate with enhanced *in vitro* release of hepatic nuclear RNA and increased nuclear NTPase and protein phosphokinase activities.[44] *In vitro* [³H]tryptophan binding to proteins of cytosols or nuclei of rat livers was decreased by the addition of cold insulin, and *in vitro* (¹²⁵I]-insulin binding to proteins of hepatic nuclei was increased when incubated with cytosols of livers of rats treated *in vivo* with tryptophan in comparison with cytosols of livers of control rats treated with water. Pretreatment of rats with puromycin before tryptophan administration prevented the increased *in vitro* binding of [³H]tryptophan to nuclear and cytosol proteins caused by cytosols of experimental rats, but it did not prevent the increased *in vitro* binding of [³H]tryptophan to nuclear proteins resulting from nuclei of experimental rats. Preincubation of hepatic nuclei with concanavalin A prevented the increased *in vitro* binding of [³H]tryptophan to nuclear proteins, prelabeled nuclear RNA release, and nuclear NTPase activity of livers of tryptophan-treated rats. The results suggest that tryptophan rapidly binds with hepatic proteins (possibly glycoproteins) associated with the nuclear membrane where there is an increase in the activities of enzymes involved in phosphorylation and dephosphorylation along with release of nuclear mRNA into the cytoplasm.

A paper by LeJohn and Stevenson[155] has cast some light on the above results and may offer an explanation for the findings described. It was reported using *Achlya* (a freshwater mold) that tryptophan binds to a cell wall membrane proteoglycan. The tryptophan uptake was considered to be a binding process, because while uptake of methionine and phenyalanine was inhibited by metabolic poisons (NaN₃, dinitrophenol, and Hg²⁺), that of tryptophan was not. What the tryptophan could be binding to was deciphered by LeJohn in the following way. When germlings were osmotically shocked, they lost their ability to take up tryptophan by a purine analog-enhanced process.[156] The proteoglycan that was isolated from the osmotic shock fluid has been shown to bind tryptophan.[157] Thus, considering these studies, hepatic cytosol protein may be considered to play a role in enhancing nucleocytoplasmic translocation of mRNA, and it may be a glycoprotein. In the livers of rats treated with hypertonic NaC1 this proteoglycan is liberated into the liver cytosol from membranes (possibly nuclear membranes) and then has the ability to stimulate nuclear transport of RNA in normal control nuclei. In the livers of rats treated with tryptophan, this proteoglycan is stimulated by increased synthesis or activation in the liver cytosol and then leads to the stimulation of nuclear RNA transport. This glycoprotein(s) may have a binding affinity for [³H]tryptophan and may be involved in nucleocytoplasmic translocation of mRNA.

Baglia and Maul[158] indicated that a glycoprotein, identified as lamin B, is a major component of the nuclear envelope and nuclear matrix. This glycoprotein may not only be a structural nuclear protein but also may have NTPase activity, which is essential in nucleocytoplasmic transport. Whether changes in the lamin B of liver nuclear envelopes of rats treated with tryptophan occurs is unclear.

4.3.4.1 Nuclear Binding

The observation that L-tryptophan binds to proteins of hepatic nuclear envelope appeared to be a major finding.[159,160] This binding of L-tryptophan is
somewhat analogous to the binding of L-tryptophan described earlier in the
E. coli system.[161,162] Also, it was suggested that this binding effect was similar
to that which occurs with a number of hormones.[141,163] The laboratory of
Sidransky and co-workers has extended the knowledge of L-tryptophan
binding to hepatic nuclear envelopes and will be reviewed.

In 1987 Kurl et al.[159] first reported that the nuclear envelopes of rat liver
specifically bind ^{3}H-tryptophan under *in vitro* conditions. This binding was
sensitive to proteolytic enzymes and to exoglycosidases, implicating glycoproteins as involved in the binding. Unlabeled L-tryptophan was an effective
inhibitor of ^{3}H-tryptophan binding to nuclear envelopes, whereas other
related compounds, including D-tryptophan, serotonin, 5-hydroxy-DL-tryp-
tophan, kynurenine, β-NAD, and niacin, had negligible effects. On Scatchard
analysis, the nuclear envelopes were found to contain two binding components for ^{3}H-tryptophan. One component had a high affinity for tryptophan
($K_D = 0.67$nM and $B_{max} = 21.3$ fmol/mg protein), whereas the second, low
affinity component had both a higher K_D (18.1 nM) and concentration
($B_{max} = 327.3$ fmol/mg protein).

Next, studies were directed toward purification of the nuclear envelope
binding protein for L-tryptophan.[160] Two affinity matrices, concanavalin A-
agarose and tryptophan-agarose, were utilized. Findings with lectin affinity
chromatography suggested that the binding entity was a glycoprotein since
it could be eluted off the column with methyl α-D-mannopryanoside (0.2M).
Elutes from both columns, when electrophoresed separately (under denaturing conditions) on polyacrylamide gels, revealed the presence of a protein
with an apparent molecular weight of approximately 33,000 to 34,000 which
was the same as that observed when covalently bound (i.e., cross linked)
^{3}H-tryptophan was analyzed on polyacrylamide gels under denaturing conditions and then autoradiographed. Polyclonal antibodies raised against the
binding protein recognized polypeptides with molecular weights of 64,000
and 33,000 to 34,000 when analyzed by the Western blot technique, suggesting that the protein was probably a dimer. Immunohistochemical studies
revealed that the antigen was localized in the nuclear membranes, thereby
corroborating the biochemical premise that the binding protein was present
in nuclear envelopes of rat liver. Further evidence of the existence of a
tryptophan-binding protein of nuclear envelopes came from a report by
Schroder et al.[164] They reported a tryptophan-binding protein of nuclear
envelopes of mouse lymphoma (L5178y) cells that was described as having
similar characteristics to those of rat hepatic nuclear envelopes. Subsequently, nuclear and nuclear envelope binding of tryptophan has been
reported in rat transplantable hepatomas (5123 and 19)[165] and in rat brain.[166]

Further studies were concerned with the relationships between the rat
hepatic nuclear receptor protein for L-tryptophan and enzymatic activity of

poly(A)polymerase of the rat hepatic nuclear envelope. First, Kurl et al.[167] reported on the identity and isolation of a protein with poly(A)polymerase activity from hepatic nuclear envelopes. It was considered to be a glycoprotein based upon its ability to bind to concanavalin A-agarose and to be eluted from the column with methyl α-D-mannopyranoside (0.2M) as well as the inhibitory effects of α-mannosidase. The enzyme had a molecular weight of 64,000 when analyzed on polyacrylamide gel electrophoresis under denaturing conditions and had a sedimentation coefficient of 4.5 S. Immunohistochemical studies using polyclonal antibodies raised against the purified enzyme revealed that the antigen was localized in the nuclear membranes.

Subsequently, Kurl et al.[168] reported on the association of poly(A)polymerase with the tryptophan receptor in rat hepatic nuclei. Experiments were conducted with two liver nuclear envelope proteins, a tryptophan receptor glycoprotein, and poly(A)polyermases, and comparisons of the structural similarities were made using affinity chromatography, sodium dodecyl sulfate-polyacrylamide gel electrophoresis (SDS-PAGE), and antibody specificity. The numerous analyses suggested that the tryptophan receptor and poly(A)polymerase shared structural homology. Further review of the relationship between the tryptophan receptor and poly(A)polymerase needs to consider some of the pertinent effects or actions of L-tryptophan. Tryptophan clearly affects RNA metabolism.[45] As early as 10 min after tryptophan administration, there is an increase in the concentration of polyadenylated mRNA transported from the cell nucleus to the cytoplasm.[85,90] A concomitant increase in the activities of enzymes, nucleoside triphosphatase,[112] and poly(A)polymerase,[169] that are involved in the polyadenylation of mRNA[170] is observed. The increase in poly(A)polymerase activity in response to tryptophan is not due to a decrease in poly(A) or poly(A)$^+$ mRNA. However, deadenylated RNA, such as rRNA, has no effect on NTPase, alluding to the essential role of polyadenylation for this transport of mRNA from the nucleus to the cytoplasm.[171] Poly(A)polymerase has been purified by both concanvalin A[167] and poly(A)sepharose columns. Using the latter column, a protein isolated from rat hepatic nuclei with a M_R of 65,000 was described.[172] Monoclonal antibodies raised against this protein inhibit the efflux of mRNA from the nucleus.[172] Thus, the physical characteristics and immunoblot analysis allude to a single polypeptide. However, definitive evidence of whether the tryptophan receptor and poly(A)polymerase are indeed the same proteins needs to be provided by the sequence of the genes encoding the two proteins.

4.3.4.1.1 Vital Areas in Tryptophan Molecule

Studies were conducted to determine whether other compounds would compete for ^{3}H-tryptophan binding to rat hepatic nuclei or nuclear envelopes.[173,174] The data of such studies made it possible to determine which sites in L-tryptophan were vital for receptor binding. The tryptophan-binding site could be mapped by analyzing the data as to which and how test compounds inhibited labeled [³H]tryptophan binding. The binding site seemed to contain four regions contributing to specific and significant binding. Figure 4.2 depicts a representation of the binding site with regions *a*, *b*, and *c* involving the amino acid component of binding and region *R* corresponding to the indole component of tryptophan binding. Region *a* seems to permit only a hydrogen atom and probably represents a loop of protein closely apposed to the ligand. Thus, an α-methyl group significantly diminished binding affinity as reflected by the lack of inhibition of labeled tryptophan binding for such compounds as α-methyl tryptophan, isobutyric acid, or amino isobutyric acid. The amino acid alanine competed effectively with tryptophan because its amino acid portion was identical to tryptophan and lacked only the indole residue. The stereoisomeric configuration was also important so that the mirror-imaged D-tryptophan or D-alanine did not bind effectively to the nuclear envelope-binding protein. The *b* region, unlike the *a* region, permitted some degree of substitution. It seemed that this region may have a partial positive charge or permit hydrogen bonding in its protein pocket. The carbonyl oxygen will have a partial negative charge and was available for dipolar or hydrogen bond interactions. If the acid group was esterified, the resultant compounds, tryptophan-methyl ester and tryptophan-ethyl ester, competed effectively as the parent ligand. However, if the moiety was an amide linkage with net positive charge, there was reduction in binding reflected by the lack of inhibition of labeled tryptophan binding. The *c* region represented the amino group in a protein pocket possessing a net negative charge. Substitutions on the amino nitrogen may not disturb the negatively charged nitrogen but inhibited binding based on steric considerations. Interestingly, *N*-substituted compounds, which inhibited tryptophan binding to nuclei, did not inhibit binding to nuclear envelopes, presumably due to enzymatic modification of the compounds. The importance of regions *b* and *c* was also appreciated by noting that compounds lacking the carbonyl oxygen or the amino group (such as tryptamine and indole-acetic acid) did not inhibit tryptophan binding. The position of the amino group, appropriately fitting into region *c*, was also crucial given that α-amino alanine was an effective inhibitor of tryptophan binding but β-amino alanine was not. Thus, regions *b* and *c* contributed significant free energy of binding, probably due to charge or hydrogen-bonding interactions. The *R* region permitted a variety of compounds that mimicked the indole group of the parent ligand. This region probably contained hydrophobic protein interactions because acidic or basic amino acids, such as aspartate and glutamate or lysine, did not bind. Particular substitutions of the indole ring seem to be important and may represent steric interactions: 4-fluoro-tryptophan and 5-fluoro-tryptophan did bind, but 6-fluoro-tryptophan did not bind, and 5-methyl-DL-tryptophan bound, but 1-, 4-, 6-, and 7-methyl-DL-tryptophan did not appreciably bind to nuclear envelopes. Interestingly, though phenylalanine and tyrosine had some degree of inhibition of labeled tryptophan binding, straight-chain or branch-chain aliphatic residues showed no such activity.

$$
\begin{array}{c}
\quad\quad a \\
\quad\quad | \\
R - CH_2 - C - C - b \\
\quad\quad | \\
\quad\quad NH \\
\quad\quad | \\
\quad\quad c
\end{array}
$$

R

Competes	Does Not Compete
Tryptophan (trp) – indole	Aspartic acid – COOH
4 or 5-fluoro trp – 4 or 5 fluoroindole	Arginine – CH$_2$CH$_2$C=NH NH
5-methyl trp – 5 methylindole	Glutamic acid – CH$_2$COOH
7-aza trp – 7 azaindole	Isoleucine – CH$_2$CH$_3$ CH$_3$
3(1-naphthyl)alanine – naphthyl	Leucine – CH-CH$_3$ CH$_3$
Alanine – H	Lysine – CH$_2$CH$_2$CH$_2$NH$_2$
Cysteine – SH	Methionine – CH$_2$SCH$_3$
Cystine – SSCH$_2$CHCOOH NH$_2$	
Homocysteine – CH$_2$SH	Serine – OH
Histidine – imidazole	Theonine – CH$_3$ OH
Phenylalanine – phenyl	Valine – CH$_3$ CH$_3$
Tyrosine – hydroxphenyl	
	Norleucine – CH$_2$CH$_2$CH$_3$
	Norvaline – CH$_2$CH$_3$
	Glutamine – CH$_2$CONH$_2$
	6-fluoro trp – 6 fluroindole
	5-methoxy trp – 5 methoxyindole
	1,4,4,-6 or 7-methyl trp – 1,4,6 or 7 methylindole

a

Competes	Does Not Compete
trp-H	α-methyl trp – CH$_3$

b

Competes	Does Not Compete
trp-OH	Tryptophamide-NH$_2$
trp methyl ester – OCH$_3$	trp β naphthylamide-naphthylamide
trp ethyl ester - OCH$_2$CH$_3$	

c

Competes	Does Not Compete
trp-H	N-formyl trp-COH
	N-acetyl trp-COCH$_3$
	N-methyl trp-CH$_3$

FIGURE 4.2

Vital areas of tryptophan molecule for binding to hepatic nuclei or nuclear envelopes. Ability of unlabeled compounds to compete with ³H-tryptophan binding to hepatic nuclei. Vital sites of L-tryptophan molecule.

4.3.4.1.2   Vital Sites in Nuclear Receptor

Sidransky and Verney[175] reported that the hepatic nuclear receptor that binds L-tryptophan contained sulfhydryl groups within its protein that were vital for the binding reaction. In this study the effects *in vitro* of selenite and selenate on nuclear L-tryptophan receptors of rat liver were investigated. Sodium selenite at 10^{-6} M inhibited the *in vitro* ^{3}H-tryptophan binding to rat liver nuclear receptors. No inhibitory effect of selenite on ^{3}H-tryptophan binding to nuclear receptor was found in the presence of 10^{-4} M dithiothreitol, a protective agent for sulfhydryl groups. Selenate as well as sulfite or sulfate did not exert an inhibitory effect on the tryptophan receptor. The results based upon *in vitro* studies indicated that selenium in the form of selenite may reversibly affect the L-tryptophan binding at the sulfhydryl sites in the nuclear receptor protein. *In vivo* administration of high (toxic) levels of selenite before or along with L-tryptophan inhibited the L-tryptophan-induced stimulation of hepatic protein synthesis.

Based upon the findings in the prior section in regard to the vital areas of the L-tryptophan molecule that bind to the hepatic nuclear receptor for tryptophan, it is likely that the carbonyl group of L-tryptophan, site *b* (Figure 4.2) reacts with the sulfhydryl groups of the receptor protein, at least at one of the vital binding sites. Interference with the sulfhydryl groups, as with selenite, caused inhibition of *in vitro* ^{3}H-tryptophan binding to hepatic nuclei.

Consideration that sulfhydryl groups on the nuclear tryptophan receptor may play a vital role in the binding reaction is justified even though the sequence of the purified receptor protein[159,160] has as yet not been performed. However, other nuclear receptors, such as the glucocorticoid receptor[176] and the 3,5,3'-triiodothyronine (T_3) receptor,[177] which responded to selenite similarly to that with the tryptophan receptor, have been demonstrated to contain functional sulfhydryl residues presumed to be in the hormone-binding domain.[141,178] Steroid and thyroid hormones may exert their effects through fundamentally similar mechanisms.[140,141] Based upon the findings,[175] it appears that the nuclear tryptophan receptor may also be related to other nuclear receptors, and the possible relationship between their actions needs to be determined.

4.4   Interrelationships with Other Components (Blood and Dietary)

4.4.1   Blood Protein

As described earlier, tryptophan is present in low levels in the diet and in the proteins of tissues and organs, as well as in the free amino acid pools, including that in the blood. In 1950, Schurr et al.[179] determined the amino acid concentrations in various tissues of the rat. If these data are used to calculate tissue-to-plasma ratios, it becomes apparent that the relative availability of plasma tryptophan to tissues is much less than that of the other amino acids.

In addition to the quantitative findings in regard to tryptophan, another early report revealed an important and unique property of tryptophan within the blood. In 1957, McMenemy et al.[180] described a unique property of tryptophan — that it was the only amino acid in plasma that was largely bound to protein. This attribute, specifically the ratio of free to bound tryptophan in the blood, has much physiological significance. For example, only the small free fraction of plasma tryptophan has access to the brain. Factors that influence the equilibrium between free and bound tryptophan in the plasma have been considered to alter the availability of tryptophan to the brain, where it has special importance as a precursor of the neurotransmitter 5-hydroxytryptamine (serotonin).[181–183] Tryptophan differs from other amino acids in that its concentration in the plasma of rats increases (30 to 40%) after fasting, after insulin administration, or after consuming a carbohydrate meal.[184]

4.4.2 Competition with Tryptophan's Binding with Hepatic Nuclear Receptor

Studies by Sidransky et al.[159,174,185,186] dealing with ^{3}H-tryptophan binding to rat hepatic nuclei *in vitro* revealed that some amino acids, such as L-alanine, L-phenylalanine, and L-tyrosine, but not others, such as L-leucine, competed for such binding. In an attempt to determine how this occurs and the consequences thereof, a number of studies have been conducted.

The aromatic and branched chain amino acids use the same major amino acid transport system.[187] Thus, alterations in branched-chain amino acid levels, particularly in the blood, can affect the actions of the aromatic amino acids, including tryptophan.

4.4.2.1 *Other Amino Acids*

4.4.2.1.1 *Alanine*

The nonessential amino acid, L-alanine, has been reported to compete with tryptophan binding to hepatic nuclei *in vitro*.[174,185] However, L-alanine is not capable of stimulating hepatic protein synthesis as does L-tryptophan.[185] Yet, L-alanine in competing with L-tryptophan for nuclear receptor binding is able to diminish or negate L-tryptophan's ability to stimulate hepatic protein synthesis.[185] Similarly, DL-β(l-naphthyl)alanine is capable of acting like L-alanine.[173] Also, L-alanine inhibited elevations of other rapidly induced metabolic reactions, such as nuclear RNA efflux and nuclear poly(A)polymerase activity, which occurred due to L-tryptophan alone. These two stimulatory responses have been considered to be involved in the process by which L-tryptophan enhanced hepatic protein synthesis.[90,102,169]

4.4.2.1.2 *Leucine*

Leucine is an essential, branched-chain amino acid that does not compete with tryptophan for nuclear tryptophan receptor binding *in vitro*.[186] However, the addition of L-leucine to unlabeled L-tryptophan caused significantly less inhibition of ^{3}H-tryptophan binding *in vitro* to hepatic nuclei than did unlabeled L-tryptophan alone.[186] Also, L-isoleucine and L-valine revealed binding effects similar to that with L-leucine. In regard to hepatic protein synthesis, L-leucine alone has no effect, yet when added with L-tryptophan, it inhibits the increase of protein synthesis due to L-tryptophan alone. The mechanisms by which L-leucine acts are not yet clear. It does not appear to be related to altered transport of L-tryptophan, as can occur with branched-chain amino acids. Although L-leucine does not stimulate hepatic protein synthesis, it has been reported to stimulate muscle protein synthesis.[188] Whether this effect of L-leucine on muscle may influence the liver response is not clear.

In view of the preceding studies with L-leucine and with L-alanine, it was appropriate to determine whether dietary imbalances induced by tube-feeding different ratios of L-alanine or L-leucine in relation to L-tryptophan would affect tryptophan's stimulatory effect on hepatic protein synthesis.[189] Mice, food-deprived overnight, were tube-fed one feeding of solution, keeping L-tryptophan constant and varying ratios of alanine to tryptophan of 0.4, 2.1, or 4.0 or ratios of leucine to tryptophan of 4.8, 7.2, or 9.6. Mice were killed after 1 h, and protein synthesis (^{14}C-leucine incorporation into proteins *in vitro* using hepatic microsomes) was assayed. Tryptophan alone stimulated hepatic protein synthesis by 83%, while alanine-to-tryptophan ratios of 2.1 or 4.0 but not of 0.4 and leucine-to-tryptophan ratios of 9.6 but not of 4.8 or 7.2 caused significant decreases in the stimulation of hepatic protein synthesis. Thus, dietary imbalances between the two selected amino acids and L-tryptophan were able to influence tryptophan's effect on hepatic protein synthesis.

4.4.2.2 **Vitamins**

In an earlier section, the close precursor association between L-tryptophan and niacin has been described. Therefore, other vitamins and their interrelationships or interactions with L-tryptophan will be considered.

4.4.2.2.1 *Ascorbic Acid (Vitamin C)*

Vitamin C is one of several vitamins considered to be dietary antioxidants. In recent years, much attention has been given to the role of antioxidants in a number of chronic disease states. Benefits from the ingestion of high levels of vitamins considered as dietary antioxidants, such as β-carotene, A, C, and E, have been expounded from many sources. However, epidemiological studies in many cases have not been conclusive.

In considering that vitamin C is an important dietary antioxidant, studies were conducted on the effects of the addition of vitamin C upon selected actions of L-tryptophan and on its ability to bind to a specific hepatic nuclear receptor for L-tryptophan and to stimulate protein synthesis.[190] The results indicated that the addition of ascorbic acid at 10^{-6} to 10^{-4} M to hepatic nuclei *in vitro* inhibited ^{3}H-tryptophan binding to the nuclei and nuclear envelopes. Also, the *in vivo* administration of ascorbic acid before or along with L-tryptophan decreased the tryptophan-induced stimulation of hepatic protein synthesis (measured *in vitro* using microsomes).

How ascorbic acid acts to inhibit *in vitro* ^{3}H-tryptophan binding to hepatic nuclei or nuclear envelopes is not clear. Some additional studies shed light on its actions. Dithiolthreitol, a protective agent for sulfhydryl groups, was unable to affect the inhibitory binding effect due to ascorbic acid.[190] This indicates that ascorbic acid does not act on thiol groups of the nuclear receptor for L-tryptophan, as was described in studies with selenite.[175] L-leucine diminishes the inhibitory binding effect of ascorbic acid. However, since the mechanism by which L-leucine acts is as yet undetermined, this does not help in understanding how ascorbic acid acts. While the additional studies do not clarify how ascorbic acid itself acts, they do indicate that the effect on tryptophan binding to hepatic nuclei can become modified by agents, which themselves act in different ways.

Of interest is that ascorbic acid inhibits other receptor binding under experimental conditions. Ascorbic acid was reported to be a potent inhibitor of the binding of both dopamine agonists (^{3}H-dopamine and ^{3}H-ADTN) and antagonists (^{3}H-spiroperidol and ^{3}H-domperidone) to neostriatal membrane preparations.[191] Ascorbic acid inhibits the specific binding of both the D1 agonist, ^{3}H-SKF38393, and the D2 agonist, ^{3}H-N-04237, at physiologically relevant concentrations.[192] These results were consistent with an allostearic effect at the level of the receptor. Ascorbic acid (0.03 to 0.33 mM) was reported to inhibit 75% of specific binding of ^{125}I-SCH 23982 to D1 dopaminergic receptors in membrane preparations from rat striatum in a dose-dependent manner. These results suggested that ascorbic acid affected the D1 dopamine receptor for function by lipid peroxidation, competition with dopamine for low-affinity sites, and reduced oxidation of dopamine.[193] Ascorbic acid generated significant lipid peroxidation under their experimental conditions using membranes from bovine cerebral cortex and also a 26% decrease in ^{3}H-serotonin receptor binding.[194] Trolox-C, a water soluble analog of vitamin E, completely blocked the ascorbate-induced loss of serotonin receptor binding in brain receptors, which they attributed to its ability to prevent ascorbate-induced lipid peroxidation.

4.4.2.2.2   Other Vitamins

Some fat-soluble vitamins, β-carotene, retinyl acetate, calciferol, α-tocopherol, and Trolox, as well as some water-soluble vitamins, thiamine and riboflavin, acted to inhibit *in vitro* ^{3}H-tryptophan binding to hepatic nuclei.[195] Dithiothreitol, a protective agent for subfhydryl groups, added along with each vitamin, decreased the vitamin's inhibitory effect on *in vitro* ^{3}H-tryptophan binding to hepatic nuclei, with the exception of riboflavin and calciferol. L-leucine addition to vitamins caused a markedly diminished inhibitory binding effect, due to thiamine, β-carotene, retinyl acetate, α-toropherol, and Trolox, but no effect on riboflavin and calciferol. The results suggest that essentially all of the antioxidant vitamins (β-carotene, retinyl acetate, α-toropherol, and Trolox) as well as some that do not have this property (calciferol, thiamine, and riboflavin) are capable of inhibiting *in vitro* ^{3}H-tryptophan binding to hepatic nuclei.

How the above described vitamins influence *in vitro* ^{3}H-tryptophan nuclear receptor binding is not clear. Based upon the experiments with added dithiothreitol, it appears that some vitamins act on the sulfhydryl groups of the receptor, which become modified, which interferes with ^{3}H-tryptophan binding. Reviews of reports by others indicate that certain vitamins can bind to hepatic nuclei. Examples include (1) ^{3}H-α-tocopherol, which has been reported to become incorporated into isolated rat liver nuclei in a nonspecific manner by binding to chromatin nonhistone chromosomal protein,[196] and (2) rat liver nuclei, which contain receptors for a folate-binding protein.[197] As yet, it is not known whether others act similarly or not. Thus, whether competitive binding to nuclei between vitamins and tryptophan occurs is not known.

4.4.3   Factors Influencing Supply of Tryptophan to Brain

Three major factors are considered as important in determining the supply of tryptophan to the brain leading to serotonin synthesis: (1) the extent of binding of tryptophan to serum albumin, which influences the pool of free (unbound) tryptophan that interacts with the amino acid carrier mechanism located at the blood–brain barrier, (2) the plasma tryptophan concentrations, and (3) the plasma concentration of other large neutral amino acids (LNAA), which compete with tryptophan for uptake into brain. Each factor can be influenced by the nutritional or hormonal status of the host and also by interorgan relationships in the metabolism of amino acids.

4.4.3.1   Extent of Binding of Tryptophan to Serum Albumin

This has been reviewed in an earlier section. Normally, the proportion of total plasma tryptophan bound to albumin is 85 to 90%. This equilibrium can be shifted under conditions which raise plasma nonesterified fatty acid (NEFA) concentrations, such as during fasting or stress.[198] Since NEFA competes with tryptophan for binding sites on albumin, the rise of NEFA concentration displaces tryptophan from albumin, raising the concentration of free tryptophan.

4.4.3.2 Plasma Tryptophan Concentration

Plasma tryptophan concentration is a function of dietary tryptophan intake as well as the extent of removal of tryptophan from blood by tissues. The liver is the main organ influencing plasma tryptophan concentration since it actively metabolizes tryptophan while nonhepatic tissues have only relatively limited ability to act in this manner. Following a meal, in the liver, tryptophan stimulates hepatic tryptophan oxygenase activity, which affects tryptophan catabolism and determines how much tryptophan enters the general circulation.

4.4.3.3 Plasma Concentration of the LNAA

The plasma concentration of LNAA competes with tryptophan for uptake into the brain. The extent of uptake and net utilization influences levels in blood. Like tryptophan, tyrosine and phenylalanine are mainly metabolized in the liver.[199] However, the branched-chain amino acids (BCAA) are taken up and metabolized mainly by skeletal muscle and little by the liver.[200] Thus, following a meal, the BCAA rise more in peripheral blood than the other LNAA and other indispensable amino acid levels that are influenced by liver metabolism. The BCAA, therefore, have the dominating effect of the LNAA as a group on brain tryptophan uptake.

4.4.3.4 Importance of the Three Factors

It is difficult to assess which of the three factors is the most important in raising brain tryptophan levels. In a 1991 review, Peters[201] discussed in detail studies undertaken to determine the importance of plasma tryptophan levels as well as plasma tryptophan levels in relation to plasma LNAA or BCAA levels and concluded that both are important. In regard to the importance of albumin binding and the fractions of plasma tryptophan as bound or free forms on brain tryptophan levels, the findings are mixed. Fernstrom et al.[202] reported that in experiments where free and bound tryptophan levels were altered by changes in the concentrations of NEFA, brain tryptophan concentration was not affected by the changes in plasma free tryptophan concentrations. Effects were better produced by the plasma ratio of tryptophan to LNAA. Bloxam et al.[203] used drugs to displace tryptophan from albumin, increasing the plasma-free pool, and indicated that this plasma-free pool was the most important determinant of tryptophan supply to the brain. It is rational to conclude that the binding of tryptophan to albumin has an influence (whether large or small) on the carrier-mediated transport of tryptophan into the brain.

4.5 Concluding Remarks

This chapter has covered a number of important aspects dealing with the effects and actions of L-tryptophan. The pathways of L-tryptophan catabolism are variable and lead to many vital and important compounds. Many enzymes are involved in these pathways. As an essential (indispensable) amino acid, L-tryptophan is vital for protein synthesis as it becomes incorporated into many proteins. The presence of L-tryptophan as a structural amino acid in many proteins seems to indicate that in certain proteins it has an essential role in the function of the protein (or enzyme). In addition, L-tryptophan appears to have a regulatory role in controlling (enhancing) protein synthesis. Aspects regarding mechanism(s) for this process appear to relate to mRNA processing in the cell nucleus. L-tryptophan binding to a specific nuclear envelope (membrane) receptor appears to be a vital step in the regulation of mRNA outflow from the nucleus into the cytoplasm. Other dietary components (amino acids and vitamins) have the ability to compete with L-tryptophan for nuclear receptor binding and the consequences thereof. L-tryptophan's unique ability to bind to serum protein (albumin) affects its flow and distribution within the blood and to tissues and organs, especially the brain. The complexity of L-tryptophan's action provides a scientific challenge to gain a full understanding of its many unique and vital functions. Much progress has been made within the past 100 years and much will occur in the years ahead.

References

1. Ikeda, M., Tsuji, H., Nakamura, S., Ichiyama, A., Nishizuka, Y., and Hayashi, O., Studies on the biosynthesis of nicotinamide adenine dinucleotide. II. A role of picolinic carboxylase in the biosynthesis of nicotinamide adenine dinucleotide from tryptophan in mammals, *J. Biol. Chem.*, 240, 1395, 1965.
2. Shimizu, T., Nomiyama, S., Hirata, F., and Hayaishi, O., Indoleamine 2, 3-dioxygenase. Purification and some properties, *J. Biol. Chem.*, 253[13], 4700, 1978.
3. Yamazaki, F., Kuroiwa, T., Takikawa, O., and Kido, R., Human indolylamine 2, 3-dioxygenase. Its tissue distribution, and characterization of the placental enzyme, *Biochem. J.*, 230[3], 635, 1985.
4. Yoshida, R., Urade, Y., Tokuda, M., and Hayaishi, O., Induction of indoleamine 2, 3-dioxygenase in mouse lung during virus infection, *Proc. Natl. Acad. Sci. U.S.A.*, 76[8], 4084, 1979.
5. Yoshida, R., Imanishi, J., Oku, T., Kishida, T., and Hayaishi, O., Induction of pulmonary indoleamine 2, 3-dioxygenase by interferon, *Proc. Natl. Acad. Sci. U.S.A.*, 78[1], 129, 1981.
6.. Ozaki, Y., Edelstein, M. P., and Duch, D. S., The actions of interferon and anti-inflammatory agents of induction of indoleamine 2, 3-dioxygenase in human peripheral blood monocytes, *Biochem. Biophys. Res. Commun.*, 144[3], 1147, 1987.

7. Werner, E. R., Werner-Felmayer, G., Fuchs, D., Hausen, A., Reibnegger, G., and Wachter, H., Parallel induction of tetrahydrobiopterin biosynthesis and indoleamine 2, 3-dioxygenase activity in human cells and cell lines by interferon-gamma, *Biochem. J.*, 262[3], 861, 1989.

8. Takikawa, O., Habara-Ohkubo, A., and Yoshida, R., IFN-gamma is the inducer of indoleamine 2, 3-dioxygenase in allografted tumor cells undergoing rejection, *J. Immunol.*, 145[4], 1246, 1990.

9. Brown, R. R., Lee, C. M., Kohler, P. C., Hank, J. A., Storer, B. E., and Sondel, P. M., Altered tryptophan and neopterin metabolism in cancer patients treated with recombinant interleukin 2, *Cancer Res.*, 49[17], 4941, 1989.

10. Carlin, J. M., Ozaki, Y., Byrne, G. I., Brown, R. R., and Borden, E. C., Interferons and indoleamine 2, 3-dioxygenase: Role in antimicrobial and antitumor effects, *Experientia*, 45[6], 535, 1989.

11. Taylor, M. W. and Feng, G. S., Relationship between interferon-gamma, indoleamine 2, 3-dioxygenase, and tryptophan catabolism, *FASEB J.*, 5[11], 2516, 1991.

12. Byrne, G. I., Lehmann, L. K., Kirschbaum, J. G., Borden, E. C., Lee, C. M., and Brown, R. R., Induction of tryptophan degradation *in vitro* and *in vivo*: A gamma-interferon-stimulated activity, *J. Interferon Res.*, 6[4], 389, 1986.

13. Kaplan, J. H. and Pitot, H. C., The regulation of intermediary amino acid metabolism in animal tissues, in *Mammalian Protein Metabolism*, Munro, H. N., Ed., Academic Press, New York, 1970, 387–443.

14. Schimke, R. T., Sweeney, E. W., and Berlin, C. M., The roles of synthesis and degradation in the control of rat liver tryptophan pyrrolase, *J. Biol.Chem.*, 240, 322, 1965.

15. Ballard, F. J. and Hopgood, M. F., Phosphopyruvate carboxylase induction by L-tryptophan. Effects on synthesis and degradation of the enzyme, *Biochem. J.*, 136[2], 259, 1973.

16. Cihak, A. L., Tryptophan action on hepatic RNA synthesis and enzyme induction, *Mol. Cell. Biochem.*, 24[3], 131, 1979.

17. Chee, P. Y. and Swick, R. W., Effect of dietary protein and tryptophan and the turnover of rat liver ornithine aminotransferase, *J. Biol. Chem.*, 251[4], 1029, 1976.

18. Deguchi, T. and Barchas, J., Induction of hepatic tyrosine aminotransferase by indole amines, *J. Biol. Chem.*, 246[23], 7217, 1971.

19. Smith, S. A. and Pogson, C. L., Tryptophan and the control of plasma glucose concentrations in the rat, *Biochem. J.*, 168[3], 495, 1977.

20. Smith, S. A., Marston, F. A., Dickson, A. J., and Pogson, C. I., Control of enzyme activities in rat liver by tryptophan and its metabolites, *Biochem. Pharmacol.*, 28[10], 1645, 1979.

21. Kenney, F. T., Hormonal regulation of synthesis of liver enzymes, in *Mammalian Protein Metabolism*, Munro, H. N., Ed., Academic Press, New York, 1970, 4, 131–176.

22. Kato, K., Selective repression of benzoate or tryptophan mediated induction of liver tyrosine aminotransferase by phentolamine in adrenalectomized rats, *FEBS Lett.*, 8, 316, 1970.

23. Schumm, D. E. and Webb, T. E., Effect of adenosine 3':5'-monophosphate and guanosine 3':5'-monophosphate on RNA release from isolated nuclei, *J. Biol. Chem.*, 253[23], 8513, 1978.

24. Brown, R. R., Metabolism and biology of tryptophan. Some clinical implications, *Adv. Exp. Med. Biol.*, 15, 398, 1995.

25. Blakesley, V. A., Kato, H., Roberts, C. T., Jr., and LeRoith, D., Mutation of a conserved amino acid residue (tryptophan 1173) in the tyrosine kinase domain of the IGF-I receptor abolishes autophosphorylation but does not eliminate biologic function, *J. Biol. Chem.*, 270[6], 2764, 1995.

26. Clackson, T. and Wells, J. A., A hot spot of binding energy in a hormone-receptor interface, *Science*, 267[5196], 383, 1995.

27. Meers, P. and Mealy, T, Phospholipid determinants for annexin V binding sites and the role of tryptophan 187, *Biochemistry*, 33[19], 5829, 1994.

28. Swamy, N., Brisson, M., and Ray, R., Trp-145 is essential for the binding of 25-hydroxyvitamin D3 to human serum vitamin D-binding protein, *J. Biol. Chem.*, 270[6], 2636, 1995.

29. Wilson, B. A., Blanke, S. R., Reich, K. A., and Collier, R. J., Active-site mutations of diphtheria toxin. Tryptophan 50 is a major determinant of NAD affinity, *J. Biol. Chem.*, 269[37], 23296, 1994.

30. Maenaka, K., Kawai, G., Watanabe, K., Sunada, F., and Kumagai, I., Functional and structural role of a tryptophan generally observed in protein-carbohydrate interaction. TRP-62 of hen egg white lysozyme, *J. Biol.Chem*, 269[10], 7070, 1994.

31. Guillot, D., Penin, F., Di Pietro, A., Sontag, B., Lavergne, J. P., and Reboud, J. P., GTP binding to elongation factor eEF-2 unmasks a tryptophan residue required for biological activity, *J. Biol.Chem.*, 268[28], 20911, 1993.

32. Guillot, D., Lavergne, J. P., and Reboud, J. P., Trp221 is involved in the protective effect of elongation factor eEF-2 on the ricin/alpha-sarcin site of the ribosome, *J. Biol. Chem.*, 268[35], 26082, 1993.

33. Faurobert, E., Otto-Bruc, A., Chardin, P., and Chabre, M., Tryptophan W207 in transducin T alpha is the fluorescence sensor of the G protein activation switch and is involved in the effector binding, *EMBO J.*, 12[11], 4191, 1993.

34. Liu, J., Chen, C. M., and Walsh, C. T., Human and *Escherichia coli* cyclophilins: Sensitivity to inhibition by the immunosuppressant cyclosporin A correlates with a specific tryptophan residue, *Biochemistry*, 30[9], 2306, 1991.

35. Baubichon-Cortay, H., Baggetto, L. G., Dayan, G., and Di Pietro, A., Overexpression and purification of the carboxyl-terminal nucleotide-binding domain from mouse P-glycoprotein. Strategic location of a tryptophan residue, *J. Biol. Chem.*, 269[37], 22983, 1994.

36. Raszka, M. and Mandel, M., Interaction of aromatic amino acids with neutral polyadenylic acid, *Proc. Natl. Acad. Sci. U.S.A.*, 68[6], 1190, 1971.

37. Toulme, J. J., Charlier, M., and Helene, C., Specific recognition of single-stranded regions in ultraviolet-irradiated and heat-denatured DNA by tryptophan-containing peptides, *Proc. Natl. Acad. Sci. U.S.A.*, 71[8], 3185, 1974.

38. Sigel, H. and Naumann, C. F., Ternary complexes in solution. XXIV. Metal ion bridging of stacked purine-indole adducts. The mixed-ligand complexes of adenosine 5'-triphosphate, tryptophan, and manganese(II), copper(II), or zinc(II), *J. Am. Chem. Soc.*, 98[3], 730, 1976.

39. Helene, C. and Dimicoli, J. L., Interaction of oligopeptides containing aromatic amino acids with nucleic acids. Fluorescence and proton magnetic resonance studies, *FEBS Lett.*, 26[1], 6, 1972.

40. Dimicoli, J. L. and Helene, C., Interactions of aromatic residues of proteins with nucleic acids. I. Proton magnetic resonance studies of the binding of tryptophan-containing peptides to poly(adenylic acid) and deoxyribonucleic acid, *Biochemistry*, 13[4], 714, 1974.

41. Stahl, N. and Prusiner, S. B., Prions and prion proteins, *FASEB J.*, 5[13], 2799, 1991.
42. Yau, W. M., Wimley, W. C., Gawrisch, K., and White, S. H., The preference of tryptophan for membrane interfaces, *Biochemistry*, 37[42], 14713, 1998.
43. Preusch, P. C., Norvell, J. C., Cassatt, J. C., and Cassman, M., Progress away from 'no crystals, no grant,' *Nat. Struct. Biol.*, 5[1], 12, 1998.
44. Sidransky, H., Murty, C. N., and Verney, E., Nutritional control of protein synthesis. Studies relating to tryptophan-induced stimulation of nucleocytoplasmic translocation of mRNA in rat liver, *Am. J. Pathol.*, 117[2], 298, 1984.
45. Sidransky, H., Tryptophan. Unique action by an essential amino acid, in *Nutritional Pathology: Pathobiochemistry of Dietary Imbalances*, Sidransky, H., Ed., Marcel Dekker, New York, 1985, 1-62.
46. Gacad, G., Dickie, K., and Massaro, D., Protein synthesis in lung: Influence of starvation on amino acid incorporation into protein, *J. Appl. Physiol.*, 33[3], 381, 1972.
47. Jorgensen, A. J. and Majumdar, A. P., Bilateral adrenalectomy: Effect of tryptophan force-feeding on amino acid incorporation into ferritin, transferrin, and mixed proteins of liver, brain and kidneys *in vivo*, *Biochem. Med.*, 16[1], 37–46. 1976.
48. Majumdar, A. P., Effects of fasting and subsequent feeding of a complete or tryptophan-free diet on the activity of DNA-synthesizing enzymes and protein synthesis in gastric mucosa of rats, *Ann. Nur. Metab.*, 26[4], 264, 1982.
49. Lin, F. D., Smith, T. K., and Bayley, H. S., A role for tryptophan in regulation of protein synthesis in porcine muscle, *J. Nutr.*, 118[4], 445–449. 1988.
50. Blazek, R. and Shaw, D. M., Tryptophan availability and brain protein synthesis, *Neuropharmacology*, 17[12], 1065, 1978.
51. Fleck, A., Shepherd, J., and Munro, H. N., Protein synthesis in rat liver. Influence of amino acids in diet on microsomes and polysomes, *Science*, 150, 628, 1965.
52. Sidransky, H., Bongiorno, M., Sarma, D. S., and Verney, E., The influence of tryptophan on hepatic polyribosomes and protein synthesis in fasted mice, *Biochem. Biophys. Res. Commun.*, 27[2], 242, 1967.
53. Sidransky, H., Sarma, D. S., Bongiorno, M., and Verney, E., Effect of dietary tryptophan on hepatic polyribosomes and protein synthesis in fasted mice, *J. Biol. Chem.*, 243[6], 1123, 1968.
54. Sox, H. C., Jr. and Hoagland, M. B., Functional alterations in rat liver polysomes associated with starvation and refeeding, *J. Mol. Biol.*, 20[1], 113, 1966.
55. Staehelin, T., Verney, E., and Sidransky, H., The influence of nutritional change on polyribosomes of the liver, *Biochim. Biophys. Acta*, 145[1], 105, 1967.
56. Webb, T. E., Blobel, G., and Potter, V. R., Polyribosomes in rat tissues. 3. The response of the polyribosome pattern of rat liver to physiologic stress, *Cancer Res.*, 26[2], 253, 1966.
57. Wilson, S. H. and Hoagland, M. B., Physiology of rat-liver polysomes. The stability of messenger ribonucleic acid and ribosomes, *Biochem. J.*, 103[2], 556, 1967.
58. Wunner, W. H., Bell, J., and Munro, H. N., The effect of feeding with a tryptophan-free amino acid mixture on rat-liver polysomes and ribosomal ribonucleic acid, *Biochem. J.*, 101[2], 417, 1966.

59. Noll, H., Staehelin, T., and Wettstein, F. O., Ribosomal aggregate engaged in protein synthesis. Ergosome breakdown and messenger ribonucleic acid transport, *Nature*, 198, 632, 1963.

60. Pronczul, A. W., Baliga, B. S., Triant, J. W., and Munro, H. N., Comparaison of the effect of amino acid supply on hepatic polysome profiles *in vivo* and *in vitro*, *Biochim. Biophys. Acta*, 157[1], 204, 1968.

61. Pamart, B., Girard-Globa, A., and Bourdel, G., Induction of tyrosine aminotransferase and depression of protein synthesis in rat liver by a tryptophan-free mixture of amino acids, *J. Nutr.*, 104[9], 1149, 1974.

62. Sidransky, H., Verney, E., and Sarma, D. S., Effect of tryptophan on polyribosomes and protein synthesis in liver, *Am. J. Clin. Nutr.*, 24[7], 779, 1971.

63. Feigelson, P., Feigelson, M., and Fancher, C., Kinetics of liver nucleic acid turnovers during enzyme induction in the rat, *Biochim. Biophys. Acta*, 32, 133, 1959.

64. Cammarano, P., Chinali, G., Gaetani, S., and Spadoni, M. A., Involvement of adrenal steroids in the changes of polysome organization during feeding of unbalanced amino acid diets, *Biochim. Biophys. Acta*, , 155[1], 302, 1968.

65. Rothschild, M. A., Oratz, M., Mongelli, J., Fishman, L., and Schreiber, S. S., Amino acid regulation of albumin synthesis, *J. Nutr.*, 98[4], 395, 1969.

66. Oravec, M. and Sourkes, T. L., Inhibition of hepatic protein synthesis by α-methyl-DL-tryptophan *in vivo*. Further studies on the glyconeogenic action of α-methyltryptophan, *Biochemistry*, 9[22], 4458, 1970.

67. Park, O. J., Henderson, L. M., and Swan, P. B., Effects of the administration of single amino acids on ribosome aggregation in rat liver, *Exp. Biol. Med.*, 142[3], 1023, 1973.

68. Jorgensen, A. J. and Majumdar, A. P., Bilateral adrenalectomy: Effect of a single tube-feeding of tryptophan on amino acid incorporation into plasma abumin and fibrinogen *in vivo*, *Biochem. Med.*, 13[3], 231, 1975.

69. Majumdar, A. P. N., Tryptophan requirement for protein synthesis. A review, *Nut. Rep. Int.*, 26, 509, 1982.

70. Pronczuk, A. W., Rogers, Q. R., and Munro, H. N., Liver polysome patterns of rats fed amino acid imbalanced diets, *J. Nutr.*, 100[11], 1249, 1970.

71. Ip, C. C. and Harper, A. E., Liver polysome profiles and protein synthesis in rats fed a threonine-imbalanced diet, *J. Nutr.*, 104[2], 252, 1974.

72. Sarma, D. S. R., Verney, E., Bongiorno, M., and Sidransky, H., Influence of tryptophan on hepatic polyribosomes and protein synthesis in non-fasted mice, *Nut. Rep. Int.*, 4, 1, 1971.

73. Munro, H. N., Role of amino acid supply in regulating ribosome function, *Fed. Proc.*, 27[5], 1231, 1968.

74. Hori, M., Fisher, J. M., and Rabinovitz, M., Tryptophan deficiency in rabbit reticulocytes: Polyribosomes during interrupted growth of hemoglobin chains, *Science*, 155[758], 83, 1967.

75. Hunt, R. T., Hunter, A. R., and Munro, A. J., The control of haemoglobin synthesis: Factors controlling the output of alpha and beta chains, *Proc. Nutr. Soc.*, 28[2], 248, 1969.

76. Rogers, Q. R., The nutritional and metabolic effects of amino acid imbalances, in *Protein Metabolism and Nutrition*, Cole, D. J. A., Ed., Butterworths, London, 1976.

77. Sidransky, H., Murty, C. N., and Verney, E., Effect of tryptophan on the inhibitory action of selected hepatotoxic agents on hepatic protein synthesis, *Exp. Mol. Pathol.*, 37[3], 305, 1982.

78. Allen, R. E., Raines, P. L., and Regen, D. M., Regulatory significance of transfer RNA charging levels. I. Measurements of charging levels in livers of chow-fed rats, fasting rats, and rats fed balanced or imbalanced mixtures of amino acids, *Biochim. Biophys. Acta*, 190[2], 323, 1969.

79. Henderson, A. R., The effect of feeding with a tryptophan-free amino acid mixture on rat liver magnesium ion-activated deoxyribonucleic acid-dependent ribonucleic acid polymerase, *Biochem. J.*, 120[1], 205, 1970.

80. Vesley, J. and Cihak, A., Enhanced DNA-dependent RNA polymerase and RNA synthesis in rat liver nuclei after administration of L-tryptophan, *Biochim. Biophys. Acta*, 204, 614, 1970.

81. Majumdar, A. P., Effect of tryptophan on hepatic nuclear free and engaged RNA-polymerases in young and adult rats, *Experientia*, 34[10], 1258, 1978.

82. Oravec, M. and Korner, A., Stimulation of ribosomal and DNA-like RNA synthesis by tryptophan, *Biochim. Biophys. Acta*, 247[3], 404, 1971.

83. Wunner, W. H., The time sequence of RNA and protein synthesis in cellular compartments following an acute dietary challenge with amino acid mixtures, *Proc. Nutr. Soc.*, 26[2], 153, 1967.

84. Murty, C. N. and Sidransky, H., The effect of tryptophan on messenger RNA of the liver of fasted mice, *Biochim. Biophys. Acta*, 262[3], 328, 1972.

85. Murty, C. N., Verney, E., and Sidransky, H., Effect of tryptophan on polyriboadenylic acid and polyadenylic acid-messenger ribonucleic acid in rat liver, *Lab. Invest.*, 34[1], 77, 1976.

86. Blatti, S. P., Ingels, C. J., Lindell, T. J., Morris, P. M., Weayer, R. F., Weinberg, F., and Rutter, W. J., Structure and regulatory porperties of eukaryotic RNA polymerase, *Cold Spring Harbor Symp. Quant. Biol.*, 35, 649, 1970.

87. Roeder, R. G. and Rutter, W. J., Specific nucleolar and nucleoplasmic RNA polymerases, *Proc. Natl. Acad. Sci. U.S.A.*, 65[3], 675, 1970.

88. Majumdar, A. P. and Jorgensen, A. J., Response of well-fed adrenalectomized rats to tryptophan force-feeding on hepatic protein and RNA synthesis, *Biochem. Med.*, 16[3], 266, 1976.

89. Majumdar, A. P., Effects of fasting and tryptophan force-feeding on the activity of hepatic nuclear RNA polymerases in rats, *Scand. J. Clin. Lab. Invest.*, 39[1], 61, 1979.

90. Murty, C. N., Verney, E., and Sidransky, H., The effect of tryptrophan on nucleocytoplasmic translocation of RNA in rat liver, *Biochim. Biophys. Acta*, 474[1], 117, 1977.

91. Sidransky, H., Verney, E., and Murty, C. N., Effect of tryptophan on hepatic polyribosomal disaggregation due to hypertonic sodium chloride, *Lab. Invest.*, 34[3], 291, 1976.

92. Sidransky, H., Verney, E., and Murty, C. N., Effect of tryptophan on hepatic polyribosomes and protein synthesis in rats treated with carbon tetrachloride, *Toxicol. Appl. Pharmacol.*, 39[2], 295, 1977.

93. Garrett, C. T., Cairns, V., Murty, C. N., Verney, E., and Sidransky, H., Effect of tryptophan on informosomal and polyribosome-associated messenger RNA in rat liver, *J. Nutr.*, 114[1], 50, 1984.

94. Brawerman, G., Eukaryotic messenger RNA, *Annu. Rev. Biochem.*, 43[0], 621–642, 1974.

95. Perry, R. P., Processing of RNA, *Annu. Rev. Biochem.*, 45, 605, 1976.
96. Smuckler, E. A. and Koplitz, R. M., Polyadenylic acid content and electrophoretic behavior of *in vitro* released RNAs in chemical carcinogenesis, *Cancer Res.*, 36[3], 881, 1976.
97. Clawson, G. A., Woo, C. H., and Smuckler, E. A., Independent responses of nucleoside triphosphatase and protein kinase activities in nuclear envelope following thioacetamide treatment, *Biochem. Biophys. Res. Commun.*, 95[3], 1200, 1980.
98. Patel, N. T., Folse, D. S., and Holoubek, V., Release of repetitive nuclear RNA into the cytoplasm in liver of rats fed 3'-methyl-4-dimethylaminoazobenzene, *Cancer Res.*, 39[11], 4460, 1979.
99. Shearer, R. W., Altered RNA transport without derepression in a rat kidney tumor induced by dimethylnitrosamine, *Chem.-Biol. Interact.*, 27[1], 91, 1979.
100. Yannarell, A., Schumm, D. E., and Webb, T. E., Age-dependence of nuclear RNA processing, *Mech. Ageing Dev.*, 6[4], 259, 1977.
101. Schumm, D. E. and Webb, T. E., Modified messenger ribonucleic acid release from isolated hepatic nuclei after inhibition of polyadenylate formation, *Biochem. J.*, 139[1], 191, 1974.
102. Murty, C. N., Verney, E., and Sidransky, H., In vivo and in vitro studies on the effect of tryptophan on translocation of RNA from nuclei of rat liver, *Biochem. Med.*, 22[1], 98, 1979.
103. Ono, H. and Terayama, H., Amino acid incorporation into proteins in isolated rat liver nuclei, *Biochim. Biophys. Acta*, 166[1], 175, 1968.
104. Ono, H., Ono, T., and Wada, O., Amino acid incorporation by nuclear membrane fraction of rat liver, *Life Sci.*, 18[2], 215, 1976.
105. Murty, C. N., Hornseth, R., Verney, E., and Sidransky, H., Effect of tryptophan on enzymes and proteins of hepatic nuclear envelopes of rats, *Lab. Invest.*, 48[3], 256, 1983.
106. Sarma, D. S., Bongiorno, M., Verney, E., and Sidransky, H., Effect of oral administration of tryptophan or water on hepatic polyribosomal disaggregation due to puromycin, *Exp. Mol. Pathol.*, 19[1], 23, 1973.
107. Sidransky, H., Verney, E., and Sarma, D. S., Effect of tryptophan on hepatic polyribosomal disaggregation due to ethionine, *Exp. Biol. Med.*, 140[2], 633, 1972.
108. Harris, J. R., The biochemistry and ultrastructure of the nuclear envelope, *Biochim. Biophys. Acta*, 515[1], 55, 1978.
109. Clawson, G. A., James, J., Woo, C. H., Friend, D. S., Moody, D., and Smuckler, E. A., Pertinence of nuclear envelope nucleoside triphosphatase activity to ribonucleic acid transport, *Biochemistry*, 19[12], 2748, 1980.
110. Agutter, P. S., McCaldin, B., and McArdle, H. J., Importance of mammalian nuclear-envelope nucleoside triphosphatase in nucleo-cytoplasmic transport of ribonucleoproteins, *Biochem. J.*, 182[3], 811, 1979.
111. Vorbrodt, A. and Maul, G. G., Cytochemical studies on the relation of nucleoside triphosphatase activity to ribonucleoproteins in isolated rat liver nuclei, *J. Histochem. Cytochem.*, 28[1], 27, 1980.
112. Murty, C. N., Verney, E., and Sidransky, H., Effect of tryptophan on nuclear envelope nucleoside triphosphatase activity in rat liver, *Exp. Biol. Med.*, 163[1], 155, 1980.
113. Lam, K. S. and Kasper, C. B., Selective phosphorylation of a nuclear envelope polypeptide by an endogenous protein kinase, *Biochemistry*, 18[2], 307, 1979.

114. Steer, R. C., Wilson, M. J., and Ahmed, K., Protein phosphokinase activity of rat liver nuclear membrane, *Exp. Cell Res.*, 119[2], 403, 1979.

115. Steer, R. C., Wilson, M. J., and Ahmed, K., Phosphoprotein phosphatase activity of rat liver nuclear membrane, *Biochem. Biophys. Res. Commun.*, 89[4], 1082, 1979.

116. McDonald, J. R. and Agutter, P. S., The relationship between polyribonucleotide binding and the phosphorylation and dephosphorylation of nuclear envelope protein, *FEBS Lett.*, 116[2], 145, 1980.

117. Aaronson, R. P. and Blobel, G., On the attachment of the nuclear pore complex, *J. Cell Biol.*, 62[3], 746-754. 1974.

118. Franke, W. W., Structure, biochemistry, and functions of the nuclear envelope, *Int. Rev. Cytol.*, Suppl. 4, 71, 1974.

119. Stuart, S. E., Clawson, G. A., Rottman, F. M., and Patterson, R. J., RNA transport in isolated myeloma nuclei. Transport from membrane-denuded nuclei, *J. Cell Biol.*, 72[1], 57, 1977.

120. Palayoor, T., Schumm, D. E., and Webb, T. E., Transport of functional messenger RNA from liver nuclei in a reconstituted cell-free system, *Biochim. Biophys. Acta*, 654[2], 201, 1981.

121. Bocker, R., Jones, I. K., and Kersten, W., Metabolism of protein and RNA in liver of rats deprived of tryptophan, *J. Nutr.*, 107[9], 1737, 1977.

122. Wannemacher, R. W., Jr., Cooper, W. K., and Yatvin, M. B., The regulation of protein synthesis in the liver of rats. Mechanisms of dietary amino acid control in the immature animal, *Biochem. J.*, 107, 615, 1968.

123. Roth, J., Peptide hormone binding to receptors: A review of direct studies *in vitro*, *Metab. Clin. Exp.*, 22[8], 1059, 1973.

124. Kahn, C. R., Membrane receptors for polypeptide hormones, *Meth. Membr. Biol.*, 3, 81, 1975.

125. Goldfine, I. D. and Smith, G. J., Binding of insulin to isolated nuclei, *Proc. Natl. Acad. Sci. U.S.A.*, 73[5], 1427, 1976.

126. Goldfine, I. D., Smith, G. J., Wong, K. Y., and Jones, A. L., Cellular uptake and nuclear binding of insulin in human cultured lymphocytes: Evidence for potential intracellular sites of insulin action, *Proc. Natl. Acad. Sci. U.S.A.*, 74[4], 1368, 1977.

127. Vigneri, R., Goldfine, I. D., Wong, K. Y., Smith, G. J., and Pezzino, V., The nuclear envelope. The major site of insulin binding in rat liver nuclei, *J. Biol. Chem.*, 253[7], 2098, 1978.

128. Goldfine, I. D., Purrello, F., Clawson, G. A., and Vigneri, R., Insulin binding sites on the nuclear envelope: Potential relationship to mRNA metabolism, *J. Cell. Biochem.*, 20[1], 29, 1982.

129. Goldfine, I. D., Clawson, G. A., Smuckler, E. A., Purrello, F., and Vigneri, R., Action of insulin at the nuclear envelope, *Mol. Cell. Biochem.*, 48[1], 3, 1982.

130. Roth, R. A. and Cassell, D. J., Insulin receptor: Evidence that it is a protein kinase, *Science*, 219[4582], 299, 1983.

131. Gorski, J. and Gannon, F., Current models of steroid hormone action: A critique, *Annu. Rev. Physiol.*, 38, 425, 1976.

132. Yamamoto, K. R. and Alberts, B. M., Steroid receptors: Elements for modulation of eukaryotic transcription, *Annu. Rev. Biochem.*, 45, 721, 1976.

133. Ballard, P. L., Baxter, J. D., Higgins, S. J., Rousseau, G. G., and Tomkins, G. M., General presence of glucocorticoid receptors in mammalian tissues, *Endocrinology*, 94[4], 998, 1974.

134. Giannopoulos, G., Hassan, Z., and Solomon, S., Glucocorticoid receptors in fetal and adult rabbit tissues, *J. Biol.Chem.*, 249[8], 2424, 1974.
135. Markovic, R. and Petrovic, J., Competition of tryptophan and hydrocortisone for receptor proteins of rat liver cytosol, *Int. J. Biochem.*, 6, 47, 1975.
136. Baker, M. E., Vaughn, D. A., and Fanestil, D. D., Competitive inhibition of dexamethasone binding to the glucocorticoid receptor in HTC cells by tryptophan methyl ester, *J. Steroid Biochem.*, 13[8], 993, 1980.
137. Majumdar, A. P. and Jorgensen, A. J., Influence of cortisol on tryptophan-mediated stimulation of hepatic protein synthesis in well-fed adrenalectomized rats, *Biochem. Med.*, 17[1], 116, 1977.
138. Verney, E. and Sidransky, H., Further enhancement by tryptophan of hepatic protein synthesis stimulated by phenobarbital or cortisone acetate, *Exp. Biol. Med.*, 158[2], 245, 1978.
139. Sap, J., Munoz, A., Damm, K., Goldberg, Y., Ghysdael, J., Leutz, A., Beug, H., and Vennstrom, B., The c-erb-A protein is a high-affinity receptor for thyroid hormone, *Nature*, 324[6098], 635, 1986.
140. Thompson, C. C. and Evans, R. M., Trans-activation by thyroid hormone receptors: Functional parallels with steroid hormone receptors, *Proc. Natl. Acad. Sci. U.S.A.*, 86[10], 3494, 1989.
141. Weinberger, C., Thompson, C. C., Ong, E. S., Lebo, R., Gruol, D. J., and Evans, R. M., The c-erb-A gene encodes a thyroid hormone receptor, *Nature*, 324[6098], 641, 1986.
142. Renkawitz, R., Kaltschmidt, C., Leers, J., Martin, B., Muller, M., and Eggert, M., Enhancement of nuclear receptor transcriptional signalling, *J. Steroid Biochem. Mol. Biol.*, 56[1-6], 39, 1996.
143. Hoppner, W., Sussmuth, W., O'Brien, C., and Seitz, H. J., Cooperative effect of thyroid and glucocorticoid hormones on the induction of hepatic phosphoenolpyruvate carboxykinase *in vivo* and in cultured hepatocytes, *Eur. J. Biochem.*, 159[2], 399, 1986.
144. Bedo, G., Santisteban, P., and Aranda, A., Retinoic acid regulates growth hormone gene expression, *Nature*, 339[6221], 231, 1989.
145. Samuels, H. H., Aranda, A., Casanova, J., Copp, R. P., Flug, F., Forman, B. M., Horowitz, Z. D., Janocko, L., Park, H. Y., and Pascual, A., Identification of the cis-acting elements and trans-acting factors that mediate cell-specific and thyroid hormone stimulation of growth hormone gene expression, *Rec. Progr. Horm. Res.*, 44, 53, 1988.
146. Fujimoto, N., Watanabe, H., and Ito, A., Up-regulation of the estrogen receptor by triiodothyronine in rat pituitary cell lines, *J. Steroid Biochem. Mol. Biol.*, 61[1–2], 79, 1997.
147. Naar, A. M., Boutin, J. M., Lipkin, S. M., Yu, V. C., Holloway, J. M., Glass, C. K., and Rosenfeld, M. G., The orientation and spacing of core DNA-binding motifs dictate selective transcriptional responses to three nuclear receptors, *Cell*, 65[7], 1267, 1991.
148. Sidransky, H. and Verney, E., Hormonal influences on tryptophan binding to rat hepatic nuclei, *Adv. Exp. Med. Biol.*, 467, 369, 1999.
149. Zhou, Y., Samson, M., Osty, J., Francon, J., and Blondeau, J. P., Evidence for a close link between the thyroid hormone transport system and the aromatic amino acid transport system T in erythrocytes, *J. Biol. Chem.*, 265[28], 17000, 1990.

150. Zhou, Y., Samson, M., Francon, J., and Blondeau, J. P., Thyroid hormone concentrative uptake in rat erythrocytes. Involvement of the tryptophan transport system T in countertransport of tri-iodothyronine and aromatic amino acids, *Biochem. J.*, 281[Pt. 1], 81, 1992.
151. Salter, M., Knowles, R. G., and Pogson, C. I., Transport of the aromatic amino acids into isolated rat liver cells. Properties of uptake by two distinct systems, *Biochem. J.*, 233[2], 499, 1986.
152. Kemp, H. F. and Taylor, P. M., Interactions between thyroid hormone and tryptophan transport in rat liver are modulated by thyroid status, *Am. J. Physiol.*, 272[5 Pt. 1], E809, 1997.
153. McMenamy, R. H., Albumin binding, in *Albumin Structure, Function and Uses*, Rosenoer, V. M., Oratz, M., and Rothschild, M. A., Eds., Pergamon Press, New York, 1977, 143–158.
154. Badawy, A. A. and Smith, M. J., Changes in liver tryptophan and tryptophan pyrrolase activity after administration of salicylate and tryptophan to the rat, *Biochem. Pharmacol.*, 21[1], 97, 1972.
155. LeJohn, H. B. and Stevenson, R. M., Inhibition of amino acid transport and enhancement of tryptophan binding in a water mold by a range of natural and synthetic cytokinins, *Can. J. Microbiol.*, 28, 1165, 1982.
156. Cameron, L. E. and Lejohn, H. B., On the involvement of calcium in amino acid transport and growth of the fungus *Achlya, J. Biol. Chem.*, 247[15], 4729, 1972.
157. Lejohn, H. B., A rapid and sensitive auxin binding system for detecting N6-substituted adenines, and some urea and thiourea derivatives, that show cytokinin activity in cell division tests, *Can. J. Biochem.*, 53[7], 768, 1975.
158. Baglia, F. A. and Maul, G. G., Nuclear ribonucleoprotein release and nucleoside triphosphatase activity are inhibited by antibodies directed against one nuclear matrix glycoprotein, *Proc. Natl. Acad. Sci. U.S.A.*, 80[8], 2285, 1983.
159. Kurl, R. N., Verney, E., and Sidransky, H., Tryptophan binding sites on nuclear envelopes of rat liver, *Nutr. Rep. Int.*, 36, 669, 1987.
160. Kurl, R. N., Verney, E., and Sidransky, H., Identification and immunohistochemical localization of a tryptophan binding protein in nuclear envelopes of rat liver, *Arch. Biochem. Biophys.*, 265[2], 286, 1988.
161. Crawford, I. P. and Stauffer, G. V., Regulation of tryptophan biosynthesis, *Annu. Rev. Biochem.*, 49, 163, 1980.
162. Somerville, R. L., Hermann, K. M., and Somerville, R. L., Eds., *Amino Acid Biosynthesis and Regulation*, Addsion-Wesley, Reading, MA, 1983, 351–578.
163. Beato, M., Herrlich, P., and Schutz, G., Steroid hormone receptors: Many actors in search of a plot, *Cell*, 83[6], 851, , 1995.
164. Schroder, H. C., Wenger, R., Gerner, H., Reuter, P., Kuchino, Y., Sladic, D., and Muller, W. E., Suppression of the modulatory effects of the antileukemic and anti-human immunodeficiency virus compound avarol on gene expression by tryptophan, *Cancer Res.*, 49[8], 2069, 1989.
165. Sidransky, H., Kurl, R. N., Holmes, S. C., and Verney, E. Tryptophan binding to nuclei of rat liver and hepatoma, *J. Nutr. Biochem.*, 6, 73, 1995.
166. Cosgrove, J. W., Verney, E., Schwartz, A. M., and Sidransky, H., Tryptophan binding to nuclei of rat brain, *Exp. Mol. Pathol.*, 57[3], 180, 1992.
167. Kurl, R. N., Holmes, S. C., Verney, E., and Sidransky, H., Nuclear envelope glycoprotein with poly(A) polymerase activity of rat liver: Isolation, characterization, and immunohistochemical localization, *Biochemistry* 27[25], 8974, 1988.

168. Kurl, R. N., Barsoum, A. L., and Sidransky, H., Association of poly(A)poly-merase with tryptophan receptor in rat hepatic nuclei, *J. Nutr. Biochem.*, 3, 366, 1992.

169. Kurl, R. N., Verney, E., and Sidransky, H., Effect of tryptophan on rat hepatic nuclear poly(A)polymerase activity, *Amino Acids* 5, 263, 1993.

170. Bardwell, V. J., Zarkower, D., Edmonds, M., and Wickens, M., The enzyme that adds poly(A) to mRNAs is a classical poly(A) polymerase, *Mol. Cell. Biol.*, 10[2], 846, 1990.

171. Bernd, A., Schroder, H. C., Zahn, R. K., and Muller, W. E., Modulation of the nuclear-envelope nucleoside triphosphatase by poly(A)-rich mRNA and by microtubule protein, *Eur. J. Biochem.*, 129[1], 43, 1982.

172. Schroder, H. C., Diehl-Seifert, B., Rottmann, M., Messer, R., Bryson, B. A., Agutter, P. S., and Muller, W. E., Functional dissection of nuclear envelope mRNA translocation system: Effects of phorbol ester and a monoclonal anti-body recognizing cytoskeletal structures, *Arch. Biochem. Biophys.*, 261[2], 394, 1988.

173. Sidransky, H., Verney, E., and Kurl, R., Comparison of effects of L-tryptophan and a tryptophan analog, D, L-beta-(1-naphthyl)alanine, on processes relating to hepatic protein synthesis in rats, *J. Nutr.*, 120[10], 1157, 1990.

174. Sidransky, H., Verney, E., Cosgrove, J. W., and Schwartz, A. M., Studies with compounds that compete with tryptophan binding to rat hepatic nuclei, *J. Nutr.*, 122[5], 1085, 1992.

175. Sidransky, H. and Verney, E., The presence of thiols in the hepatic nuclear binding site for L-tryptophan: Studies with selenite, *Nutr. Res.*, 16, 1023, 1996.

176. Tashima, Y., Terui, M., Itoh, H., Mizunuma, H., Kobayashi, R., and Marumo, F., Effect of selenite on glucocorticoid receptor, *J. Biochem.*, 105[3], 358, 1989.

177. Brtko, J. and Filipcik, P., Effect of selenite and selenate on rat liver nuclear 3, 5, 3'-triiodothyronine (T3) receptor, *Biol. Trace Element Res.*, 41[1-2], 191, 1994.

178. Miesfeld, R., Rusconi, S., Godowski, P. J., Maler, B. A., Okret, S., Wikstrom, A. C., Gustafsson, J. A., and Yamamoto, K. R., Genetic complementation of a glucocorticoid receptor deficiency by expression of cloned receptor cDNA, *Cell*, 46[3], 389, 1986.

179. Schurr, P. E., Thompson, H. T., Henderson, L. M., and Elvehjem, C. A., Deter-mination of free amino acids in rat tissues, *J. Biol.Chem.*, 182, 39, 1950.

180. McMenemy, R. M., Lund, C. C., and Oncley, J. L., Unbound amino acid con-centrations in human blood plasmas, *J. Clin. Invest.*, 36, 1672, 1957.

181. Tagliamonte, A., Biggio, G., Vargiu, L., and Gessa, G. L., Free tryptophan in serum controls brain tryptophan level and serotonin synthesis, *Life Sci., Pt. 2– Biochem. Gen. Mol. Biol.*, 12[6], 277, 1973.

182. Knott, P. J. and Curzon, G., Free tryptophan in plasma and brain tryptophan metabolism, *Nature*, 239[5373], 452, 1972.

183. Curzon, G., The control of brain tryptophan concentration, *Acta Vitaminol. Enzymol.*, 29[1-6], 69, 1975.

184. Fernstrom, J. D. and Wurtmen, R. J., Elevation of plasma tryptophan by insulin in rat, *Metab. Clin. Exp.*, 21[4], 337, 1972.

185. Sidransky, H. and Verney, E., Influence of L-alanine on effects induced by L-tryptophan on rat liver, *J. Nutr. Biochem.*, 7, 200, 1996.

186. Sidransky, H. and Verney, E., Influence of L-leucine of L-tryptophan binding to rat hepatic nuclei, *J. Nutr. Biochem.*, 8, 592, 1997.

187. McGivan, J. D. and Pastor-Anglada, M., Regulatory and molecular aspects of mammalian amino acid transport, *Biochem. J.*, 299 (Pt. 2), 321, 1994.
188. Li, J. B. and Odessey, R., Regulation of protein turnover in heart and skeletal mucle by branched-chain amino acid and the keto acids, in *Problems and Potential of Branched-Chain Amino Acids in Physiology and Medicine*, Odessey, R., Ed., Elsevier, New York, 1986, 83–106.
189. Sidransky, H. and Verney, E., Effect of amino acid imbalances on the stimulatory effect of L-tryptophan on hepatic protein synthesis, *Amino Acids*, 12, 205, 1997.
190. Sidransky, H. and Verney, E., Effects of ascorbic acid on hepatic nuclear binding of L-tryptophan, *Nutr. Res.*, 20, 865, 2000.
191. Heikkila, R. E., Cabbat, F. S., and Manzino, L., Differential inhibitory effects of ascorbic acid on the binding of dopamine agonists and antagonists to neostriatal membrane preparations: Correlations with behavioral effects, *Res. Commun. Chem. Pathol. Pharmacol.*, 34[3], 409, 1981.
192. Tolbert, L. C., Morris, P. E., Jr., Spollen, J. J., and Ashe, S. C., Stereospecific effects of ascorbic acid and analogues on D1 and D2 agonist binding, *Life Sci.*, 51[12], 921, 1992.
193. Kimura, K. and Sidhu, A., Ascorbic acid inhibits 125I-SCH 23982 binding but increases the affinity of dopamine for D1 dopamine receptors, *J. Neurochem.*, 63[6], 2093, 1994.
194. Britt, S. G., Chiu, V. W., Redpath, G. T., and VandenBerg, S. R. Elimination of ascorbic acid-induced membrane lipid peroxidation and serotonin receptor loss by Trolox-C, a water soluble analogue of vitamin E, *J. Receptor Res.*, 12[2], 181, 1992.
195. Sidransky, H. and Verney, E., Effects of vitamins on hepatic nuclear binding of L-tryptophan, *Amino Acids*, 20, 123, 2001.
196. Patnaik, R. N. and Nair, P. P., Studies on the binding of d-alpha-tocopherol to rat liver nuclei, *Arch. Biochem. Biophys.*, 178[2], 333, 1977.
197. da Costa, M., Rothenberg, S. P., and Beckman, S. J., Rat liver nuclei contain receptors for a folate binding protein, *Exp. Biol. Med.*, 174[3], 350, 1983.
198. McMenamy, R. H. The binding of indole analogues to human serum albumin: Effects of fatty acids, *J. Biol. Chem.*, 240, 4235, 1965.
199. Miller, L. L., The role of liver and the non-hepatic tissues in the regulation of free amino acid levels in the blood, in *Amino Acid Pools*, Holden, J. T., Ed., Elsevier, Amsterdam, 1962, 708–721.
200. Harper, A. E., Miller, R. H., and Block, K. P., Branched-chain amino acid metabolism, *Annu. Rev. Nutr.*, 4, 409, 1984.
201. Peters, J. C., Tryptophan nutrition and metabolism: An overview, in *Kynurenine and Serotonin Pathways*, Schwartz, R. et al., Eds., Plenum Press, New York, 1991, 345–358.
202. Fernstrom, J. D., Hirsch, M. J., Madras, B. K., and Sudarsky, L., Effects of skim milk, whole milk and light cream on serum tryptophan binding and brain tryptophan concentrations in rats, *J. Nutr.*, 105[10], 1359, 1975.
203. Bloxam, D. L., Tricklebank, M. D., Patel, A. J., and Curzon, G., Effects of albumin, amino acids, and clofibrate on the uptake of tryptophan by the rat brain, *J. Neurochem.*, 34[1], 43, 1980.
204. Jorgensen, A. J. and Majumdar, A. P., Influence of tryptophan on the level of hepatic microsomal cytochrome P-450 in well-fed normal, adrenalectomized, and phenobarbital-treated rats, *Biochim. Biophys. Acta*, 444[2], 453, 1976.

205. Sidransky, H., Verney, E., and Murty, C. N., Effect of elevated dietary tryptophan on protein synthesis in rat liver, *J. Nutr.*, 111[11], 1942, 1981.
206. Evarts, R. P. and Mostafa, M. H., Effects of indole and tryptophan on cytochrome P-450, dimethylnitrosamine demethylase, and arylhydrocarbon hydroxylase activities, *Biochem. Pharmacol.*, 30[5], 517, 1981.
207. Evarts, R. P. and Mostafa, M. H., The effect of L-tryptophan and certain other amino acids on liver nitrosodimethylamine demethylase activity, *Food Cosmetics Toxicol.*, 16[6], 585, 1978.
208. Sidransky, H., Murty, C. N., Myers, E., and Verney, E., Tryptophan-induced stimulation of hepatic ornithine decarboxylase activity in the rat, *Exp. Mol. Pathol.*, 38[3], 346, 1983.

5

Blood and Hormonal Responses to Tryptophan (Deficiency or Excess)

CONTENTS

5.1   Blood Tryptophan Levels

5.1.1   Introduction

Since L-tryptophan is of importance in the metabolism of many organs, it is understandable that numerous studies have been directed toward determining blood levels of L-tryptophan in humans and in experimental animals under normal and abnormal conditions. These studies have been concerned with learning about conditions whereby blood L-tryptophan levels became altered. Such studies have established normal blood levels in humans and animals and also have revealed blood changes in a variety of altered states. These findings have served to stimulate further investigations into why blood levels of L-tryptophan change and into the possible mechanisms responsible. In this chapter, some human diseases where blood L-tryptophan levels become altered are reviewed, and a few selected examples are cited to stress how this change may occur. Also, a number of experimental animal studies whereby species and agents affect blood L-tryptophan levels are reviewed and possible mechanisms involved are considered.

5.1.2   Normal

In 1950, Schurr et al.[1] determined the amino acid concentrations in various tissues of the rat. When these data were used to calculate tissue/plasma ratios, it became apparent that the relative availability of plasma tryptophan to tissues was much less than that of the other amino acids. In 1957, McMenemy et al.[2] described a unique property of tryptophan: It was the only amino acid in human plasma that was largely bound to protein. This attribute, specifically the ratio of free to bound tryptophan in the blood, has much physiological significance. For example, only the small free fraction of plasma tryptophan has access to the brain. Factors that influence the equilibrium between free and bound tryptophan in the plasma have been considered to alter the availability of tryptophan to the brain, where it has special importance as a precursor of the neurotransmitter 5-hydroxy-tryptamine (serotonin).[3-5] Tryptophan differs from other amino acids in that its concentration in plasma of rats increases (30 to 40%) after fasting, after insulin administration, or after consuming a carbohydrate meal.[6]

Wide daily fluctuations in the concentrations of plasma tryptophan, as well as of other amino acids, occur in healthy humans.[7] Feigin et al.[8] reported a diurnal rhythm for total whole-blood amino acid levels in healthy humans. Daily fluctuations have been observed for all of the nutritionally important amino acids.[9,10] A number of investigators have studied factors that may influence diurnal fluctuations of plasma tryptophan in humans.[11,12] Many reports cite marked variations, usually decreased levels, of plasma tryptophan, under a variety of disease states. However, it is difficult to assess the importance of these observations.

Kirwin et al.[13] reported on plasma and cerebral spinal fluid (CSF) tryptophan levels in healthy subjects. They observed variations over time (30-h period) but failed to show diurnal fluctuation. In this study, they used continuous CSF sampling via an indwelling lumbar catheter to study CSF neurochemistry.

5.1.3   Abnormal

The literature contains many reports about changes in serum tryptophan levels in patients with a variety of illnesses. In some cases, investigators have attached much significance to these alterations in serum tryptophan levels. However, at present, in most cases it is difficult to interpret the significance of these findings. Yet one should be aware of correlations between certain diseases and serum tryptophan levels. It is appropriate to cite some examples of diseases where serum tryptophan levels have been found to be diminished or increased.

In many of the illnesses where serum tryptophan levels are diminished, it is evident that there is usually enhanced activity along the kynurenine pathway, often involving indoleamine-2,3-dioxygenase (IDO). This has a negative effect on the serotonin pathway. Indeed, many patients receiving interferon-γ

(IFN-γ), which activates and leads to expression of IDO and decreased plasma tryptophan levels, may develop evidence of depression, dementia, as well as fatigue and weakness, findings not uncommon in conditions having enhanced immune system activity, such as AIDS, infection, autoimmune diseases, and related conditions.

5.1.3.1   HIV Infection

Since neurologic dysfunction and destruction are frequent complications of human immunodeficiency virus type 1 (HIV-1) infection, the mechanisms involved by which the symptoms, such as dementia or polyneuropathy, occur have been researched. Fuchs et al.[14] suggested that disturbance of tryptophan metabolism may be responsible, since reduced tryptophan together with increased kynurenine, as well as reduced serotonin concentrations, were reported to occur frequently in the sera of advanced HIV-1 infected patients.[15,16] Fuchs et al.[17] described a significant association between low tryptophan concentration and neurologic/psychiatric symptoms in HIV-1 patients. Also, there was a negative correlation of tryptophan with kynurenine and neopterin concentrations, which indicated activity of indoleamine 2,3-dioxygenase (IDO) in patients. IDO can be induced by cytokines and, therefore, low tryptophan levels may result from chronic immune stimulation in HIV-1 seropositive patients. Fuchs et al.[18,19] also described that serum (IFN-γ) concentrations were increased along with increases in serum and CSF neopterin levels and decreases of serum and CSF levels of tryptophan in patients with HIV-1 infections compared to healthy HIV-1 seronegative persons. Thus, tryptophan concentrations correlated negatively to neopterin concentrations and serum neopterin concentrations correlated positively to IFN-γ concentrations in HIV-1 infected patients.

The decreased tryptophan levels found simultaneously with increased kynurenine levels in HIV-1 infected patients indicated active degradation of tryptophan via induction of IDO. The expression of IDO as well as activation of the enzyme can be induced by IFN-γ.[20] In addition, IFN-γ correlates positively to neopterin concentrations. Increased neopterin levels reflect induction of GTP-cyclohydrolase I, which is inducible by IFN-γ *in vitro*.[21] Of interest is that the decrease of tryptophan concentration is much greater than the increase of kynurenine.[19] Also, the correlations between INF-γ and neopterin were much stronger with tryptophan than with kynurenine. This can be attributed to the rapid metabolism of kynurenine. Quinolinic acid, a tryptophan metabolite, was found to be increased during HIV-1 infection.[22] Reports by Heyes et al.[23-25] have attached much significance to the finding that quinolinic acid, a neurotoxic kynurenine-pathway metabolite derived from L-tryptophan, is elevated in HIV-1 patients, especially in those with marked neurological damage. It is a neurotoxic convulsant metabolite of tryptophan that is activated by INF-γ. It remains elevated for extended periods with HIV and increases as much as 100-fold over controls in patients with AIDS dementia complex. It may be a possible cause and marker of neurological damage in HIV-infected patients. Kerr et al.[26] reported that in *in vitro* studies, inhibition of quinolinic acid synthesis by 6-chloro-D-tryptophan (an inhibitor of quinolinic acid biosynthesis) reduced toxicity of cultured HIV-infected cells.

Gisslen et al.[27] described that tryptophan concentrations increased in CSF and blood after zidovudine treatment of patients with HIV-1 infection. Their data suggested an association between decreased immune stimulation and reduced tryptophan degradation in patients treated with zidovudine. A decrease in neopterin during the antiviral treatment correlated with an increase in tryptophan.

It seems probable that the wasting in AIDS patients is due at least in part to a chronic depletion of tryptophan. Although in AIDS patients blood tryptophan levels are low, other amino acids are not reduced to the same extent.[28] This pattern is similar to that found in pellagra due to poor tryptophan intake.[29] Nutrition and anthropometric studies on AIDS patients indicate that protein is lost but fat is little changed. Administration of excessive dietary tryptophan may relieve the tryptophan deficiency but may increase quinolinic acid levels, which would likely worsen the AIDS dementia. Conceivably, a better approach to improve tryptophan levels would be to utilize inhibitors of IDO, which would also decrease the levels of quinolinic acid. Such approaches with inhibitors of IDO *in vitro* have been investigated.[30–33]

5.1.3.2　Systemic Sclerosis

Csipo et al.[34] have described decreased serum tryptophan and elevated neopterin levels in patients with systemic sclerosis. Signs of chronic activation of cell-mediated immunity in systemic sclerosis were demonstrated by elevated neopterin levels.[35] Neopterin is a biologically stable metabolite that reflects the increased synthesis of interferon-γ. Interferon-γ induces a decrease in serum tryptophan levels via the induction of IDO, so that the detection of a decrease in serum tryptophan levels seems to serve as a tool for evaluating activation of cellular immunity.[36] Of interest is that the serum interferon-γ level itself was not increased in systemic sclerosis.[37,38]

5.1.3.3　Diseases with Defects in Absorption

Defects in the gastrointestinal absorption of L-tryptophan can cause diminished blood tryptophan levels and influence the health of patients.

5.1.3.3.1　Hartnup Disease

Hartnup disease is an inherited autosomal recessive disease that manifests itself in malabsorption of neutral amino acids, including tryptophan, in the gastrointestinal tract and also in deficient reabsorption of these amino acids in the renal tubules. The deficient uptake of tryptophan can result in a pellagra-like condition, which may include mental manifestations such as ataxia, emotional lability, nystagmus, hallucinations, and depression.[39,40] Tryptophan ethyl ester, a lipid-soluble tryptophan derivative, is effective at circumventing defective gastrointestinal neutral amino acid transport and may be useful in the treatment of Hartnup disease.[41]

5.1.3.3.2   Crohn's Disease

In Crohn's disease, serum tryptophan is often found to be low in patients. Beeken[42] reported that tryptophan absorption in patients with Crohn's disease had distinctly subnormal results (13 patients) while 19 patients had normal tryptophan absorption values (compared to 16 healthy controls). The patients with abnormal results ate less, lost more weight, and had lower serum albumin levels than those with normal absorption.

5.1.3.3.3   Celiac Disease

In children and adults with celiac disease, with impaired absorption of nutrients from the gastrointestinal tract, the availability of tryptophan to the brain, as indicated by the plasma ratio of tryptophan to other large neutral amino acids (LNAA), is low, especially in those with depression.[43,44]

5.1.3.3.4   Anorexia in Cancer

Krause et al.[45] reported a correlation between anorexia and brain levels of tryptophan and serotonin in tumor-bearing animals. Therefore, it was proposed that an increase in brain serotonin synthesis may be, at least in part, responsible for the onset of cancer anorexia.[46] That this hypothesis based upon animal studies may also hold true in humans was suggested by data reported by Fanelli et al.[47] Using a questionnaire, they investigated the feeding behavior of 45 patients with various types of cancer and 13 control subjects. Plasma levels of free tryptophan were significantly increased in anorectic cancer patients and seemed to confirm that free tryptophan may play an important role in cancer anorexia in humans. Plasma ratio of free tryptophan to competing neutral amino acids, which might better predict brain tryptophan levels, was significantly higher in anorectic cancer patients than in controls or in nonanorectic cancer patients. That serotonin and its precursor tryptophan from blood appear to be good candidates for physiological regulation of feeding behavior has been reported.[48] The pathogenesis of anorexia in cancer is probably multifactorial, directly influenced by psychological, metabolic, and therapeutic factors. Yet the role of tryptophan and serotonin in blood and brain merits consideration.

5.1.3.3.5   Exercise

Free plasma tryptophan increased significantly after 40 to 60 min of exercise (bicycle), but total tryptophan did not reveal a significant change.[49] Prolactin levels correlated with free plasma tryptophan throughout the tests. The induced increase in free plasma tryptophan was probably mediated by nonesterified fatty acids that competed with tryptophan for binding sites on albumin.[50]

5.1.3.4 Concluding Comments

Low blood concentrations of tryptophan can be caused by low levels of dietary tryptophan, by tryptophan malabsorption, or by excessive metabolism of tryptophan. Examples of each have been cited in the preceding paragraphs and in Chapter 2. Overall, studies of patients with inadequate intake of tryptophan due to low levels in the diet or due to malabsorption demonstrate that tryptophan deficiency causes a number of symptoms. Decreased protein synthesis due to decreased regulation of protein synthesis or to limited tryptophan for incorporation into or synthesis of protein, as well as low levels of niacin and serotonin, may be important in initiating many of the symptoms. For example, depression is a symptom often associated with many of the cited conditions or diseases, and its etiology may be related to low levels of serotonin.[51] Excessive metabolism of tryptophan may best be related to HIV infection, where immune activation is associated with elevated interferon-γ, which may have pathophysiological significance in relation to the induction of indoleamine-2,3-dioxygenase.

5.1.4 Experimental Animal Studies

5.1.4.1 Species Differences

In considering the normal blood levels of L-tryptophan in animals, it is important to realize that there are differences among the various animal species. Badawy and Evans[52] reported on the liver and serum-total and serum-free tryptophan levels in various species: group 1 included rat, mouse, pig, turkey and chicken, and group 2 included cat, frog, guinea pig, hamster, gerbil, ox, sheep, and rabbit. In general, group 1 species had similar values, but distinctly higher levels in all three parameters than in group 2 species. The differences were attributed to the absence of the apoenzyme for liver tryptophan 2,3-dioxygenase in group 2 species. Species lacking the apoenzyme or the hormonal induction mechanism have a deficient kynurenine pathway. It is speculated that these species (group 2) are sensitive to the toxicity of tryptophan. Indeed, the frog and hamster showed increased toxicity (sign of poisoning) due to tryptophan administration.

5.1.4.2 Agents or Conditions Causing Decreases in Blood Tryptophan Levels

5.1.4.2.1 Rats

5.1.4.2.1.1 Isoprenaline — The administration of isoprenaline intraperitoneally to rats caused a significant decrease in plasma concentration of tryptophan as well as tyrosine.[53] Since propranolol, the β-adrenergic antagonist, inhibited the decrease in plasma tryptophan level, the decrease was considered to be mediated via adrenergic β-receptors.

5.1.4.2.1.2　Toluene — Toluene, after intraperitoneal injections or after inhalation, caused a decrease in rat plasma concentrations of tryptophan as well as of tyrosine.[54] The mechanism for this is not clear. It may be related to the direct effect of toluene on the liver cell membranes, with a subsequent increase in liver cell uptake of amino acids.

5.1.4.2.1.3　Tryptophan-Free Diet — Rats were trained to eat their normal daily diet in a period of 2 h for 20 days. On the 21st day, they received a tryptophan-free diet. Serum tryptophan (free) was decreased by 90% (maximal within 2 h after food presentation and persisted for more than 24 h).[55] Brain tryptophan levels were also decreased. The mechanisms for the fall in serum tryptophan was considered probably to be due to a rapid removal of endogenous tryptophan from the circulation by liver and other tissues and its incorporation into proteins. Similar results were reported by Gessa et al.[56]

Moja et al.[57] treated rats with cycloheximide, an inhibitor of protein synthesis, and then fed a tryptophan-free mixture. The cycloheximide treatment largely prevented the marked decrease of plasma tryptophan (total and free). These data supported the hypothesis that protein synthesis was the mechanism through which the ingested tryptophan-free mixture decreased blood tryptophan levels. However, this interpretation was not consistent with the findings of Wunner et al.[58] and Sidransky et al.,[59] who observed a low rate of polyribosome formation and low incorporation of labeled amino acids in the livers of rodents previously fasted and then acutely fed a tryptophan-free amino acid mixture.

It is of interest that Moja et al.[60] reported that healthy humans receiving a tryptophan-free amino acid mixture revealed a decrease of plasma tryptophan levels.

5.1.4.2.1.4　Rapid Tryptophan Depletion Experiments — Studies with rapid tryptophan depletion, which causes diminished blood tryptophan levels, have been conducted with a variety of neuropsychiatric conditions in humans and also in experimental animal studies. These findings are reviewed in detail in Chapter 7.

5.1.4.3　Agents or Conditions Causing Increases in Blood Tryptophan Levels

5.1.4.3.1　Rabbits

5.1.4.3.1.1　Haloperiodol and Chlorpromazine — Chronic administration of haloperidol and chlorpromazine to rabbits led to significant increases in plasma tryptophan compared to saline-treated controls.[68] The results suggested that tryptophan in plasma is poorly transported in the brains of rabbits treated with chlorpromazine, and that treatment with haloperidol

or chlorpromazine may lead to a reduced tryptophan flux into the kynurenine pathway.

5.1.4.3.2 Rats

5.1.4.3.2.1 Amitriptyline — Chronic amitriptyline administration intraperitoneally resulted in a significant increase in serum-free tryptophan but no
effect on total serum tryptophan.[62] It is felt that amitriptyline possibly competes with tryptophan for albumin binding and thereby leads to a rise in
free tryptophan.

5.1.4.3.3 Mice

5.1.4.3.3.1 Obese (ob/ob) Mice — Genetically obese hyperglycemic mice
(*ob/ob*) were compared with their nonlittermate lean controls and were
reported to have increased levels of plasma-total and -free tryptophan levels.[63] Also, brain serotonin, pituitary ACTH content, and plasma insulin
levels were increased, but plasma TSH, T_3, and T_4 were not different in the
obese mice.

5.2 Hormones

5.2.1 Introduction

Endocrine function is impaired by dietary protein deficiency.[64] However,
much less is known about the effects of individual amino acid deficiencies
on the endocrine system. Overall, reduced growth and changes in body
composition are major consequences of protein and amino acid deficiencies,
and among the hormones possibly involved are thyroid hormones, growth
hormone, insulin, and sex steroids.

Findings with ingestion of tryptophan-deficient diets are of special interest
because tryptophan is an obligatory dietary precursor of brain amines that
regulate hormonal function in the central nervous system. Early studies have
revealed that tryptophan-deficient rats have low brain levels of serotonin[55]
and appear to remain in an arrested state of growth and maturation.[65]

5.2.2 Hormonal Changes in Experimental Animals Involving Tryptophan (Deficient Dietary or Administered Excess Tryptophan)

5.2.2.1 Broiler Chicks

Using broiler chicks fed a tryptophan-deficient diet, Carew et al.[66] reported
that the chicks grew less efficiently than pair-fed controls and had
decreased plasma thyroxine (T_4) and increased plasma triiodothyronine
(T_3) and growth hormone (GH) levels. Plasma testosterone was little

affected. They suggested that the tryptophan deficiency led to decreases in brain serotonin levels, which influenced the response of other hormones, being a negative modulator of the synthesis or release of plasma GH and T_3 in chickens.

5.2.2.2 Pigs

Montgomery et al.[67] fed pigs alternately a tryptophan-deficient diet and the same diet supplemented with tryptophan. The deficient diet depressed food intake, caused changes in plasma amino acid pattern, increased plasma glucose levels, and increased plasma urea levels per unit food intake. Plasma levels of insulin and growth hormone were somewhat elevated after 2 days of feeding the deficient diet.

Brameld et al.[68] used a pig hepatocyte culture system to investigate the effect of adding individual amino acids on the expression of growth hormone receptor and insulin-like growth factor-I mRNA. First, removal of tryptophan inhibited the stimulation of insulin-like growth factor-I expression that was induced by T_3, dexamethosone, and growth hormone, with decreases in growth hormone receptor in some cases. Tryptophan addition had a stimulatory effect that was dose-dependent on expression of class 1 transcripts of insulin-like growth factor I, but had no effect on growth hormone receptor or class 2 transcripts of insulin-like growth factor I.

5.2.2.3 Terrestial Slug Limax Maximus

The slug *Limax maximus* has been shown to reduce its food intake, as do other species, when fed a diet devoid of tryptophan.[69,70] Because tryptophan is the precursor of serotonin and the supply of the precursor is generally the limited factor in serotonin synthesis,[71] Gietzen et al.[72] studied the effect of a tryptophan-devoid diet on the control of food intake in an invertebrate species, *Limax maximus*. While food intake was depressed by a tryptophan-devoid diet, the serotonergic metacerebral giant cell was still functional after 2 weeks. Neither brain serotonin nor plasma tryptophan concentrations were affected. These data suggested that in the slug, unlike in the rat, there is protection of tryptophan levels by some metabolic manipulation. This apparent protection of the concentration of tryptophan in the slug appears to be undertaken at the cost of a considerable imbalance of the remaining plasma amino acids rather than due to a simple starvation response, as was seen in the pair-fed group that showed more consistent decreases in plasma amino acid levels. Thus, in the slug, the continued depression in feeding seen in the tryptophan-devoid group probably resulted from an imbalanced amino acid profile or some metabolic consequence thereof, rather than the decrease in tryptophan concentration or any diminution of serotonin function from a decrease in precursor levels. Thus, one may conclude that in the slug, diet intake appears to be regulated by factors other than serotonin action.

5.2.2.4 Rats

Clemens et al.[73] fed rats a tryptophan-free diet and determined the effects on serum prolactin and corticosterone levels. The tryptophan-free diet lowered brain serotonin concentrations to about half of normal. While basal serum prolactin levels in rats fed the tryptophan-free diet were the same as those found in control rats, when given serotonin, the rats fed the tryptophan-free diet revealed a significant release of prolactin compared to controls. Similarly, a marked supersensitivity to the corticosterone-releasing property of serotonin was observed in the tryptophan-deficient rats.

Yokogoshi and Yoshida[74] have reported that fasted (48 h) rats tube-fed tryptophan for 2 h revealed no change in serum insulin levels but increases in serum glucocorticoid.

Tsiolakis and Marks[75] gave L-tryptophan to fasted rats intragastrically or intravenously and observed increased plasma insulin levels (greater increase by intragastric route) after 10, 30, and 45 min. Intragastric tryptophan raised plasma pancreatic glucagon levels over those in controls given saline. A similar marked and sustained increase in plasma glucagon in rats after administration of L-tryptophan had been reported by Lloyd et al.[76]

5.2.3 Hormonal Changes in Humans

A number of studies with humans have been concerned with whether tryptophan may affect the secretion of hormones.

5.2.3.1 Insulin

Ajdukiewicz et al.[77] reported that nonfasted humans showed a significant rise in plasma insulin 30 min after ingesting tryptophan. Floyd et al.[78] reported a small rise in plasma insulin following intravenous tryptophan. Fahmy et al.[79] demonstrated that oral tryptophan induced an elevation of plasma insulin in normal subjects and in adult-onset diabetes.

5.2.3.2 Adrenal Hormones

Modlinger et al.[80,81] reported that tryptophan administration to fasted patients induced elevations in blood levels of aldosterone, cortisol, ACTH, and renin.

5.2.3.3 Growth Hormone and Prolactin

Winokur et al.[82] infused L-tryptophan intravenously into 11 healthy male subjects and studied plasma hormone levels. Significant increases were observed in plasma growth hormone and prolactin concentrations after L-tryptophan was given compared to saline-infused controls. No alterations in cortisol or thyrotropin levels were noted. Also, in experimental animals,

L-tryptophan and serotonin are powerful releasers of prolactin and have been shown to be involved in some physiological states in which prolactin is released, i.e., during suckling, stress, etc.[83] Hypothalamic regulations of prolactin secretion in animals (mammals) and humans have been reported to be similar.

5.2.3.4 Glucagon

Tryptophan administration orally to 14 normal subjects induced a rise in plasma glucose accompanied by a rise in plasma glucagon levels and also by increased concentrations of circulating insulin and growth hormone.[84] The increase in plasma glucose due to tryptophan in humans differs from the reported hypoglycemic effect in rats.

5.2.3.5 Serotonin and Other Hormones

Since tryptophan is a precursor of serotonin, it was appropriate to investigate the role of serotonin in the secretion of anterior pituitary hormones via effects on hypothalamic hypophyseal releasing and release-inhibiting factors. Direct or indirect pharmacological evidence exists that the secretion of prolactin, growth hormone, luteinizing-releasing hormone, thyrotropin, corticotropin, and perhaps also aldosterone, beta-endorphin, and renin may be influenced by serotonergic mechanisms in some species.[85]

5.2.4 Relationships between Hormones and Tryptophan in Regard to Protein Synthesis

Since the administration of single amino acids elicits certain metabolic reactions indirectly via stimulation through hormones from the adrenal cortex, a number of studies were conducted using adrenalectomized animals to determine whether or not tryptophan administration would still stimulate hepatic protein synthesis. Using adrenalectomized mice, stimulation of hepatic protein synthesis due to tryptophan was independent of adrenal cortical hormones.[59] Other studies[86,87] using well-fed adrenalectomized and adrenalectomized diabetic rats, reported that the tube-feeding of tryptophan stimulated amino acid incorporation into plasma albumin, transferrin, and fibrinogen and into liver ferritin *in vivo*. However, Cammarano et al.[88] reported that the adrenal steroids were involved in the changes of hepatic polyribosome organization during feeding of high levels of tryptophan. Also, it has been reported that tryptophan administration to rats that had hepatic protein synthesis stimulated by the administration of cortisone acetate showed further enhanced stimulation of hepatic protein synthesis and a shift of hepatic polyribosomes toward heavier aggregation.[89]

Since availability of tryptophan to cells is vital in protein synthesis, investigation directed toward hormonal influence on tryptophan transport was conducted. Blondeau et al.[90] used cultured astrocytes to study the relationship between the transport of thyroid hormone and that of amino acids, including tryptophan. T_3 inhibited tryptophan uptake, which was attributed to an effect on the L1 system.

5.2.5 Hormones and Hepatic Nuclear Tryptophan Receptor Binding

A number of studies have indicated that the nuclear tryptophan receptor plays an important role in the sequence of events by which tryptophan acts to stimulate hepatic protein synthesis.[91-93] Therefore, it was important to investigate whether certain hormones may influence the affinity of hepatic nuclear receptor tryptophan binding. 3,5,3'-Triiodothyronine (T_3) and glucocorticoid, two hormones that are part of a group of nuclear proteins, and "ligand-responsive transcriptions factors," that belong to the same superfamily as steroid receptors[94,95] were used. Also, insulin, which has a different superfamily of receptors, was studied. These studies[96] revealed that T_3 (10^{-4} to 10^{-10} mol/L) appreciably inhibited *in vitro* ³H-tryptophan binding to rat hepatic nuclei, and T_3 (10^{-16} to 10^{-4} mol/L) appreciably ameliorated the inhibiting effect of unlabeled L-tryptophan on *in vitro* ³H-tryptophan binding. *In vivo* administration of T_3 plus tryptophan inhibited the stimulated hepatic protein synthesis that occurred with tryptophan alone. *In vitro* addition of hydrocortisone had no effect, and addition of insulin had only a small inhibitory effect on *in vitro* ³H-tryptophan binding to hepatic nuclei, but each when added to unlabeled L-tryptophan diminished the inhibitory effect of unlabeled L-tryptophan alone.

Other studies using selenite, a catalyst of the oxidation of sulfhydryl groups, have been of interest. Selenite had an inhibitory effect on hepatic nuclear binding of tryptophan,[97] which was similar to the inhibitory effect for T_3[98] and glucocorticoid[99] binding to nuclei. This suggests that L-tryptophan and also hormones, such as T_3 and glucocorticoid, may bind, at least in part, to sulfhydryl sites in its receptor protein.

5.2.6 Concluding Comments

Many studies reveal that there appears to be a functional relationship between L-tryptophan and a number of hormones. Data from several studies suggest the L-tryptophan may act on receptors of some hormones and vice versa. Also, the absence or excess of dietary tryptophan appears to affect hormone levels in blood. Speculation as to how this comes about is that the close relationship of levels of L-tryptophan and especially of serotonin is involved. Thus, serotonin probably acts to influence the secretion of anterior pituitary hormones via effects on hypothalamic hypophyseal releasing and release-inhibitory factors.

References

1. Schurr, P. E., Thompson, H. T., Henderson L. M., and Elvehjem, C. A., Determination of free amino acids in rat tissues, *J. Biol. Chem.*, 182, 39, 1950.
2. McMenemy, R. M., Lund, C. C., and Oncley, J. L., Unbound amino acid concentrations in human blood plasmas, *J. Clin. Invest.*, 36, 1672, 1957.
3. Tagliamonte, A., Biggio, G., Vargiu, L., and Gessa, G. L., Free tryptophan in serum controls brain tryptophan level and serotonin synthesis, *Life Sci. Pt. 2 Biochem. Gen. Mol. Bio.*, 12, 277, 1973.
4. Knott, P. J. and Curzon, G., Free tryptophan in plasma and brain tryptophan metabolism, *Nature*, 239, 452, 1972.
5. Curzon, G., The control of brain tryptophan concentration, *Acta Vitaminol. Enzymol.*, 29, 69, 1975.
6. Fernstrom, J. D. and Wurtmen, R. J., Elevation of plasma tryptophan by insulin in rat, *Metab. Clin. Exp.*, 21, 337, 1972.
7. Eynard, N., Flachaire, E., Lestra, C., Broyer, M., Zaidan, R., Claustrat, B., and Quincy, C., Platelet serotonin content and free and total plasma tryptophan in healthy volunteers during 24 hours, *Clin. Chem.*, 39, 2337, 1993.
8. Feigin, R. D., Lainer, A. S., and Beisel, W. R., Circadian periodicity of blood amino acids in adult men, *Nature*, 215, 512, 1967.
9. Feigin, R. D., Klainer, A. S., and Beisel, W. R., Factors affecting circadian periodicity of blood amino acids in man, *Metab. Clin. Exp.*, 17, 764, 1968.
10. Wurtman, R. J., Rose, C. M., Chou, C., and Larin, F. F., Daily rhythms in the concentrations of various amino acids in human plasma, *New Engl. J. Med.*, 279, 171, 1968.
11. Young, V. R., Hussein, M. A., Murray, E., and Scrimshaw, N.S., Tryptophan intake, spacing of meals, and diurnal fluctuations of plasma tryptophan in men, *Am. J. Clin. Nutr.*, 22, 1563, 1969.
12. Fernstrom, J. D., Wurtman, R. J., Hammarstrom-Wiklund, B., Rand, W. M., Munro, H. N., and Davidson, C. S. Diurnal variations in plasma concentrations of tryptophan, tryosine, and other neutral amino acids: Effect of dietary protein intake, *Am. J. Clin. Nutr.*, 32, 1912, 1979.
13. Kirwin, P. D., Anderson, G. M., Chappell, P. B., Saberski, L., Leckman, J. F., Geracioti, T. D., Heninger, G. R., Price, L. H., and McDougle, C. J., Assessment of diurnal variation of cerebrospinal fluid tryptophan and 5-hydroxyindoleacetic acid in healthy human females, *Life Sci.*, 60, 899, 1997.
14. Fuchs, D., Werner, E. R., Dierich, M. P., and Wachter, H., Cellular immune activation in the brain and human immunodeficiency virus infection [letter], *Ann. Neurol.*, 24, 289, 1988.
15. Werner, E. R., Fuchs, D., Hausen, A., Jaeger, H., Reibnegger, G., Werner-Felmayer, G., Dierich, M. P., and Wachter, H., Tryptophan degradation in patients infected by human immunodeficiency virus, *Biol. Chem. Hoppe-Seyler*, 369, 337, 1988.
16. Launay, J. M., Copel, L., Callebert, J., Corvaia, N., Lepage, E., Bricaire, F., Saal, F., and Peries, J., Decreased whole blood 5-hydroxytryptamine (serotonin) in AIDS patients, *J. Acquir. Imm. Defic. Syndr.*, 1, 324, 1988.
17. Fuchs, D., Moller, A. A., Reibnegger, G., Stockle, E., Werner, E. R., and Wachter, H., Decreased serum tryptophan in patients with HIV-1 infection correlates with increased serum neopterin and with neurologic/psychiatric symptoms, *J. Acquir. Imm. Defic. Syndr.*, 3, 873, 1990.

18. Fuchs, D., Forsman, A., Hagberg, L., Larsson, M., Norkrans, G., Reibnegger, G., Werner, E. R., and Wachter, H., Immune activation and decreased tryptophan in patients with HIV-1 infection, *J. Interferon Res.,* 10, 599, 1990.

19. Fuchs, D., Moller, A. A., Reibnegger, G., Werner, E. R., Werner-Felmayer, G., Dierich, M. P., and Wachter, H., Increased endogenous interferon-gamma and neopterin correlate with increased degradation of tryptophan in human immunodeficiency virus type 1 infection, *Immunol. Lett.,* 28, 207, 1991.

20. Yoshida, R., Imanishi, J., Oku, T., Kishida, T., and Hayaishi, O., Induction of pulmonary indoleamine 2,3-dioxygenase by interferon, *Proc. Natl. Acad. Sci. U.S.A.,* 78, 129, 1981.

21. Wachter, H., Fuchs, D., Hausen, A., Reibnegger, G., and Werner, E. R., Neopterin as marker for activation of cellular immunity: Immunologic basis and clinical application, *Adv. Clin. Chem.,* 27, 81, 1989.

22. Heyes, M. P., Rubinow, D., Lane, C., and Markey, S. P., Cerebrospinal fluid quinolinic acid concentrations are increased in acquired immune deficiency syndrome, *Ann. Neurol.,* 26, 275, 1989.

23. Heyes, M. P., Saito, K., and Markey, S. P., Human macrophages convert L-tryptophan into the neurotoxin quinolinic acid, *Biochem. J.,* 283, 633, 1992.

24. Heyes, M. P., Gravell, M., London, W. T., Eckhaus, M., Vickers, J. H., Yergey, J. A., April, M., Blackmore, D., and Markey, S. P., Sustained increases in cerebrospinal fluid quinolinic acid concentrations in rhesus macaques (*Macaca mulatta*) naturally infected with simian retrovirus type-D, *Brain Res.,* 531, 148, 1990.

25. Heyes, M. P., Jordan, E. K., Lee, K., Saito, K., Frank, J. A., Snoy, P. J., Markey, S. P., and Gravell, M., Relationship of neurologic status in macaques infected with the simian immunodeficiency virus to cerebrospinal fluid quinolinic acid and kynurenic acid, *Brain Res.,* 570, 237, 1992.

26. Kerr, S. J., Armati, P. J., Pemberton, L. A., Smythe, G., Tattam, B., and Brew, B. J., Kynurenine pathway inhibition reduces neurotoxicity of HIV-1-infected macrophages, *Neurology,* 49, 1671, 1997.

27. Gisslen, M., Larsson, M., Norkrans, G., Fuchs, D., Wachter, H., and Hagberg, L., Tryptophan concentrations increase in cerebrospinal fluid and blood after zidovudine treatment in patients with HIV type-1 infection, *AIDS Res. Hum. Retroviruses,* 10, 947, 1994.

28. Hortin, G. L., Landt, M., and Powderly, W. G. Changes in plasma amino acid concentrations in response to HIV-1 infection, *Clin. Chem.,* 40, 785, 1994.

29. Truswell, A. S., Hansen, J. D., and Wannenburg, P., Plasma tryptophan and other amino acids in pellagra, *Am. J. Clin. Nutr.,* 21, 1314, 1968.

30. Peterson, A. C. and LaLoggia A. J., Evaluation of substituted B-carbolines as noncompetitive indole 2,3-dioxygenase inhibitors, *Med. Chem. Res.,* 3, 473, 1993.

31. Peterson, A. C., Migawa, M. T., LaLoggia, A. J. et al., Evaluation of functionalized tryptophan derivatives and related compounds as competitive inhibitors of indoleamine 2,3-dioxygenase, *Med. Chem. Res.,* 3, 531, 1994.

32. Salter, M., Beams, R. M., Critchley, M. A., Hodson, H. F., Iyer, R., Knowles, R. G., Madge, D. J., and Pogson, C. I., Effects of tryptophan 2,3-dioxygenase inhibitors in the rat, *Adv. Exp. Med. Biol.,* 294, 281, 1991.

33. Cady, S. G. and Sono, M., 1-Methyl-DL-tryptophan, beta-(3-benzofuranyl)-DL-alanine (the oxygen analog of tryptophan), and beta-[3-benzo(b)thienyl]-DL-alanine (the sulfur analog of tryptophan) are competitive inhibitors for indoleamine 2,3-dioxygenase, *Arch. Biochem. Biophys.,* 291, 326, 1991.

34. Csipo, I., Czirjak, L., Szanto, S., Szerafin, L., Sipka, S., and Szegedi, G., Decreased serum tryptophan and elevated neopterin levels in systemic sclerosis, *Clin. Exp. Rheumatol.*, 13, 269, 1995.

35. Clements, P. J., Peter, J. B., Agopian, M. S., Telian, N. S., and Furst, D. E., Elevated serum levels of soluble interleukin 2 receptor, interleukin 2 and neopterin in diffuse and limited scleroderma: Effects of chlorambucil, *J. Rheumatol.*, 17, 908, 1990.

36. Byrne, G. I., Lehmann, L. K., Kirschbaum, J. G., Borden, E. C., Lee, C. M., and Brown, R. R., Induction of tryptophan degradation *in vitro* and *in vivo*: A gamma-interferon-stimulated activity, *J. Interferon Res.*, 6, 389, 1986.

37. Needleman, B. W., Wigley, P. M., and Stair, R. W., Interleukin-1, interleukin-2, interleukin-4, interleukin-6, tumor necrosis factor alpha, and interleukin-gamma levels in sera from patients with scleroderma, *Arthritis Rheum.* 35, 67, 1992.

38. Prior, C. and Haslam, P.L., *In vivo* levels and *in vitro* production of interferon-gamma in fibrosing interstitial lung diseases, *Clin. Exp. Immunol.*, 88, 280, 1992.

39. Lehmann, J., Mental and neuromuscular symptoms in tryptophan deficiency, *Acta Psychiatr. Scand.* (Suppl.), 237, 1, 1972.

40. Rosenberg, L. E. and Scriver C. R., Disorders of amino acid metabolism, in *Duncan's Diseases of Metabolism: Genetics and Metabolism*, Bondy, P. K. and Rosenberg, L. E., Eds., W. B. Saunders, Philadelphia, 1974, 465–633.

41. Jonas, A. J. and Butler, I. J., Circumvention of defective neutral amino acid transport in Hartnup disease using tryptophan ethyl ester, *J. Clin. Invest.*, 84, 200, 1989.

42. Beeken, W. L., Serum tryptophan in Crohn's disease, *Scand. J. Gastroenterol.*, 11, 735, 1976.

43. Hallert, C., Astrom, J., and Sedvall, G., Psychic disturbances in adult coeliac disease. III. Reduced central monoamine metabolism and signs of depression, *Scand. J. Gastroenterol.*, 17, 25, 1982.

44. Hernanz, A. and Polanco, I., Plasma precursor amino acids of central nervous system monoamines in children with coeliac disease, *Gut*, 32, 1478, 1991.

45. Krause, R., James, J. H., Ziparo, V., and Fischer, J. E., Brain tryptophan and the neoplastic anorexia-cachexia syndrome, *Cancer*, 44, 1003, 1979.

46. Krause, R., Humphrey, C., von Meyenfeldt, M., James, H., and Fischer, J. E., A central mechanism for anorexia in cancer: A hypothesis, *Cancer Treat. Rep.*, 65 (Suppl. 5), 15, 1981.

47. Fanelli, F. R., Cangiano, C., Ceci, F., Cellerino, R., Franchi, F., Menichetti, E. T., Muscaritoli, M., and Cascino, A., Plasma tryptophan and anorexia in human cancer, *Eur. J. Cancer Clin. Oncol.*, 22, 89, 1986.

48. Fernstrom, J. D. and Wurtman, R. J., Brain serotonin content: Increase following ingestion of carbohydrate diet, *Science*, 174, 1023, 1971.

49. Fischer, H. G., Hollmann, W., and De Meirleir, K., Exercise changes in plasma tryptophan fractions and its relationship with prolactin, *Int. J. Sports Med.*, 12, 487, 1991.

50. McMenemey, R. H., Lund, C. C., Van Marcke, J., and Oncley, J. L., The binding of L-tryptophan to human plasma at 37°C, *Arch. Biochem.*, 93, 135, 1961.

51. Meltzer, H. Y. and Lowy, M. T., The serotonin hypothesis of depression, in *Psychopharmacology: The Third Generation of Progress*, Meltzer, H. Y., Ed., Raven Press, New York, 1987, 513–526.

52. Badawy, A. A. and Evans, M., Animal liver tryptophan pyrrolases: Absence of apoenzyme and of hormonal induction mechanism from species sensitive to tryptophan toxicity, *Biochem. J.*, 158, 79, 1976.
53. Eriksson, T. and Carlsson, A., Adrenergic influence on rat plasma concentrations of tyrosine and tryptophan, *Life Sci.*, 30, 1465, 1982.
54. Voog, L. and Eriksson T., Toluene-induced decrease in rat plasma concentrations of tyrosine and tryptophan, *Acta Pharmacol. Toxicol.*, 54, 151, 1984.
55. Biggio, G., Fadda, F., Fanni, P., Tagliamonte, A., and Gessa, G. L., Rapid depletion of serum tryptophan, brain tryptophan, serotonin and 5-hydroxyindoleacetic acid by a tryptophan-free diet, *Life Sci.*, 14, 1321, 1974.
56. Gessa, G. L., Biggio, G., Fadda, F., Corsini, U., and Tagliamonte, A., Effect of the oral administration of tryptophan-free amino acid mixtures on serum tryptophan, brain tryptophan, and serotonin metabolism, *J. Neurochem.*, 22, 869, 1974.
57. Moja, E. A., Restani, P., Corsini, E., Stacchezzini, M. C., Assereto, R., and Galli, C. L., Cycloheximide blocks the fall of plasma and tissue tryptophan levels after tryptophan-free amino acid mixtures, *Life Sci.*, 49, 1121, 1991.
58. Wunner, W. H., Bell, J., and Munro, H. N., The effect of feeding with a tryptophan-free amino acid mixture on rat-liver polysomes and ribosomal ribonucleic acid, *Biochem. J.*, 101, 417, 1966.
59. Sidransky, H., Sarma, D. S., Bongiorno, M., and Verney, E., Effect of dietary tryptophan on hepatic polyribosomes and protein synthesis in fasted mice, *J. Biol. Chem.*, 243, 1123, 1968.
60. Moja, E. A., Stoff, D. M., Gessa, G. L., Castoldi, D., Assereto, R., and Tofanetti, O., Decrease in plasma tryptophan after tryptophan-free amino acid mixtures in man, *Life Sci.*, 42, 1551, 1988.
61. Hussein, L. and Goedde, H. W., Diurnal rhythm in the plasma level of total and free tryptophan and cortisol in rabbits. Effect of haloperidol and chlorpromazine, *Res. Exp. Med.*, 176, 123, 1979.
62. Kim, J. S., Schmid-Burgk, W., Claus, D., and Kornhuber, H. H., Effects of amitriptyline on serum glutamate and free tryptophan in rats, *Arch. Psych. Nervenkrankheiten*, 232, 391, 1982.
63. Garthwaite, T. L., Kalkhoff, R. K., Guansing, A. R., Hagen, T. C., and Menahan, L. A., Plasma free tryptophan, brain serotonin, and an endocrine profile of the genetically obese hyperglycemic mouse at 4–5 months of age, *Endocrinology*, 105, 1178, 1979.
64. Leathem, J. H., Hormones and protein nutrition, *Rec. Progr. Hormone Res.*, 14, 141, 1958.
65. Segall, P. E. and Timiras, P. S., Patho-physiologic findings after chronic tryptophan deficiency in rats: A model for delayed growth and aging, *Mech. Aging Dev.*, 5, 109, 1976.
66. Carew, L. B., Jr., Alster, F. A., Foss, D. C., and Scanes, C. G., Effect of a tryptophan deficiency on thyroid gland, growth hormone and testicular functions in chickens, *J. Nutr.*, 113, 1756, 1983.
67. Montgomery, G. W., Flux, D. S., and Greenway, R. M., Tryptophan deficiency in pigs: Changes in food intake and plasma levels of glucose, amino acids, insulin and growth hormone, *Hormone Metab. Res.*, 12, 304, 1980.
68. Brameld, J. M., Gilmour, R. S., and Buttery, P. J., Glucose and amino acids interact with hormones to control expression of insulin-like growth factor-I and growth hormone receptor mRNA in cultured pig hepatocytes, *J. Nutr.*, 129, 1298, 1999.

69. Delaney, K. and Gelperin, A., Post-ingestive food-aversion learning to amino acid deficient diets by the terrestrial slug *Limax maximus*, *J. Comp. Physiol. A Sensory Neural Behav. Physiol.*, 159, 281, 1986.

70. Lee, J. H. and Chang, J. J., Learning of post-ingestive food-aversion by the land slug, *Inciloaria fruhstorferi daiseniana* to amino acid deficient diets, *Soc. Neurosci.*, 12, 39, 1986.

71. Fernstrom, J. D., Aromatic amino acids and monoamine synthesis in the central nervous system: Influence of the diet, *J. Nutr. Biochem.*, 1, 508, 1990.

72. Gietzen, D. W., Harris, A. S., Carlson, S., and Gelperin, A., Amino acids and serotonin in *Limax maximus* after a tryptophan devoid diet, *Comp. Biochem. Physiol. A Comp. Physiol.*, 101, 143, 1992.

73. Clemens, J. A., Bennett, D. R., and Fuller, R. W., The effect of a tryptophan-free diet on prolactin and corticosterone release by serotonergic stimuli, *Hormone Metab. Res.*, 12, 35, 1980.

74. Yokogoshi, H. and Yoshida A., Effect of feeding or intubation of tryptophan or methionine and threonine in hepatic polysome profiles in rats under meal-feeding or fasting conditions, *Agric. Biol. Chem.*, 47, 373, 1983.

75. Tsiolakis, D. and Marks, V., The differential effect of intragastric and intravenous tryptophan on plasma glucose, insulin, glucagon, GLI and GIP in the fasted rat, *Hormone Metab. Res.*, 16, 226, 1984.

76. Lloyd, P., Smith, S. A., Stribling, D., and Pogson, C. I., Factors affecting tryptophan-induced hypoglycaemia in rats, *Biochem. Pharmacol.*, 31, 3563, 1982.

77. Ajdukiewicz, A. B., Keanse, P., Pearson, J., Read, A. E., and Salmon, P. R., Insulin releasing activity of oral L-tryptophan in fasting and non-fasting subjects, *Scand. J. Gastroenterol.*, 3, 622, 1968.

78. Floyd, J. C., Jr., Fajans, S. S., Conn, J. W., Knopf, R. F., and Rull, J., Stimulation of insulin secretion by amino acids, *J. Clin. Invest.*, 45, 1487, 1966.

79. Fahmy, K. A., Moustapha, S. M., Salama, M. K., Khattab, M., and Basta, H. G., Tryptophan — an insulinotropic nutrient, *Nutr. Rep. Int.*, 653, 1983.

80. Modlinger, R. S., Schonmuller, J. M., and Arora, S. P., Stimulation of aldosterone, renin, and cortisol by tryptophan, *J. Clin. Endocrinol. Metab.*, 48, 599, 1979.

81. Modlinger, R. S., Schonmuller, J. M., and Arora, S. P., Adrenocorticotropin release by tryptophan in man, *J. Clin. Endocrinol. Metab.*, 50, 360, 1980.

82. Winokur, A., Lindberg, N. D., Lucki, I., Phillips, J., and Amsterdam, J. D., Hormonal and behavioral effects associated with intravenous L-tryptophan administration, *Psychopharmacology*, 88, 213, 1986.

83. Meites, J., Neuroendocrine control of prolactin in experimental animals, *Clin. Endocrinol.*, 6 (Suppl.), 9S, 1977.

84. Hedo, J. A., Villanueva, M. L., and Marco, J., Elevation of plasma glucose and glucagon after tryptophan ingestion in man, *Metab. Clin. Exp.*, 26, 1131, 1977.

85. Meltzer, H. Y., Witta, B., Tricou, B. J., Simonovic, H. M., Fang, V., and Manov, G., Effect of serotonin precursors and serotonin agonists on plasma hormone levels, *Adv. Biochem. Psychopharmacol.*, 34, 117, 1982.

86. Jorgensen, A. J. and Najumdar, A. P., Bilateral adrenalectomy: Effect of tryptophan force-feeding on amino acid incorporation into plasma albumin and fibrinogen *in vivo*, *Biochem. Med.* 13, 231, 1975.

87. Jorgensen, A. J. and Majumdar, A. P., Bilateral adrenalectomy: Effect of tryptophan force-feeding on amino acid incorporation into ferritin, transferrin, and mixed proteins of liver, brain and kidneys *in vivo*, *Biochem. Med.*, 16, 37, 1976.

88. Cammarano, P., Chinali, G., Gaetani, S., and Spadoni, M. A., Involvement of adrenal steroids in the changes of polysome organization during feeding of unbalanced amino acid diets, *Biochim. Biophys. Acta*, 155, 302, 1968.

89. Verney, E. and Sidransky, H., Further enhancement by tryptophan of hepatic protein synthesis stimulated by phenobarbital or cortisone acetate, *Exp. Biol. Med.*, 158, 245, 1978.

90. Blondeau, J. P., Beslin, A., Chantoux, F., and Francon, J., Triiodothyronine is a high-affinity inhibitor of amino acid transport system L1 in cultured astrocytes, *J. Neurochem.*, 60, 1407, 1993.

91. Sidransky, H. and Verney, E., Influence of L-alanine on effects induced by L-tryptophan on rat liver, *J. Nutr. Biochem.*, 7, 200, 1996.

92. Sidransky, H. and Verney, E., Differences in tryptophan binding to hepatic nuclei of NZBWF1 and Swiss mice: Insight into mechanism of tryptophan's effects, *J. Nutr.*, 127, 270, 1997.

93. Sidransky, H., Verney, E., Cosgrove, J. W., and Schwartz, A. M., Studies with compounds that compete with tryptophan binding to rat hepatic nuclei, *J. Nutr.*, 122, 1085, 1992.

94. Weinberger, C., Thompson, C. C., Ong, E. S., Lebo, R., Gruol, D. J., and Evans, R. M., The c-erb-A gene encodes a thyroid hormone receptor, *Nature*, 324, 641, 1986.

95. Sap, J., Munoz, A., Damm, K., Goldberg, Y., Ghysdael, J., Leutz, A., Beug, H., and Vennstrom, B., The c-erb-A protein is a high-affinity receptor for thyroid hormone, *Nature*, 324, 635, 1986.

96. Sidransky, H. and Verney, E., Hormonal influences on tryptophan binding to rat hepatic nuclei, *Metab. Clin. Exp.*, 48, 144, 1999.

97. Sidransky, H. and Verney, E., The presence of thiols in the hepatic nuclear binding site for L-tryptophan: Studies with selenite, *Nutr. Res.*, 16, 1023, 1996.

98. Brtko, J. and Filipcik, P., Effect of selenite and selenate on rat liver nuclear 3,5,3'-triiodothyronine (T3) receptor, *Biol. Trace Element Res.*, 41, 191, 1994.

99. Tashima, Y., Terui, M., Itoh, H., Mizunuma, H., Kobayashi, R., and Marumo, F., Effect of selenite on glucocorticoid receptor, *J. Biochem.*, 105, 358, 1989.

6

Tryptophan Effects or Influences on Biological Processes

CONTENTS

6.1   Introduction

For many years, tryptophan has been considered an important nutrient that may affect a number of biological processes in animals and humans. The implication that tryptophan itself may act on or influence important processes merits review. In some cases, the results suggest that tryptophan may act directly, in others it may act indirectly, and in some it may not act at all. This chapter reviews data available on tryptophan's possible involvement in pregnancy and infant development, on aging, alcoholism, cardiovascular diseases, liver disease, and cancer.

6.2   Pregnancy, Fetal and Infant Development

6.2.1   Pregnancy and Fetal Development

6.2.1.1   *Blood Tryptophan in Pregnancy*

Schrocksnadel et al.[1] reported on the levels of blood tryptophan in uncomplicated pregnancy (45 healthy pregnant women, 15 in each trimester). In healthy pregnant women, plasma tryptophan values decreased during pregnancy (median 1st trimester: 72 µmol/L; 2nd trimester: 51 µmol/L; 3rd trimester: 46 µmol/L). In the puerperium (15 women), the median value was 60 µmol/L. In addition, an inverse correlation existed between the concentrations of neopterin and of tryptophan. They concluded that the decreased tryptophan levels during normal pregnancy might be related to immune activation phenomena.

6.2.1.2   *Dietary Deprivation of Tryptophan*

Zamenhof et al.[2] studied the effect of dietary deprivation of tryptophan on rats during the second half of pregnancy. The omission of tryptophan from a chemically defined amino acid diet caused a drop in maternal body weight and liver weight. In the neonate, there were decreases in body weight and in cerebral parameters (weight, DNA, and protein). Similar changes also were observed with the dietary omission of lysine or methionine. These findings were essentially similar to those produced by total dietary protein deprivation in the comparable period of pregnancy.[3] Thus, it appears that the absence of a single dietary essential amino acid, such as tryptophan, even during half of pregnancy may be as harmful as total absence of dietary proteins during this period, at least as far as prenatal brain development is concerned. However, this study did not indicate any effects specific for dietary deficiency of tryptophan.

Sanfilippo et al.[4] studied the effects of a tryptophan-deprived diet on rats starting at day 1 and day 14.5 after conception and continuing until birth. Then this feeding was continued uninterruptedly in the litter after birth, and during lactation and postnatal development. The litters of day 1 and day 14.5 started mothers showed underdevelopment at birth that worsened during postnatal development, more so in the former group. At 30 days postnatally, the male rats but not the female rats showed decreased sexual development (testes were not descended and there was no spermatogenesis).

6.2.1.3 Effect of an Excess of Tryptophan

Matsueda and Niiyama[5] studied the effects of diets (6% casein), each with an excess (5%) of one essential amino acid, on the maintenance of pregnancy and reproductive performance, including fetal growth in rats from day 1 to day 14 or 21 of pregnancy. Judging from the total food consumption and body weight gain during pregnancy, they found that methionine had the most severe effects, followed by leucine and tryptophan. In comparison with pair-fed controls, pregnant rats fed the excess tryptophan diet had a 20% loss of fetuses and of maintained nitrogen balance, carcass protein, and fat; they also had lowered weights of females and decreased fetal brain weights and amounts of DNA, RNA, and protein. Excess dietary tryptophan induced no appreciable changes in maternal plasma-free amino acids but two- to three-fold increases in acidic and aromatic amino acids in the fetal brain. The results of experiments of feeding diets with excess of a single essential amino acid, such as tryptophan, have been considered in connection with studies on inborn errors of amino acid metabolism. The influences of hyperaminoacidemia on fetal development in pregnant animals, especially on neuronal development, merit further exploration.

Meier and Wilson[6] have reported that added dietary tryptophan during pregnancy reduces embryo and neonate survival in the golden hamster. When using 1.8 to 3.7% tryptophan in a high (23%)-protein diet or using 8.0% tryptophan in a moderate (16%)-protein diet during pregnancy, litter size and neonate weights were reduced and mortality of neonates after 1 week was increased in comparison with controls. Although the mechanism by which increased dietary tryptophan acts on the embryo and neonate is not clear, consideration has been given that it may be related to the elevation of serotonin. Exogenous serotonin has been reported to cause abortions in several vertebrate species, to reduce litter sizes, to increase stillbirths and neonate abnormalities, and otherwise to influence pregnancy adversely.[7–9] Since the availability of tryptophan is probably the most important rate-limiting factor in serotonin synthesis[10] and since studies have revealed that increases[11] or decreases[12] of dietary tryptophan lead to concomitant changes in serotonin levels, it is likely that tryptophan may act via serotonin. Currently, many humans use tryptophan to decrease appetite[13] and to promote sleep[14] and, therefore, it may be important to determine whether or not increased tryptophan intake during pregnancy may be potentially harmful. Further studies are needed to clarify if this danger exists.

The effect of the administration of L-tryptophan (30 mg per 100 g body weight) on hepatic polyribosomes and protein synthesis in pregnant rats and their fetuses and in lactating rats and their pups has been investigated.[15] Pregnant rats tube-fed tryptophan 1 h before killing revealed increased hepatic protein synthesis but essentially unmodified polyribosomal aggregation of maternal livers while no changes were observed in fetal livers in comparison to controls (water treated). Lactating rats tube-fed tryptophan 1 h before killing revealed increased polyribosomal aggregation and protein synthesis of the livers in comparison to controls. Pups of those mothers that received tryptophan (3.8 mg) intraperitoneally 1 h before killing did not reveal a significant change in the hepatic polyribosomes or protein synthesis. In an attempt to explain why the tube-feeding of tryptophan to pregnant rat stimulated hepatic protein synthesis in the mother but not in the fetal liver, the presence of different levels of tryptophan in the blood in the two (maternal and fetal) circulations was considered. It has been reported that the level of most amino acids is considerably higher in fetal than in maternal blood.[16-18] Tryptophan, as well as total amino acid concentration, in plasma decreases significantly with pregnancy,[18] while in the fetus (21 days) the plasma tryptophan level is higher (65 to 91%) than in the mother.[18,19] This suggests that the plasma tryptophan level in the fetus may already be high, so an additional elevation via the maternal ingestion of tryptophan may not have a further stimulatory effect. In general, it has been reported that there is a faster turnover of tissue proteins in the fetus than in the adult.[20] Also, it is known that the fetal liver is involved in active hematopoiesis, and the numerous hematopoietic cells alter the cellular population in the fetal liver. These cells may not be responsive to tryptophan. The reason why the livers of young (8- to 13-day-old) pups do not respond to the administration of tryptophan with enhanced hepatic protein synthesis is not known, but it is possible that such young pups still react like fetuses and may have altered (high) circulating tryptophan levels in the livers. Indeed it has been reported that the intracellular concentrations of free amino acids in the rat liver are low at time of birth, but by the 10th day they increase and peak at 19 days.[21] Measurement of the concentration of free tryptophan shows a similar trend.[21] Thus, an increase of hepatic level of tryptophan by intraperitoneal injection may be unable to further stimulate the already elevated protein synthesis that has been induced in response to the high liver free amino acid pools, including that of tryptophan. However, the administration of tryptophan to mature animals in which hepatic protein synthesis has already been stimulated by dietary[22,23] or hormonal[24] means, as well as following partial hepatectomy,[25] has been demonstrated to further enhance hepatic protein synthesis. Thus, one must search for other reasons, possibly such as immaturity or endocrine alterations, to account for the resistance of pups or fetuses to the stimulatory effect of tryptophan on the livers.

Arevalo et al.[26] reported that the oral administration of tryptophan to pregnant rats induced a dose-related increase of tryptophan concentrations in different fetal tissues, including brain. The increase in tryptophan tissue concentration was detected for low doses (50 mg/kg) and remained unsaturated after administration of high doses (1000 mg/kg). Tryptophan concentration in the brain was 300% higher than in the carcass and 600% higher than in the placenta. Thus, tryptophan is not affected by the placental barrier and tryptophan becomes concentrated in brain tissue.

The effect of tryptophan administration to pregnant rats was studied on the development of serotonergic systems and serotonin-related hormones in the offspring.[27] The male offspring of rats treated with tryptophan (20 mg per 100 g body weight per day) during the second half of gestation revealed a four- to seven-fold increase in serum prolactin 40 and 70 days after birth and a two-fold increase in serum luteinizing hormone 70 days after birth. An increase in serotonin and 5-hydroxyindole-acetic acid levels was present in the forebrain of adult offspring of tryptophan-treated rats. Thus, it appears that tryptophan regulates serotonergic differentiation during early development.

Earlier, Hernandez-Rodriguez and Chagoya[28] reported on the effect of prenatal tryptophan supplementation on serotonin synthesis and the activity of Na^+,K^+-ATPase in the rat cerebral cortex during postnatal development, from birth up to day 30. Elevated levels of both were observed in comparison to controls.

Henderson and Kitos[29] studied the effect of tryptophan on organophosphate insecticide-induced teratogenic signs in chicken embryos. Fertile chicken eggs at 3 days of incubation were treated with a teratogenic dose of the organophosphate insecticide, diazinon, in the presence or absence of exogenous L-tryptophan. By day 10 of development, the insecticide reduced the NAD^+ content of the hind limbs of the embryos to less than 20% of normal and by day 15 it caused severe type I and type II teratogenic responses. The co-presence of tryptophan served to maintain the NAD^+ levels of the treated embryos close to or above normal and significantly alleviated the symptoms of type I teratisms. These findings supported the concept that the insecticide acts to decrease the availability of tryptophan to the embryo. On the other hand, Snawder and Chambers[30] used *Xenopus laevis* embryos exposed to the organophosphorus insecticide, malathion, with or without tryptophan treatment. They found that tryptophan increased the NAD^+ levels but did not influence the severity or incidence of defects. Thus, the reduction of NAD^+ does not seem to be responsible for the effects seen in *Xenopus* or account for some defects in avian species.

6.2.1.4 Brain Development (Prenatal and Postnatal)

In searching for the most important site that may be affected by L-tryptophan in fetal development, it was appropriate to investigate the brain. Studies with experimental animals have demonstrated that the nutritional status relative to the amount of dietary protein during prepartum and also post-partum development has an important role in determining subsequent brain tryptophan metabolism. Indeed, alterations in brain tryptophan, serotonin, and 5-hydroxyindoleacetic acid concentrations occurred in rats as a consequence of dietary protein insufficiencies during prenatal and/or postnatal development.[31,32] Because the availability of tryptophan to brain and peripheral tissues may be a limiting factor in protein synthesis during early development,[33,34] alterations in the utilization of this essential amino acid under conditions of prenatal and postnatal protein malnutrition have been considered to possibly cause permanent alterations in the organism. The influence of prepartum and postpartum nutritional status on brain indolamine metabolism indicated that both play important roles in determining this process.[31,32,35] The increased brain levels of tryptophan and serotonin as a consequence of protein inadequacies can best be related to the increased amounts of free plasma tryptophan available for their brain metabolism, even while total plasma tryptophan levels are decreased. These rats seem to be shunting more tryptophan to the brain at the expense of the periphery. From a teleological viewpoint, the increases in brain serotonin and 5-hydroxyindoleacetic acid may be only the consequence of a need to assure the availability of tryptophan for adequate brain protein synthesis and development in early life.

In determining the ontogenesis of tryptophan in rat brain, Hamon and Bourgoin[36] described that during the first 3 postnatal weeks levels of brain tryptophan are exceptionally high, two to four times those found in adult rats. This was considered to be related to two peculiarities concerning tryptophan transport in young animals: (1) lack of tryptophan binding to serum albumin, which allows its diffusion from plasma to tissues earlier for the early life period and (2) the greater capacity of synsptosomes from neonates to accumulate tryptophan.

Bourgoin et al.[37] explained that the high free-serum tryptophan levels in the first period of postnatal life were due to relative lack of binding to serum albumin. Factors responsible for this were (1) lower concentration of serum albumin, the binding protein; (2) the inhibition of binding by nonesterified fatty acids, which were at a high level in the serum of young rats until weaning; and (3) the decreased number of available binding sites for tryptophan on the defatted serum albumin, whereas the apparent association constant of tryptophan binding to serum albumin was similar in newborn and adult.

6.2.2   Infant Development

6.2.2.1   *Tryptophan Deficiency*

The effects of tryptophan deficiency during human development were described by Jaeger et al.[38] They reported on a tragic incident where tryptophan had been left out of a commercially available dietetic formula used for children with phenylketonuria. Such children suffered from lethargy, hair loss, skin lesions, loss of appetite, diarrhea, and neurological disturbances. Most of the symptoms resolved after a return to adequate diet, but some neurological symptoms, visual impairment, optic atrophy, ataxia, and spastic paresis of the legs persisted.

6.2.2.2   Blood Tryptophan Levels

De Antoni et al.[39] determined the levels of total and free serum tryptophan in newborn babies at birth, 1 day later, and 5 days after birth. As also described by others,[40] total and free tryptophan levels were very high in the umbilical cord at birth, decreased quickly and significantly 24 h after birth, and showed a slight increase 5 days after birth.

A number of studies have reported that the plasma free tryptophan levels in infants are indicative of brain serotonin synthesis.[41,42] They also reported that in gestationally malnourished rats or human infants the plasma free tryptophan was elevated and considered that an increased transport of tryptophan to the brain caused a possible enhancement of serotonin synthesis.

Findings by Zammarchi et al.[43] on blood free tryptophan levels in jaundiced newborn infants during phototherapy are of interest. They reported a significant decrease in free tryptophan levels 24 h after phototherapy. This was explained by the decrease in nonesterified fatty acids (NEFA) during phototherapy. Since both tryptophan and NEFA are bound to serum albumin and NEFA can displace tryptophan from their binding sites, the decrease in free tryptophan may be secondary to the change in NEFA levels.

6.2.3   Effects on Piglets

Cortamira et al.[44] reported on the effect of dietary tryptophan on liver, muscle, and whole-body protein synthesis in weaned piglets. Using weaned, 10-day-old piglets, they fed *ad libitum* or force-fed a tryptophan-deficient or tryptophan-adequate (control) diet for 2 weeks and measured protein synthesis rates *in vivo* 2 h after a meal. In the *ad libitum* feeding experiment, tryptophan deficiency as compared with tryptophan adequacy significantly decreased food intake, growth performance, and fractional protein synthesis rates (using a "flooding dose" of ^{3}H-phenylalanine) of liver and muscle (longissimus dorsi and semitendinous). In the force-feeding experiment, piglets were tube-fed tryptophan-deficient and adequate diets at two feeding levels from a previous *ad libitum* feeding experiment. Both tryptophan-adequate and feeding levels (mainly higher levels) significantly increased growth performance and fractional protein synthesis rates. The liver maximum protein synthesis rate occurred in the tryptophan-adequate plus the higher intake group. At 30 min after a meal, plasma insulin levels were higher in both experimental and control groups fed the higher diet intake. They concluded that dietary tryptophan deficiency decreased liver and muscle protein synthesis rates, and this may be related to a post-prandial release of insulin following a decreased rate of nutrient absorption. However, in a later study, Ponter et al.[45] could not establish a relationship between plasma insulin and muscle synthesis rates in piglets treated under similar conditions.

In another study, Lin et al.[46] reported that there was a depressive effect of tryptophan deficiency on protein synthesis rate in pig muscle. Also, earlier studies revealed that, among the essential amino acids, tryptophan was one of the most critical at weaning on the effect of its deficiency on the appetite of piglets[47] in the same way that its deficiency affected the appetite of older pigs.[48]

Ponter et al.[45] reported on the effects of dietary tryptophan (deficient, adequate, or excess) with high carbohydrate or fat diet on liver, muscle, skin, femur, pancreas, stomach, and whole-body protein synthesis in weaned piglets. They used piglets weaned at 10 days of age and infused diets directly into the stomach through an indwelling gastric catheter for 27 days. They measured fractional protein synthesis rate using a "flooding dose" of ³H-phenylalanine via jugular catheter. Tryptophan supplementation globally augmented the fractional protein synthesis rate linearly in the liver, semitendinous muscle, skin, and whole body, while it had quadratic effects in longissimus dorsi muscle (highest in tryptophan-adequate diet groups) and jejunal mucosa (lowest in tryptophan-adequate diet groups). Pancreatic fractional protein synthesis was increased by tryptophan addition up to a plateau. The fractional synthesis rate was highest after the high fat diets in the digestive tissues and femur, while in skin and longissimus dorsi muscle the fractional protein synthesis rate was highest after the high-carbohydrate diets. In general, adequate or excess tryptophan diets did not appreciably change the fractional protein synthesis rates of duodenal mucosa and jejunal mucosa, but small increases occurred in stomach. This study confirmed the depressive effects of a tryptophan-deficient diet on fractional protein synthesis rates, RNA activity, and growth. Also, it could not establish a relationship between plasma insulin and muscle fractional protein synthesis rate in this study.

6.2.4 Summary

This section has reviewed the effects of a tryptophan-deficient diet or of tryptophan administration or supplementation on pregnancy, on the fetus, and on postnatal animals or humans. It is apparent that tryptophan does play a role in the fetal state and postnatally. Its effects are probably through the levels of blood free tryptophan levels in the mother, the fetus, and the infant. The blood free tryptophan levels influence the brain tryptophan levels and also the brain serotonin levels. Thus, blood tryptophan levels can influence protein synthesis in various tissues, especially in the brain, along with serotonin synthesis, in the fetus and in the infant. Other amino acids can also affect protein synthesis, but tryptophan is unique in its effect on serotonin levels.

6.3 Tryptophan and Aging

6.3.1 Tryptophan Ingestion and Longevity

6.3.1.1 Long-Term Ingestion of a Tryptophan-Deficient Diet

Dietary manipulation has been utilized as a possible means for altering the rate of mammalian aging. Indeed, many experimental studies (early and recent) have demonstrated a life-extending effect of calorie restriction, whereby the rate of aging appears to become retarded.[49-54] In regard to tryptophan and aging, a quarter of a century ago, Segall and Timiras[55] undertook experimental studies to evaluate the effect of long-term dietary tryptophan restriction on the process of aging in the rat. The maturational and growth arrest for long periods under their experimental conditions was attributed to the ability of the tryptophan-deficient diet to lower brain serotonin levels. Along with a slight increase in the average life span at late ages of the experimental animals, they observed a delay in the age of onset of visible tumors. However, their pair-fed controls, as did the findings with calorie-restricted rats in experimental studies reported by others,[49-52] demonstrated a prolonged life span and a delayed onset of tumors. Ooka et al.[56] reported that diets containing tryptophan in concentrations 30 and 40% of those fed to controls from weaning to 24 to 30 months could delay aging in Long-Evans female rats. Mortality among low-tryptophan rats was greater in the juvenile period but substantially less than controls at late ages. Increased longevity in mice fed a low tryptophan diet has also been reported.[57] Low levels of tryptophan in the diet cause voluntary restriction of food intake[55] as well as hormonal alterations.[58] Thus, in the absence of clear quantitative assessment of findings due to a tryptophan-deficient diet compared with those due to decreased diet (energy) intake, it is difficult to attribute prolonged longevity specifically to low intake of tryptophan per se. At present, the effect could more likely be attributed to the general response pattern of decreased *ad libitum* diet consumption due to the ingestion of a deficient diet.[59]

6.3.1.2 Blood, Brain, Intestinal Tract, and Renal Tryptophan Levels and Aging

6.3.1.2.1 Blood

Normally, free plasma amino acid concentrations show relatively little variation.[60] However, a number of reports indicated that plasma total tryptophan levels are lower in the older than in the younger population for both sexes.[61] Also, a number of reports have indicated that serum tryptophan levels were decreased in some disease states.[62,63] A number of hypotheses have been proposed as an explanation. Clearly, under certain conditions the serum tryptophan levels become altered, but the full consequences thereof remain unknown.

6.3.1.2.2   Brain

Tang and Melethil[64] studied the kinetics of blood–brain barrier uptake of tryptophan in rats as affected by aging and reported that aging decreases the ability of the blood–brain barrier to transport tryptophan. Yeung and Friedman[65] reported that age-related reduction of cortical tryptophan and plasma ratio of tryptophan to large neutral amino acids in old animals was attenuated by chronic diet restriction. The results of their study using young (6 months) and old (24 months) male Fischer-344 rats suggested that serotonergic neurons were more susceptible to change during aging than were the catecholaminergic neurons. Demling et al.[61] speculated that the age-dependent decrease in plasma tryptophan might contribute to the metabolic basis of affective disorders in elderly people. Their data support the hypothesis that lower tryptophan levels and tryptophan ratios (total or free tryptophan concentrations divided by the sum of the other large neutral amino acids) in plasma, with the consequences of a decreased influx of tryptophan into the brain and diminished synthesis of serotonin, may act as a vulnerability factor for depressed states in older age.

6.3.1.2.3   Intestinal Tract

Navab and Winter[66] investigated the effect of aging on intestinal absorption of tryptophan *in vitro* in the rat. Using whole-thickness everted jejunal rings to measure L-tryptophan uptake, they observed that uptake was reduced in older (2-year-old) rats compared with that in younger (6-month-old) rats.

6.3.1.2.4   Kidney

Fleck[67] reported that the plasma concentrations of tryptophan were lower in young (10-day-old) than in an adult (2-month-old) male Wistar rats, and the renal clearance of the amino acid was lower in young rats, but the effective tubular reabsorption capacity was higher in young rats.

The above observations deal with the consequences of aging on tryptophan levels in different components or areas of the body. Whether and how these changes in levels of tryptophan may in themselves influence the process of aging is not clear.

6.3.1.3   Tryptophan Metabolism with Aging

Tryptophan 2,3-dioxygenase is the main hepatic enzyme in the metabolism of L-tryptophan. Levels of this enzyme in the liver have been investigated in the rat during various phases of the life span. In general, the level of this enzyme shows no significant change until adulthood but decreases significantly thereafter with increasing age. Induction of the activity of this enzyme increases significantly due to hydrocortisone treatment in rats of all ages. Yet, the effect of such treatment is highest in the mature rat.[68] Whether and how the activity of this important enzyme may play a role in regulating blood tryptophan levels at different ages are not clear.

6.3.1.4 Tryptophan Effects via Hormones

Because a number of hormonal changes occur during the aging process, it has been thought that L-tryptophan may act upon hormonal actions to affect aging. Some of the possible relationships have been considered, especially relating to the liver.

6.3.1.4.1 Age-Dependent Regulation of Glucocorticoid Receptors in Liver

Glucocorticoids act on a variety of cellular and metabolic effects. Alterations in the adaptive responsiveness to hormones have been reported to be age related, as have the changes in the induction of many enzymes.[69] The hormone-mediated responses are controlled by binding to specific intracellular receptors. Age-related changes in the steroid receptor-binding sites occur in most animal tissues.[70] Increased numbers of binding sites for glucocorticoid receptors in liver have been reported at the weanling stage compared to the mature state of Long-Evans rats[71] and for 3-month-old vs. 12-month-old Sprague-Dawley rats.[72] This suggests that the glucocorticoid receptor level and some of its physiochemical properties vary at different ages of rats, and these differences may lead to functional changes in tissue response as a function of age. Age-related changes in glucocorticoid receptors in a number of organs have been described.[73]

6.3.1.4.2 Age-Dependent Regulation of Thyroxine and Triiodothyronine Receptors in Liver

Aging has often been defined as an altered state of tissue responsiveness to hormonal signals and/or as altered synthetic and secretory processes of the endocrine glands. Since thyroxin (T_4) and triiodothyronine (T_3) have diverse effects on metabolic processes, they may especially be important components of the aging process. Altered thyroid function with aging has been reported.[74] Although *in vitro* binding of T_3 to liver nuclear receptor suggests that the density of the receptor does not change with aging,[75,76] alterations in receptor-controlled cellular functions could still occur with aging and may be indirectly induced through changes in availability of cellular T_4 and T_3 and, consequently, in receptor saturation. Margarity et al.[77] studied the effects of aging on the *in vivo* subcellular distribution and binding of T_3 and T_4 to hepatic nuclei as well as on the process of T_4 to T_3 conversion in Long-Evans rats. They observed that with aging *in vivo* nuclear T_3 binding did not change significantly, but nuclear T_3 binding derived from T_4 was decreased as a consequence of reduced T_4 to T_3 conversion and also T_4 binding was depressed.

6.3.1.4.3 Tryptophan and Regulation of Hormone Receptors in Liver

Since L-tryptophan has been demonstrated to have a specific nuclear receptor in liver,[78–80] it was important to consider whether its receptor may be similar or related to other hormone-related hepatic nuclear receptors. Triiodothyronine (T_3) receptors and glucocorticoid receptors are part of a group of nuclear proteins, "ligand responsive transcription factors," that belong to the same protein super-family as steroid receptors.[81,82] The steroid hormone nuclear receptors have been extensively investigated, and the complexity of their actions on a vast number of physiologic and pathologic processes is apparent.[83] In an attempt to determine whether the hepatic nuclear receptor for L-tryptophan may possibly be related to those hormonal receptors, some experimental studies searching for possible similarities have been conducted. Some recent findings[84] have suggested that the nuclear L-tryptophan receptor may possibly be related to hormone-related nuclear receptors, and possible commonalities between their actions may exist. Such commonalities may relate hormonal effects on the aging process. Speculations in this regard have been reviewed.[85]

6.3.1.4.4 Melatonin and Aging

Melatonin is a hormone secreted mainly by the pineal gland. It is synthesized from tryptophan, and its characteristic circadian rhythm is ruled by light. Touitou et al.[86] have reviewed the relationship of melatonin and aging. Since the circulating levels of melatonin decrease with aging, questions arise regarding its origin and/or the consequences of this condition, which may be related to the availability of tryptophan.

6.3.1.5   Rationale for Considering Tryptophan in Relation to Aging

The rationale for exploring whether specific amino acids, especially L-tryptophan, may play a role in influencing the process of aging is a justifiable one. Altered expression of genes must indeed influence longevity. Studies and hypotheses for amino-acid-dependent regulation of gene expression in mammalian cells have been reported.[87] It is vital to gain a definition of the molecular steps whereby the cellular concentration of individual amino acids can regulate gene expression, and this may contribute to our understanding of metabolic control in mammalian cells during the lifetime of the host.

Whether L-tryptophan may play a role in aging is currently not known. Some of the recent investigative findings regarding L-tryptophan suggest that it could be involved. This may be related to L-tryptophan's ability to bind to a specific hepatic nuclear receptor, which is somewhat similar to that which occurs with a number of steroid hormones. Based upon earlier findings, it has been speculated that the nuclear tryptophan receptor protein may be involved in gene regulation,[79] possibly in a manner similar to that demonstrated for several steroid receptors that regulate gene transcription.[88–90] Supportive findings that NZBWF$_1$ mice have a significantly diminished nuclear tryptophan receptor affinity in liver in comparison to that of other mouse strains is of great interest.[91] NZBWF$_1$ mice are autoimmune-susceptible and have a relatively short life span with many features of accelerated aging.[92] In NZBWF$_1$ mice, the decreased nuclear receptor affinity for L-tryptotophan in liver appeared to be diminished even more in young

(6.5-week-old) than in older (30-week-old) mice.[93] An explanation for the latter finding is not clear but possibly represents some minor adaptation in the 30-week-old mice over that in the 6.5-week-old mice. Nonetheless, both age groups of NZBWF$_1$ mice clearly have significantly less nuclear tryptophan receptor affinity than that in Swiss mice.

At the present time, no definitive evidence exists that L-tryptophan per se is involved in the process of aging. The early reports that animals fed a tryptophan-deficient diet had an increase in longevity should most likely be attributed to decreased diet intake. Since some similarities between the specific nuclear receptor for L-tryptophan and the nuclear receptors for steroid hormones appear to exist, it has been speculated that under some circumstances L-tryptophan may possibly act like steroid hormones, which have been demonstrated to play roles in the aging process.[73] Such speculation should stimulate further investigation concerning how L-tryptophan acts as a regulatory control of protein metabolism normally and during aging.

6.4   Tryptophan and Alcohol

6.4.1   Introduction

Ethanol consumption is probably one of the most important and widespread environmental factors in inducing human liver disease throughout the world. It is recognized that ethanol is a potent hepatotoxic agent, although a full understanding of the mechanism by which it acts upon the liver is still not completely clear. A review regarding the effects of ethanol on hepatic protein synthesis is available.[94] As described in this review and in another later report,[95] it appears that most of the more recent experimental studies have demonstrated that a single administration of ethanol causes a decrease in hepatic protein synthesis in experimental animals. In this section, the possible influences of tryptophan in relation to ethanol's effect on the liver, especially relating to hepatic protein synthesis in experimental studies, will be reviewed.

Tryptophan is the most extensively studied amino acid in relation to alcohol and alcoholism. This is probably because it is the precursor of serotonin. Serotonin levels as altered by ethanol could have a role in disturbances in mood, clinical features of alcohol dependence, and alcohol withdrawal states. The control of alcohol consumption itself by serotonin has been considered.[96] Accounts of the effects of ethanol on tryptophan and serotonin metabolism have been reviewed.[97,98] This section limits itself to selected aspects of ethanol and tryptophan metabolism in experimental animals and in humans. How these changes may secondarily affect serotonin metabolism is mentioned.

6.4.2   Review of Influential Factors on Liver Injury

6.4.2.1   *Influence of Nutritional Status and Tryptophan on Ethanol-Induced Liver Injury*

In 1968, Lucas et al.[99] reported that the ability of rats to tolerate ethanol varied with the nature of their dietary protein. When rats were fed a diet that promoted better growth, they generally became less intoxicated as compared with rats fed a diet that was not as effective in growth promotion. Later studies using single amino acids along with ethanol were concerned with their influence on toxicity. Special attention was given to dietary tryptophan since this essential amino acid had been demonstrated to have a unique effect in regulating and stimulating hepatic protein synthesis.[100,101] Jarowski and Ward[102] reported that 30 min of pretreatment with L-tryptophan (165 mg intraperitoneally) before a 2 g/kg intraperitoneal dose of 95% ethanol in nonfasted rats (130 g) produced a significant potentiation of the acute depressant effects of ethanol as measured by changes in the LD_{50}, and sleeping and immobility times. The rationale for the use of L-tryptophan as supplementation was based upon the fasting essential amino acid profile of blood plasma, which has been useful in predicting the relative dietary value of proteins.[103] Ward et al.[104] reported that oral or intraperitoneally lysine administration 30 min prior to ethanol administration did not increase the LD_{50}. Breglia et al.[105] demonstrated that there was no significant alteration of the ethanol LD_{50} with pretreatment or with simultaneous administration of selected amino acids, L-lysine, L-arginine, L-ornithine, and glycine. Dubroff et al.[106] reported that the ethanol LD_{50} value increased significantly only for rats fed a lysine- and tryptophan-supplemented ration for 30 days. These findings were consistent with the view expressed earlier by Lucas et al.[99] that reduction in toxicity can probably be attributed to an improvement in the biological value of the diet by supplementation. Also, Jeejeebhoy et al.[107] reported a decrease in albumin synthesis in rats when given ethanol (4 to 8 mg/kg) orally, which was prevented by the simultaneous administration of a complete mixture of amino acids but not by tryptophan. Rothschild et al.[108,109] reported that the addition of tryptophan to isolated perfused rabbit livers treated with ethanol aided in the recovery of albumin synthesis. The above-described experimental studies indicate that protein and amino acids, including L-tryptophan, can be shown to influence the toxicity of ethanol. However, the results are difficult to evaluate and interpret, especially in relation to the acute studies with tryptophan, where in most cases the doses used were markedly unphysiologic. Earlier, Gullino et al.[110] reported that the LD_{50} of L-tryptophan alone is 160 mg per 100 g body weight.

6.4.2.2   *Consideration of the Possible Action of Ethanol via Changes in Circulatory Amino Acids*

In an early study, Badawy and Evans[111] reported that the acute administration (2 to 10 h) of ethanol (0.5 g per 100 g body weight) to rats led to a rapid decrease in serum total tryptophan levels with a biphasic response in serum free tryptophan levels and in liver tryptophan levels (elevations at 2 to 4 h with decreases at 7 to 8 h). Also, Stowell and Morland[112] reported that the acute administration (0.25 to 8 h) of ethanol (0.4 g per 100 g body weight) led to a rapid rise after 15 min but a marked drop from 4 to 8 h in plasma free tryptophan and liver tryptophan levels. Plasma total tryptophan levels increased after 15 min but fell from 30 min onward. This suggested that ethanol administration caused a change in tryptophan availability and utilization. Eriksson et al.[113] found that rats treated with ethanol (0.2 g per 100 g body weight) for 1 h revealed marked decreases in the plasma concentrations of almost every amino acid compared to controls, and plasma total tryptophan decreased by 30%. Subsequently, these investigators[114] reported similar findings in humans. Also, in the rat, this effect of ethanol was partly inhibited by the β-adrenergic antagonist (-)-propranolol, partly by adrenalectomy or hypophysectomy, and almost completely by a combination of adrenalectomy with (-)-propranolol. This suggested an involvement of both β-adrenergic mechanisms and steroids from the adrenal cortex in the ethanol-induced decrease in plasma amino acids. Cobb and Van Thiel[115] have reviewed data relating to the effect of ethanol on adrenal gland hypersecretion. Sidransky[94] observed tryptophan levels in the serum and liver after ethanol treatment which resemble those reported by others:[111,112] with serum tryptophan, total tryptophan levels decreased after 1 h, and the decrease continued progressively for 4 h; with liver tryptophan, levels increased after 1 h and then decreased progressively for 4 h. These studies suggested that tryptophan, its needs, requirements, availability, and metabolism, may become altered due to ethanol and that supplementation with tryptophan before, during, or after ethanol may possibly prove to have a beneficial effect.

6.4.2.3 Comparing Mechanisms by which Tryptophan and Ethanol Act on Nucleocytoplasmic Translocation of mRNA in the Liver

It has been reported by Khawaja[116] that prolonged (10 weeks) ethanol ingestion by rats led to increased nucleocytoplasmic transport of RNA in liver when assayed *in vitro*. This suggested a partial loss of nuclear restrictive control. The effect was mediated through factors present in the cytosol as well as in the nuclear fraction. This effect appears to be comparable to that produced when rats are treated acutely with L-tryptophan[117] or with phenobarbitone.[118] Sidransky[94] assayed for the *in vitro* RNA release from hepatic nuclei of rats that had been treated with ethanol (0.75 g per 100 g body weight) for 0.25, 0.50, 1, 2, or 3 h before killing. The results suggested that within 1 h there was a marked enhancement of nuclear RNA release, which was due mainly to the nuclei of livers of ethanol-treated rats. The effect was much less at 2 and 3 h. Since the above enhanced nuclear RNA release due to ethanol preceded or coincided along with decrease in protein synthesis in the liver, it was different than that which occurred after L-tryptophan or phenobarbitone, each of which caused increased hepatic protein synthesis.

The acute administration[94] and also the chronic administration[116] of ethanol and the acute administration of tryptophan[119,120] induced enhanced nuclear RNA release, yet ethanol (acute or chronic) led to inhibition of protein synthesis, while tryptophan stimulated hepatic protein synthesis. Thus, it appears that the alteration of RNA release in each case was probably different. The ethanol effect was most likely due to its induction of altered or abnormal permeability of the nuclear membrane, while the tryptophan effect was considered to be due to its enhancing effect on the physiologic transport mechanism.[121] Reports have indicated that the physiologically relevant concentrations of ethanol may increase membrane fluidity.[122] This fluidity can perturb the function of membrane transport enzymes and membrane-bound enzymes.[123] Attention has been given to membrane pathology derived by ethanol consumption for long intervals.[124,125] Conceivably, nuclear membranes may also become altered.

6.4.3   Review of the Effects of Ethanol on Tryptophan and Serotonin Metabolisms

Several reviews have been published relating to tryptophan and serotonin metabolism in alcoholism.[97,98,126] Here some essential features are presented.

6.4.3.1   Acute Effects

6.4.3.1.1   Animal Studies

In the rat, the most often studied animal species, whose tryptophan metabolism resembles closely that of humans, acute ethanol administration, as described earlier, induces a biphasic effect on serum tryptophan levels, an initial increase followed by a later inhibition. Similarly, acute ethanol administration exerts a biphasic effect on brain serotonin synthesis and turnover, an initial enhancement followed by a later inhibition.[111] The initial enhancement is caused by an increase in circulating free tryptophan availability to brain, probably secondary to a catecholamine-dependent lipolysis and a nonesterified fatty acid-mediated displacement of the albumin-bound amino acid, whereas the later inhibition of serotonin synthesis and turnover is the result of a decrease in circulating free and albumin-bound tryptophan availability to the brain secondary to activation of hepatic tryptophan 2,3-dioxygenase (TP) by the earlier increase in free tryptophan to the liver. The activation of hepatic TP by acute ethanol administration, which is substrate (tryptophan) mediated, has been described in rats by Badawy and Evans.[111,127,128]

6.4.3.1.2   Human Studies

Studies in humans have been limited and have been conducted only in normal volunteers and in nonabstinent alcohol-dependent subjects. Davis et al.[129] first described the decrease in urinary excretion of the major serotonin metabolite 5-HIAA and the concomitant rise in that of 5-hydroxytryptophan as a consequence of the shift of serotonin degradation from its major oxidative to its minor reductive pathway in normal humans after acute ethanol intake. Badawy et al.[130] reported that acute ethanol intake in normal men caused a 25% decrease in total and free tryptophan levels. Also, the blood tryptophan-to-CAA ratio was down by 20%, thus lowering tryptophan availability to the brain and hence in serotonin synthesis.

6.4.3.2 Chronic Effects

6.4.3.2.1 Animal Studies

Badawy et al.[131] attributed the enhanced rat brain serotonin synthesis and turnover by chronic ethanol administration to the increased circulating tryptophan availability to the brain secondary inhibition of hepatic TP activity (NAD(P)H-dependent allosteric inhibition).

6.4.3.2.2 Human Studies

Walsh et al.[132] first described that urinary excretion of tryptophan metabolites of the hepatic kynurenine-nicotinic acid pathway was decreased after oral tryptophan loading of chronic alcoholic subjects within 1 day of cessation of ethanol intake. This suggests inhibition of hepatic TP activity in his subjects. Friedman et al.[133] subsequently showed that serum kynurenine levels after oral tryptophan loading were high in alcoholics after 1 month of abstinence. This finding of inhibition of liver TP activity should result in increased availability of circulating tryptophan to the brain for serotonin synthesis. However, further experimentation is still needed to establish fully the above interpretation.

6.4.4 Summary

Acute and chronic ethanol administration or intake and its subsequent withdrawal in experimental animals and in humans exert major effects on tryptophan and serotonin metabolism. The serotonin status is disturbed in animal models of alcoholism and in alcohol-dependent patients characterized by a higher preference for alcohol consumption. A few experimental studies have suggested that some aspects of ethanol toxicity may be improved by the administration of tryptophan.[108,109] These preliminary findings suggested the possibility of a beneficial effect of added tryptophan on hepatic protein synthesis in ethanol-treated rats, but whether tryptophan administration may be of therapeutic value needs to be established by further investigative studies.

6.5   Cardiovascular Disease

6.5.1   Hypertension

6.5.1.1   Rat Models of Hypertension

A number of studies have demonstrated that an elevated dietary intake of L-tryptophan can lower blood pressure in several rat models of hypertension.[134–140]

Squadrito et al.[141] reported that indolepyruvic acid, a keto analog of tryptophan, at 100 mg per kg per day orally for 10 days, significantly decreased systolic blood pressure in three rat models (spontaneously hypertensive, DOCA + salt hypertensive, and Grollman hypertensive) but had no effect in normotensive rats. Such treatment caused enhanced levels of tryptophan in the cortex and diencephalon and enhanced brainstem serotonin content. Their results suggested that indolepyruvic acid lowered blood pressure in different rat models of hypertension, and the effect seemed to be correlated with an increase in cerebral serotonin metabolism.

Tang et al.[142] studied the effect of chronic hypertension on brain uptake of tryptophan in chronic hypertensive rats and found that brain tryptophan levels were five-fold greater than in normotensive rats. Also, the brain uptake index values for tryptophan were two-fold higher in the experimental rats.

In regard to serotonin (5-HT), significant alterations in brain serotonin content and metabolism were present in the spontaneously hypertensive rat (SHR)[143] and in the DOCA/NaCl hypertensive rat,[144] but not in Dahl salt-resistant (DS) rats.[145] Chronic treatment with L-5-hydroxytryptophan, the immediate precursor of serotonin reduced the elevated blood presence of DS rats on a 4% NaCl diet.[146] Patterson et al.[147] investigated plasma tryptophan levels in DS and Dahl salt-resistant (DR) rats for 1 to 6 weeks on a high salt diet, which produced significant elevation in blood pressure in the DS rats after 4 and 6 weeks. Plasma tryptophan was significantly lower in the DS rats when compared to the DR rats after 4 and 6 weeks on the high salt diet. Also, no differences in plasma tryptophan were observed in DOCA salt-induced, hypertensive, spontaneously hypertensive (SHR), stroke-prone SHR, or fructose-induced hypertensive rats compared to their normotensive controls. Thus, only DS rats appeared to have a selective salt-related defect in peripheral tryptophan regulation.

A decrease in circulating tryptophan levels may be of importance in some models of hypertension. The DS rat is an example of this. The reduction in plasma tryptophan was clearly associated with the excess intake of NaCl and concomitant elevation in blood pressure. Mechanisms that could account for the reduction in plasma tryptophan could include a decrease in gastrointestinal absorption of tryptophan, an increase in urinary tryptophan excretion, increased oxidation of tryptophan by tryptophan oxygenase, and aberrant regulation (hormonal, nutrient, plasma protein) of tryptophan availability. It is indeed known that elevated 18-OH-DOC occurs, which could influence the overall effects. Insulin level changes could be involved. Alterations of levels of other amino acids in plasma may be of importance. Thus, the effects of many interacting agents or conditions may be involved. Additional studies using different experimental hypertension models may help us understand the mechanism(s) by which altered circulating tryptophan levels may be implicated. Considering the overall complexities in the etiology of different forms of hypertension, much is still to be learned about how tryptophan may be primarily or secondarily involved.

Fregly and Fater,[136] Fregly et al.,[148] and Fregly and Cade[149] have been concerned with the effect of chronic dietary administration of tryptophan in the prevention of the development of DOCA-induced hypertension in rats. They reported that the chronic administration of pyridoxine in combination with chronic administration of tryptophan had greater protection than either alone.[149] Similar findings occurred by combination of tryptophan with nicotinic acid.[150] Also, Fregly et al.[151] reported that the chronic dietary administration of tryptophan reduced the elevated systolic blood pressure of spontanously hypertensive(SH) rats. Reisselmann et al.[139] studied the effect of chronic tryptophan administration on the development of hypertension in rats during chronic exposure to cold (5 to 6°C). Their findings consisted of prevention of elevation of blood pressure attenuated cardiac hypertrophy with the chronic administration of tryptophan (850 mg per day) compared to controls. Of interest, Fregly and Cade[149] stressed an important fact regarding the antihypertensive effect of tryptophan: This amino acid has either prevented or attenuated all major types of experimentally induced hypertension in rats. No other compound has been shown to do this. This suggests that a factor in common among all these types of hypertension is related to a relative tryptophan deficiency, which results in failure to produce either enough serotonin or one or more of the compounds in the kynurenine metabolic pathway. However, it is possible that even without a relative tryptophan deficiency, tryptophan administration may still be able to stimulate serotonin production as well as kynurenine pathway metabolites. The findings based upon tryptophan's effect on hepatic protein synthesis and the mechanisms involved in this process indicate that they occur without the need of tryptophan deficiency.[152,153]

6.5.1.2 Human Studies

Treatment with tryptophan has been shown to reduce blood pressure in humans with mild to moderate essential hypertension.[154,155] The exact mechanisms by which dietary tryptophan blunts the development of hypertension or lowers blood pressure in humans are not clear. Furthermore, it is not known whether tryptophan lowers blood pressure due to peripheral or central nervous system mechanisms or if tryptophan conversion to serotonin (5-HT) is involved.[156] Wolf and Kuhn[156] reported that L-tryptophan but not D-tryptophan produced an antihypertensive effect in spontaneously hypertensive rats. Yet both isomers of tryptophan increased brain tryptophan to the same extent. Therefore, they concluded that the antihypertensive effects of L-tryptophan did not appear to be mediated by brain serotonin.

Tomoda et al.[157] reported on altered renal response to enhanced endogenous serotonin after tryptophan administration in essential hypertension in human subjects. The altered renal response (renal plasma flow, glomerular filtration rate) to tryptophan found in essential hypertension was considered to be partly related to the exaggerated efferent arteriolar constriction induced by endogenously formed serotonin. In essential hypertension, there was a baseline overproduction of renal serotonin, which may have contributed to a reduction in renal excretory capability.

6.5.1.3   Comments Regarding Mechanism

The metabolism of tryptophan to serotonin has been postulated to play an important role in cardiovascular regulation.[158,159] Serotonin effects on cardiovascular actions are complex due to the anatomical complexity of the central serotonergic systems involved in cardiovascular control and the presence of multiple subtypes of serotonin receptors.[160,161] Also, peripheral cardiovascular actions of serotonin further complicate the interpretation of studies using systemically administered serotonin agonists and precursors such as tryptophan.[159] Since tryptophan is oxidized via the kynurenine pathway, accounting for greater than 90% of tryptophan metabolism,[162] the formed tryptophan metabolites (kynurenine, quinolinic acid, nicotinic acid, etc.) have biologic activity.[137,163,164] The importance of these compounds is complicated. These inherent problems exist in the interpretation and possible significance of many studies, which showed that increased dietary tryptophan could lower blood pressure and attenuate the development of hypertension.

The possible relationship between tryptophan and sodium ions has been considered in a number of studies. Herken and Weber[165] reported that under certain conditions tryptophan injections intraperitoneally to rats led to a reduction of elimination of Na^{++}. Subsequently, Reuter et al.[166] analyzed the alterations of water and electrolyte balances by the use of clearance experiments. The fractional Na^{++} reabsorption increases, with no increase in the absolute tubular sodium transport rate since the significant reduced plasma-sodium concentration led to a decreased sodium load. The most probable cause of the decreased plasma–sodium concentrations seemed to be retention of sodium-free water under the conditions of infusion. The water retention is compatible with the antidiuretic effect of serotonin. Another relationship between tryptophan and sodium has been reported on the effects of each agent alone or together *in vivo* or *in vitro*, on *in vitro* hepatic nuclear tryptophan receptor binding and hepatic protein synthesis.[167,168] This has been considered in detail in Chapter 4.

6.5.2 Arteriosclerosis

6.5.2.1 Introduction

Sidransky[169] reviewed experimental studies dealing with aspects pertaining to the possible influence of dietary protein and amino acids on the development of hypercholesterolemia, which is considered to be intimately associated with arteriosclerosis. This review of the extensive data collected over many years from numerous experimental studies revealed unfortunately that understanding how dietary components, particularly proteins and amino acids, may act in the pathogenesis of this process is not clear. Speculation was presented that the dietary-induced alterations in serum cholesterol levels by proteins and amino acids may be related to nutritional imbalances induced by unbalanced dietary intake and/or internal derangements. The complexity of the problem was further enhanced because species variability was observed in experimental studies. In general, humans appeared to be more resistant to alterations due to changes in dietary proteins and amino acids than were other species.

6.5.2.2 Studies with L-Tryptophan

Although many studies have investigated the effects of single amino acids on decreases or increases of serum cholesterol levels in a number of animal species and humans,[169] no mention is made about tryptophan alone and its effect. In 1975, Raja and Jarowski[170] reported that the administration of capsules containing L-tryptophan (69 mg) and L-lysine monohydride (205 mg) three times daily after meals resulted in a significant drop in plasma cholesterol and triglyceride levels in six human cases.

From 1952 to 1962, several experimental studies using rats fed a choline-deficient diet reported the development of aortic arteriosclerosis.[171–173] Using rats fed a choline-deficient diet, Sidransky et al.[174] reported that elevated (2%) dietary tryptophan affected the elevated serum lipid levels of rats fed the choline-deficient diet for 1 week. Within 1 week the added dietary tryptophan to the choline-deficient diet caused a return in serum cholesterol, HDL cholesterol, and triglyceride values to levels present in rats fed the choline-supplemented diet. The significance of the alterations in serum lipids due to added dietary tryptophan was unknown, but it stressed that a specific amino acid (L-tryptophan) excess created a further nutritional imbalance, which could influence the altered circulating serum lipids due to choline deficiency. The alterations in serum lipid due to choline deficiency were thought to influence the development of arteriosclerosis in the rat, and possibly the added dietary tryptophan was able to prevent the effect. Further experimental studies are needed to determine whether this speculation was valid.

Since high plasma cholesterol levels and plasma lipid peroxidation are associated with arteriosclerosis, Aviram et al.[175] studied the effect of high dietary tryptophan on plasma lipid peroxidation in rats fed an atherogenic diet (containing coconut oil and cholesterol) and a control diet (soybean oil). Tryptophan supplementation did not affect the elevated plasma cholesterol concentration in the rats fed the atherogenic diet, yet dietary tryptophan supplementation further increased (21%) the increased (67%) lipid peroxidation in the atherogenic diet group. Under their experimental conditions, they concluded that excessive dietary tryptophan might be atherogenic since it enhanced plasma lipid peroxidation in hypercholesterolemic rats and also increased macrophage uptake of plasma cholesterol.

A number of studies were concerned with the possible relationship of serotonin and cholesterol levels. Heron et al.[176] reported that by increasing the cholesterol content in the synaptic membranes of mouse brain, serotonin receptors increased markedly. In contrast, in lowering the cholesterol concentration, the number of serotonin receptors and binding of serotonin to brain membranes decreased. These findings were consistent with the concept that serum cholesterol may influence the function of serotonin in the central nervous system.[177]

Baldo-Enzi et al.[178] investigated the serum tryptophan content and its possible binding to lipoproteins, which are the transport system in blood. Using the sera of 16 patients subjected to surgical endoarterectomies, they measured the levels of total cholesterol, cholesterol bound to LDL and HDL lipoproteins, and tryptophan. Also, the total cholesterol and tryptophan levels in atheromatous plaques excised from the carotid artery were assayed in the same patients. They also measured the total serum cholesterol and cholesterol bound to LDL and HDL_2 lipoproteins in 13 healthy women. These subjects revealed a slight hypercholesterolemia (233 mg/dl) and slightly high total HDL cholesterol levels. Tryptophan was found in LDL and HDL_2 lipoprotein fractions. Of the serum total tryptophan levels, approximately 1.6% was bound to each of the LDL and HDL_2 fractions. It appears that HDL_2 transports about four times more tryptophan than does LDL when the ratios between tryptophan bound to each lipoprotein and the cholesterol present in the same lipoprotein are considered. In the 16 endarterectomized patients, the patients did not have hypercholesterolemia while HDL cholesterol was decreased and serum tryptophan levels were in the normal range. In the athermatous plaques, the cholesterol was 12 mg/g and tryptophan was 6.3 µg/g of tissue. These preliminary data indicate that tryptophan is not only present in the athermanous plaques of the carotid arteries but also appears to be bound to LDH and HDL_2 lipoprotein fractions. Normally, blood tryptophan is transported mostly bound to albumin (80 to 90%) and only a small fraction is in the free form (10 to 20%).[179] The interesting findings by Baldo-Enzi et al.[178] need to be repeated and extended before speculation as to their importance emerges. Meanwhile, however, they speculate that tryptophan in serum lipoproteins may be interpreted either as an amino acid necessary for the rebuilding of damaged connective tissue, or, in the case of that transported by the LDL fraction, as a source for serotonin biosynthesis in platelets. Some tryptophan appears to be prevalently transported by HDL_2 lipoproteins, which suggests that the possible role of HDL_2 lipoprotein is for tryptophan removal, decreasing the availability of this precursor for serotonin biosynthesis.

Studies by Thomas and Stocker[180] and Christen et al.[181] indicated that the formation and release of the aminophenolic antioxidant 3-hydroxyanthranilic acid (3-HAA) via the kynurenine pathway are responsible for the ability of interferon-γ-primed human macrophages to inhibit the oxidation of low-density lipoprotein (LDL), an event implicated as an important event in atherogenesis. 3-HAA efficiently inhibits LDL oxidation by acting as an aqueous oxidant scavenger and a synergist for LDL-associated vitamin E.

6.5.3 Concluding Remarks

In regard to hypertension, a number of experimental animal models of hypertension have been shown to respond to the administration of L-tryptophan with a lowering of blood pressure. Also, in some human studies with essential hypertension, L-tryptophan administration has been beneficial. In considering the mechanism, the tryptophan-induced elevation of serotonin has been speculated to be of vital importance. However, other routes of action of tryptophan have also been considered and consist of effects of other tryptophan metabolites and due to changes in sodium ion concentrations in blood.

In regard to atherosclerosis, a number of studies have been concerned with the effect of tryptophan on cholesterol and lipoprotein metabolism. These studies are of much interest but unfortunately do not establish any clear connection between tryptophan and the development of atherosclerosis.

6.6 Liver in Responses to Injury and Drugs

In view of L-tryptophan's effects and actions on the livers of normal animals, it is of interest to review how L-tryptophan may act on livers of animals subjected to acute or chronic liver injury.

6.6.1 Acute Toxic Liver Injury

The influence or effects of L-tryptophan administration on the livers of animals pretreated or posttreated with hepatotoxic chemicals or drugs have been investigated in many studies. Selected studies with a number of commonly used toxic agents are cited. The review deals mainly with biochemical changes rather than with morphologic changes.

6.6.1.1   *CCl₄*

Many reports years ago dealt with the toxic effect of carbon tetrachloride on the liver of experimental animals.[182,183] Among the biochemical changes in the liver following the administration of carbon tetrachloride are disaggregation of hepatic polyribosomes and inhibition of hepatic protein synthesis.[184–186]

Sidransky et al.[187] studied the effect of tryptophan in rats on the disaggregation of hepatic polyribosomes and on the inhibition of hepatic protein synthesis due to the acute administration of CCl_4. Overnight fasted rats were treated intraperitoneally with CCl_4 before (0.5 and 1.5 h before killing) or after (0.25 and 0.75 h before killing) receiving L-tryptophan intraperitoneally. Rats that received CCl_4 alone showed marked hepatic polyribosomal disaggregation and decreased *in vitro* hepatic protein synthesis. Rats that received tryptophan before or after CCl_4 showed an improvement in *in vitro* hepatic protein synthesis, but only the former group revealed an improvement in hepatic polyribosomes. Studies in which rats received [¹⁴C]orotic acid to prelabel hepatic RNA before receiving tryptophan and CCl_4 revealed that tryptophan treatment increased the availability of poly(A)-mRNA in the cytoplasm of livers of CCl_4-treated rats. In another study, Sidransky et al.[188] used different time intervals and reported that rats treated with L-tryptophan 0.25 h before CCl_4 and 0.75 h before kill off showed improved hepatic polyribosomal aggregation and protein synthesis (*in vitro*). Thus, based upon the results of both studies, it appeared that the main effect of L-tryptophan on CCl_4 toxicity deals with prevention more than with curative action.

Rothschild et al.[109] found that the addition of tryptophan to isolated perfused livers of rabbits treated with CCl_4 aided in the recovery of albumin synthesis. This study is consistent with the findings that tryptophan had a beneficial effect on hepatic polyribosomes and protein synthesis in rats treated with CCl_4. Thus, tryptophan may be a useful therapeutic agent for the livers of experimental animals injured with CCl_4.

De Ferreyra et al.[189,190] and De Toranzo et al.[191] have for many years been concerned with CCl_4-induced hepatic necrosis and its prevention by selected amino acids. Although aspartic acid, cysteine, and tyrosine were effective when given as late as 6 h after CCl_4, the protective effects were no longer evident when observations of CCl_4-induced necrosis were made at 72 h, except for cysteine, which retained its protective potential.[191] Cysteine given 6 h after CCl_4 exerted a weak preventative effect on CCl_4-induced liver necrosis while tryptophan did not.[190] However, when both amino acids were given together, a marked protective effect was observed.[190] Based upon these findings, they speculated that cysteine may influence glutathione synthesis, which in turn may lead to the protection of cell membranes against peroxides and free radicals.[192,193] Also, they speculated that, since tryptophan stimulates hepatic protein synthesis, cysteine might also become involved in this process to the benefit of the liver. Another study was directed toward obtaining more information in regard to how cysteine and tryptophan acted in preventing CCl_4-induced hepatic necrosis.[194] Rats received CCl_4 (1 ml/kg intraperitoneally) followed 6 h later by tryptophan (300 mg/kg) and/or cysteine (950 mg/kg) via stomach tube, and rats were killed after 24 h. Treatment with tryptophan, cysteine, or both reduced the degree of hepatic necrosis observed histologically. While CCl_4 caused polyribosomal disaggregation and decreased [^{14}C]leucine incorporation into liver proteins *in vitro* and *in vivo*, treatment with tryptophan, cysteine, or both caused a shift in polyribosomes toward heavier aggregation, and protein synthesis was increased. Serum activities of lactic dehydrogenase (LDH), glutamate oxaloacetate transaminase, glutamate pyruvate transaminase, and γ-glutamyltranspeptidase were markedly increased after CCl_4 alone, but after subsequent treatment with cysteine or with tryptophan and cysteine appreciable decreases occurred. Glutathione concentration decreased but the total amount remained constant in the livers of CCl_4-treated rats, while subsequent treatment with cysteine alone or together with tryptophan elevated both levels of glutathione. Using isolated hepatocytes, CCl_4 caused decreases in cell viability, in release of LDH, and in [^{14}C]leucine incorporation into protein. Treatment with CCl_4 and tryptophan and/or cysteine revealed that cysteine alone or with tryptophan improved cell viability and decreased LDH release of the cells, while tryptophan alone or with cysteine improved protein synthesis. Upon cytologic evaluation, the isolated hepatocytes revealed membrane distortions after CCl_4 alone, but these were less marked after CCl_4 plus tryptophan, cysteine, or both (most improvement). Thus, tryptophan and cysteine act in a beneficial manner against CCl_4-induced hepatic injury in the rat. In this study, tryptophan itself was observed to have a beneficial effect against CCl_4-induced hepatic necrosis. This finding disagrees with those of De Ferreyra et al.,[190] who described no improvement due to tryptophan alone. This discrepancy may be related in part to their use of acidified solutions of amino acids in many of their experimental studies.[191,195] They mention that in many of their experimental studies the amino acids used were dissolved in water adjusted to pH ~ 1 with HCl.[191,195] On the other hand, Wang et al.[194] found that acidified solutions of tryptophan or cysteine were less effective than the solutions of each amino acid in water alone.

It is of interest that Ohta et al.[196] reported on the preventative effect of melatonin, normally synthesized from tryptophan by the pineal gland, on the progression of CCl_4-induced acute liver injury in rats (1 ml/kg body weight after 6 h and progressed at 24 h). Melatonin (50 or 100 mg/kg body weight) was administered 6 h after CCl_4 ingestion, and it prevented the increase in liver lipid peroxide content and decrease in liver reduced glutathione content in the liver injury progression that occurred after CCl_4 alone. The melatonin effect was thought to be through its antioxidant action.

6.6.1.2 Ethionine

Sidransky et al.[197] reported that mice or rats fasted overnight and treated intraperitoneally for 2 to 3 h with ethionine, a hepatotoxic agent that inhib-

ited hepatic protein synthesis, revealed hepatic polyribosomal disaggregation and decreased *in vitro* hepatic protein synthesis. Tube-feeding
L-tryptophan after ethionine treatment and 1 h before killing caused a corrective effect on hepatic polyribosomes and protein synthesis. Simultaneous
administration of ethionine and tryptophan to fasted rats 1 h before killing
induced a shift of hepatic polyribosomes toward heavier aggregation, similar
to that observed after tube-feeding tryptophan alone.

In another study, Sidransky et al.[188] reported that treatment with L-tryptophan 0.5 h before treatment with ethionine and 2.5 h before killing offered
no improvement in hepatic polyribosomes and hepatic protein synthesis
(*in vitro*). However, tube-feeding L-tryptophan 1 h after ethionine and 2 h
before killing revealed improvement in hepatic polyribosomes and protein
synthesis (*in vitro*) compared to the ethionine alone group. Thus, L-tryptophan had a curative effect but not a preventative effect due to ethionine.

6.6.1.3   Actinomycin D

Sidransky and Verney[198] investigated the effect of L-tryptophan on hepatic
polyribosomal disaggregation after actinomycin D, an agent that interferes
with DNA-dependent RNA synthesis. The disaggregation of hepatic polyribosomes in fasted rats 6 h after actinomycin treatment returned toward
normal, becoming reaggregated by the tube-feeding of L-tryptophan 2 h
before killing. However, pretreatment twice with L-tryptophan followed by
actinomycin D (5 and 1 h later) did not improve the polyribosome disaggregation. Thus, L-tryptophan was curative but not preventative in its action
on the hepatic polyribosomes.

6.6.1.4   Puromycin

Sarma et al.[199] reported that the tube-feeding of L-tryptophan (10 min) after
puromycin treatment (20 min) had a corrective effect on the state of hepatic
polyribosomes and on protein synthesis. In another study, Sidransky et al.[188]
reported that pretreatment with L-tryptophan (0.5 h) before puromycin
(20 min before kill) improved hepatic polyribosomal aggregation and protein
synthesis. Thus, L-tryptophan was preventative as well as curative in regard
to puromycin action.

6.6.1.5   Cycloheximide

Cycloheximide, an inhibitor of hepatic protein synthesis, was investigated
to determine whether it would affect *in vitro* ^{3}H-tryptophan binding to isolated rat hepatic nuclei or nuclear envelopes.[200] The addition of cycloheximide, but not of heat-treated cycloheximide, which loses its activity *in vitro*,
inhibited ^{3}H-tryptophan binding to hepatic nuclei or nuclear envelopes. *In
vivo* treatment of rats with cycloheximide diminished *in vitro* ^{3}H-tryptophan
binding to hepatic nuclei of treated rats compared to controls. *In vivo* treatment of puromycin, another inhibitor of protein synthesis, also diminished

in vitro ³H-tryptophan binding, but when puromycin was added *in vitro*, it did not affect ³H-tryptophan binding to hepatic nuclei. The mechanism by which cycloheximide acted *in vitro* was considered to probably be by its structural effect on the receptor. Four cycloheximide-related compounds, 4-phenacylpyridine-N-oxide monohydrate, 4-(2-phenylethyl)-pyridine, 4-chlorophenyl-4-phenethyl)-piperdine ketone, and 2-3,4-dimethoxy-phenyl)-3-oxo-3-pyridin-4-YL-propionitrile, likewise had inhibitory effects on *in vitro* ³H-tryptophan binding to hepatic nuclei, suggesting that structural effects are active. The effect of cycloheximide administered *in vivo* may also be in part by inhibiting protein synthesis, as was the case with puromycin.

6.6.1.6 Hypertonic NaCl

One important physiologic process that rapidly influences hepatic protein synthesis is the tonicity of the cellular environment. Administration of hypertonic solutions such as hypertonic NaCl to animals rapidly diminishes hepatic protein synthesis, whereas the administration of hypotonic solutions rapidly stimulates hepatic protein synthesis.[201–205] These responses have been correlated with alterations in cell volume; hyperosmotic cell shrinkage induces stimulation of catabolic pathways, whereas hypoosmotic cell swelling enhances anabolic pathways.[201,202] Cell volume regulation is fast (generally within minutes) but leaves cells with disturbed intracellular inorganic ion concentrations that are in most cases disadvantageous. The effects on hepatic protein synthesis of altered tonicity alone[203,205] or combined with the influence of L-tryptophan were studied. The inhibition of hepatic protein synthesis due to the administration of hypertonic salt could be negated or reversed by the administration of L-tryptophan together with the hypertonic NaCl.[168]

Subsequent studies[188] reported that the administration of L-tryptophan before (0.5 h) or after (0.5 h) hypertonic NaCl (1 h before kill off) improved hepatic polyribosomal aggregation and protein synthesis compared to controls receiving hypertonic NaCl alone.

In another study, Sidransky et al.[167] were concerned with the effects of NaCl administered *in vivo* or added *in vitro* to isolated nuclei on [³H]tryptophan binding to rat hepatic nuclei assayed *in vitro*. Hypertonic (10.7%) NaCl administered *in vivo* to rats caused at 10 min a marked decrease in *in vitro* binding (total and specific) of [³H]tryptophan to hepatic nuclei. *In vitro* incubation of isolated hepatic nuclei but not of isolated nuclear envelopes with added NaCl (particularly at 0.125×10^{-4} M and 0.25×10^{-4} M) revealed significant inhibition of [³H]tryptophan binding. However, isolated hepatic nuclear envelopes prepared after *in vitro* incubation of isolated nuclei with added NaCl did show inhibition of [³H]tryptophan binding (total and specific) compared with controls. Other salts (KCl, $MgCl_2$, $NaHCO_3$, $NaC_2H_3O_2$, NaF, or Na_2SO_4) at similar concentrations to those of NaCl, except for $MgCl_2$, when added to isolated nuclei did not appreciably inhibit nuclear tryptophan binding. Kinetic studies of *in vitro* nuclear [³H]tryptophan binding in the presence of 0.125×10^{-4} M NaCl revealed that binding decreased at 0.5 h and continued to 2 h compared with nuclear [³H]tryptophan binding with controls (without NaCl addition). The results obtained *in vivo* in rats and those obtained *in vitro* with isolated hepatic nuclei revealed NaCl-induced inhibitory effects on [³H]tryptophan binding to hepatic nuclei. Although the inhibitory effects were similar under the two different experimental conditions, the mechanism for each may be different in that the NaCl concentration in hepatic cells after administration of NaCl *in vivo* was appreciably higher than the low levels added *in vitro* to the isolated hepatic nuclei.

6.6.1.7   α-Amanitin

α-Amanitin, an inhibitor of RNA polymerase II activity[206] and of poly(A) mRNA synthesis,[188] was investigated in experiments where rats were tube-fed L-tryptophan before (0.5 h) or after (0.5 h) administering α-amanitin (0.5 or 1 h before killing).[188] Under these conditions, L-tryptophan had a preventative and curative effect in regard to α-amanitin on hepatic polyribosomal aggregation and protein synthesis.

6.6.1.8   Sparsomycin

Sparsomycin, a sulfur-containing antibiotic, inhibits protein synthesis in mammalian and bacterial cells. Tryptophan administration before or after sparsomycin did not affect the hepatic polyribosomal disaggregation or the decreased protein synthesis due to sparsomycin.[188] A possible explanation for the lack of effect by tryptophan may be due to sparsomycin's ability to cause fall-off ribosomes, which are defective as indicated by the decreased formation of polyphenylalanine when assayed *in vitro* with poly(U).[207]

6.6.1.9   Lead Acetate and Selected Metal Salts

Toxicity related to a number of metals has been reported. Metallic salts may affect a number of organs including liver and brain. It is of interest that a number of transition metals and their anions, such as lead, zinc, cadmium, arsenite, and selenite, have been demonstrated to affect nuclear binding of glucocorticoid.[208–211] Sidransky and Verney[212] investigated whether such salts would affect nuclear tryptophan binding. Lead salts and other salts of cadmium, zinc, mercury, and molybdenum, when added alone, had only small effects on ³H-tryptophan binding to rat hepatic nuclei *in vitro*. However, each of the salts, when added along with unlabeled L-tryptophan (excess 10^{-4} M), caused significantly less inhibition of ³H-tryptophan binding to hepatic nuclei than did unlabeled L-tryptophan alone. Rats receiving a high dose of lead acetate before being tube-fed L-tryptophan displayed a decrease in hepatic protein synthesis compared to the stimulating response connected with L-tryptophan alone.

The effects of lead acetate closely resemble those reported with L-leucine.[213] In each case, the compound itself does not appear to inhibit *in vitro* ^{3}H-tryptophan binding to hepatic nuclei. However, when each is added together with unlabeled L-tryptophan, it abrogates the inhibiting effect that the unlabeled L-tryptophan alone had on binding. This type of reaction pattern seems to be compatible with a response of an allosteric nature. Currently, no explanation for the effect of either compound is available.

6.6.1.10   Cordycepin

Cordycepin (3'-deoxyadenosine), an agent that suppresses polyadenylation with a marked reduction of mRNA in cytoplasmic polyribosomes, was investigated with L-tryptophan. Administration of L-tryptophan to fasted rats (1 h before kill) pretreated (2 h) with cordycepin induced a shift in hepatic polyribosomes toward heavier aggregation and an increase in *in vitro* protein synthesis.[120] Also, treatment with L-tryptophan (2.5 h before killing) and cordycepin 0.5 h later enhanced hepatic polyribosomal aggregation and protein synthesis.[188] Thus, L-tryptophan acted in a preventative and curative manner.

6.6.1.11   NaF

NaF is an inhibitor of glycolysis and negatively affects the adenylate cyclase system. Pretreatment (0.5 h) and posttreatment (1 h) with L-tryptophan before but not after NaF (1 to 2 h before kill) led to marked improvement of hepatic polyribosomal aggregation and protein synthesis.[188]

6.6.1.12   Ethanol

Ethanol has long been implicated in inducing toxic liver disease. Many studies have been concerned with ethanol's effect on hepatic protein synthesis.[94] Rothschild et al.[108] reported that the addition of L-tryptophan to isolated perfused livers of rabbits treated with ethanol aided in the recovery of albumin synthesis.

6.6.1.13   Choline Deficiency

Rats fed a choline-deficient diet rapidly develop a fatty liver. It was of interest to investigate whether rats fed such a choline-deficient diet would respond to treatment with L-tryptophan. Rats fed the control (choline-supplemented) diet but not the choline-deficient diet for 1 week and tube-fed L-tryptophan 10 min before being killed revealed enhanced labeled hepatic nuclear RNA release *in vitro*.[174] When rats were fed elevated L-tryptophan (2%) in the diets (choline-deficient (CD) or choline-supplemented (CS)) for 1 week, labeled hepatic nuclear RNA release was increased with the CS + tryptophan diet but not with the CS + tryptophan diet groups. ^{3}H-tryptophan binding to hepatic nuclei *in vitro* revealed no change in the CS + tryptophan group, decreased in the CD group, and markedly increased in the CD + tryptophan group in comparison with the control (CS) group. Hepatic nuclear nucleoside triphosphatase activity was increased only in the CS + tryptophan group, while hepatic nuclear poly(A)polymerase activity was increased in the CS + tryptophan and in the CD + tryptophan groups. The results are summarized in Table 6.1.

TABLE 6.1

Rats Fed *ad Libitum* A Choline-Deficient (CD) or A Choline-Supplemented (CS) Diet without or with Added (2%) L-tryptophan for 1 Week

	Groups			
Parameters	CS	CS + TRP	CD	CD + TRP
Liver				
Weight (fatty change)	N	N	+++	+++
Labeled nuclear RNA release	N	+	–	–
After tube-feeding TRP (10 min)	+++		N	
Nuclear NTPase activity	N	++	N	+
Nuclear poly(a)polymerase activity	N	+	+	++
^{3}H-TRP nuclear binding	N	N	–	+++
Cellular for TRP level	N	N	N	N
Nuclear for TRP level	N	N	++	++
Serum				
Free-TRP levels	N	N	N	N
Triglycerides	N	N	–	N
Cholesterol	N	N	–	N
HDL cholesterol	N	N	–	–

Note: Normal or baseline, N; decrease –; increase +.

Feeding a choline-deficient diet has been reported to induce structural and functional changes in cell membranes of microsomes,[214] of smooth endoplasmic reticulum,[215] and of mitochondria.[215] Hepatic nuclear changes have been described in choline-deficient diet-fed animals.[216] Also, hepatocyte receptors for epidermal growth factor[217] and for insulin[218] have been reported to be decreased in rats fed a choline-deficient diet. The findings of decreased liver nuclear L-tryptophan binding *in vitro* in choline-deficient diet-fed rats is consistent with nuclear membrane alterations. However, the increased hepatic nuclear L-tryptophan binding *in vitro* in the CD + tryptophan diet-fed rats is difficult to explain.

Overall, the altered responses of hepatic nuclei of rats fed a CD diet to tryptophan are difficult to explain. Nevertheless, several findings merit comments. The failure of the livers of rats fed the CD diet to show increases in [^{14}C]orotate-labeled nuclear RNA release in response to tryptophan (either tube-fed acutely or added to the diet) is consistent with the lack of increase in nuclear NTPase activity in the feeding experiments. This enzyme has been demonstrated to show increased activity in hepatic nuclei of normal animals exposed to tryptophan,[121,219,220] and this response is consistent with active nucleocytoplasmic translocations of RNA.[221] Nuclear poly(A)polymerase activity becomes enhanced in the livers of normal rats treated acutely with tryptophan[222] or fed elevated dietary tryptophan. Similar elevations occur in rats fed a CD diet that is further enhanced by elevated dietary tryptophan. Thus, it appears that enhanced polyadenylation occurs due to both conditions (elevated dietary tryptophan and CD diet). Hepatic nuclear free tryptophan levels are increased in rats fed the CD diet or the CD + tryptophan diet in comparison to controls (CS or CS + tryptophan groups). On the other hand, [^{3}H]tryptophan binding to hepatic nuclei *in vitro* is decreased in rats fed the CD diet but markedly increased in rats fed the CD + tryptophan diet. Whether the alterations in the free tryptophan levels in hepatic nuclei and in the nuclear binding capacities in the livers of rats fed the CD diet are possibly related is unclear. Also, the ability of the tryptophan in the CD + tryptophan diet to increase the serum triglyceride and cholesterol levels that are lowered by the CD diet suggests that tryptophan may overcome the disturbance in lipoprotein transport out of the liver into the serum.

6.6.1.14 Other Agents (Aflatoxin B₁, Dimethylnitrosamine, Galactosamine)

Sidransky et al.[188] expanded the information concerning tryptophan and its effects on other hepatotoxic agents, aflatoxin B_1, dimethylnitrosamine, and galactosamine in rats. In these experiments a curative effect was found due to tryptophan with aflatoxin B_1, dimethylnitrosamine, and galactosamine. Also, Kroger et al.[223] had reported that the administration of D-galactosamine-HCl induced alterations in livers of normal or adrenalectomized rats, histologically resembling hepatitis and that pretreatment with DL-tryptophan could prevent this effect.

6.6.1.15 Concluding Remarks

In some experiments concerned with the mechanism by which tryptophan acted to improve hepatic protein synthesis after toxic injury, the ability of tryptophan to stimulate hepatic mRNA synthesis, nucleocytoplasmic translocation of RNA *in vitro*, and nuclear envelope nucleoside triphosphatase activity after hepatotoxic injury was measured.[188] Nucleoside triphosphatase (Mg^{2+}-dependent adenosine triphosphatase, EC 3.6.1.3.1) was assayed since it is present in mammalian liver nuclear envelopes,[224] and there is evidence that this enzyme is involved in nucleocytoplasmic translocation of RNA.[221] All of these parameters were elevated significantly by tryptophan after agents such as actinomycin D, cordycepin, ethionine, puromycin, and hypertonic NaCl demonstrated a curative effect by tryptophan, but not after tryptophan following CCl_4, NaF, and sparsomycin demonstrated no improvement with tryptophan. These findings emphasized the importance of the role that tryptophan plays in stimulating the availability of cytoplasmic mRNA, and this effect occurred even after liver injury by certain toxic agents. On the other hand, it is unclear why after CCl_4, NaF, or sparsomycin this effect on hepatic mRNA, as well as on hepatic polyribosomes and protein synthesis, was absent.

In attempting to determine why tryptophan acted only in a preventative manner but not in a curative manner with CCl_4 and NaF, the data merited review. With CCl_4, tryptophan administration after CCl_4 treatment did not improve hepatic polyribosomal aggregation but did improve somewhat *in vitro* hepatic protein synthesis. It is probable that some aspects of the curative effect of tryptophan after CCl_4 treatment were still operative while others were not. In this case, the ribosomes injured by CCl_4 may not have become recycled, as suggested by Farber et al.,[185] based upon studies with cyclohex-imide. Nonetheless, the increased stimulation by tryptophan of new rRNA (as reported by Oravec and Korner[225] using fasted animals receiving tryp-tophan) may still be sufficient to allow for a small increase in *in vitro* hepatic protein synthesis with only a minimal change in the polyribosomal pattern. With NaF, tryptophan administration before NaF (30 min) may have caused enough stimulation of hepatic polyribosomes and protein synthesis so that the subsequent (30 min) effect of the NaF was proportionally reduced such that the end result after 60 min was one of improvement. The results after simultaneous administration of NaF and tryptophan revealed complete inhi-bition of the tryptophan effect on hepatic polyribosomes and protein syn-thesis *in vitro*, similar to that found in the curative study.

Many hepatotoxic agents, with different mechanisms of action, have been investigated in regard to whether L-tryptophan can improve the state of hepatic protein synthesis in the animals that had been treated with each toxic agent before or after L-tryptophan. The results are summarized in Table 6.2. With only a rare exception, sparsomycin, L-tryptophan administered orally seems to improve hepatic protein synthesis. This is consistent with L-tryp-tophan's action in stimulating hepatic protein synthesis in normal (fasted or fed) animals.[152,226] In studies with selected hepatotoxic agents, L-tryptophan's ability to act in a beneficial manner toward hepatic protein synthesis in the toxic agent-induced liver injury, parameters such as hepatic polyribosomal aggregation, *in vitro* nuclear RNA efflux, and nuclear nucleoside triphos-phatase activity were also studied. In general, these limited experiments indicated that hepatic metabolic changes due to L-tryptophan were similar to those described in normal animals receiving L-tryptophan.

Thus, overall, one may speculate that livers with injury due to many toxic agents are generally still capable of responding to L-tryptophan. This raises the possibility that L-tryptophan may become a therapeutic agent under certain acute pathologic states.

6.6.2   Chronic Toxic Liver Injury

The effects of the administration of tryptophan on toxic cirrhosis induced by intermittent carbon tetrachloride (CCl_4) intoxication in the rat were

TABLE 6.2

Effect of L-Tryptophan before or after Treatment with Hepatotoxic Compounds or Drugs on Hepatic Protein Synthesis (Status of Polyribosomes and *in Vitro* Protein Synthesis)

	Effect of L-Tryptophan	
Test Compound	Before (Preventive)	After (Curative)
Hepatotoxic Agents		
Actinomycin D	0	+
α-Amanitin	+	+
CCl$_4$	+	0
Cordycepin	+	+
Ethanol		+
Ethionine	0	+
Lead Acetate		+
Puromycin	+	+
Hypertonic NaCl	+	+
NaF	+	0
Sparsomycin	0	0

investigated.[227] Rats received CCl$_4$ (0.45 ml per 100 g body weight intraperitoneally) twice weekly for 10 to 14 weeks. Tryptophan (30 mg per 100 g body weight) by stomach tube was administered 1 h before killing. Tryptophan improved hepatic polyribosomal aggregation and [^{14}C]leucine incorporation into protein *in vitro* of control rats as well as long-term CCl$_4$-treated rats that had developed toxic cirrhosis. However, the effects were more marked in control than in experimental rats. Tryptophan administration induced an increase in labeled nuclear RNA release *in vitro* and a decrease in labeled tryptophan binding to nuclear protein *in vitro* of livers of rats receiving long-term CCl$_4$ and of control rats. The results indicate that the stimulatory effects of a single administration of tryptophan in toxic cirrhotic livers are similar to but somewhat less than those that occur in livers of normal, control rats.

Ohta et al.[228] studied whether L-tryptophan would alleviate CCl$_4$-induced chronic liver injury and related dysfunction in rats. Rats received a daily intraperitoneal injection of L-tryptophan (50 mg/kg) for 2 weeks after 6 weeks of subcutaneous injections of CCl$_4$ (1 mg/kg) twice weekly. In the rats treated with CCl$_4$ alone, the concentration of serum albumin and liver protein and the activity of liver protein synthesis *in vitro* decreased. The rats that also received L-tryptophan revealed that L-tryptophan alleviated these changes. They speculated that the latter finding alleviated the liver injury changes.

Aspects of tryptophan and chronic toxic liver injury are covered in the next section about tryptophan and cancer.

6.6.3   Tryptophan and Drug Effects

6.6.3.1   Demoxepam

Demoxepam, the N-desalkylated compound of chlordiazepoxide, has been reported to have an inhibiting effect on *in vitro* ^{3}H-binding to rat hepatic nuclei and had an apparent $K_D \sim 22$ μM.[229] Based upon the above results, it became of interest to consider whether L-tryptophan would also influence binding to the benzodiazepine receptors. Specific receptors for benzodiazepines have been demonstrated on neurons in the CNS of all higher vertebrates.[230] The benzodiazepine receptor possesses a high specificity for benzodiazepines and related agents. L-tryptophan has been reported as an ineffective agent on benzodiazepine recognition sites. L-tryptophan at 1900 μM gave 50% inhibition of specific binding.[231] This contrasts to the 60 μM level of demoxepam, which gave 50% inhibition of specific tryptophan binding.

6.6.3.2   Other Benzodiazepines

Other benzodiazepines, chlordiazepoxide, diazepam, prazepam, flurazepam, nordazepam, N-desalkylflurazepam, temazepam, oxazepam, lorazepam, or 4-chlorodiazepam had little influence on the L-(5-^{3}H) tryptophan binding to hepatic nuclei when added *in vitro*.[232] Only the addition of demoxepam, the N-desalkylated compound of chlordiazepoxide, caused marked competition with ^{3}H-tryptophan binding to hepatic nuclei *in vitro*. When chlordiazepoxide (1 mg per 100 g body weight) was administered intraperitoneally 20 min before killing, the isolated hepatic nuclei revealed decreased specific L-tryptophan binding compared to controls. Also, rats pretreated with chlordiazepoxide intraperitoneally before tube-feeding L-tryptophan revealed diminished tryptophan-induced hepatic nuclear RNA efflux and protein synthesis. The results suggested that chlordiazepoxide, possibly by itself or through a metabolite, can act to affect hepatic nuclear binding of L-tryptophan and to inhibit the stimulatory effect of L-tryptophan on hepatic protein synthesis.

6.6.3.3   Metyrapone

Metyrapone (2-methyl-1,2-di-3-pyridyl-1-propanone), an inhibitor of endogenous adrenal corticosteroid synthesis via inhibition of cytochrome P-450-mediated steroid hydroxylation, was evaluated for its influence on the binding of L-tryptophan to rat hepatic nuclei or nuclear envelopes.[233] The results indicated that the addition of metyrapone *in vitro* had little influence on L-(5-^{3}H)tryptophan binding to hepatic nuclei or nuclear envelopes. On the other hand, when metyrapone (1 mg per 100 g body weight) was tube-fed 30 min before killing, the isolated hepatic nuclei show decreased specific L-tryptophan binding (total binding minus nonspecific binding (using 2,000-fold excess of unlabeled L-tryptophan)) compared with controls. Also, addition of metyrapone *in vitro* to rat liver before homogenization and preparation of nuclei caused the nuclei to show decreased specific tryptophan binding compared with controls. Under these *in vitro* conditions, SKF 525A, another inhibitor of hydroxylation, showed inhibitory effects similar to those of metyrapone. Thus, metyrapone interfered with rat liver nuclear envelope receptor binding to L-tryptophan, and possibly acted via its effects on hydroxylation. At high doses, metyrapone (20 mg per 100 g body weight) appeared to inhibit tryptophan-induced stimulation of hepatic protein synthesis.

6.6.3.4 Valproic Acid

Valproic acid, a branched-chain fatty acid, which has been used in the treatment of seizures and which under certain conditions is hepatotoxic, was studied for its influence on the binding of L-tryptophan to rat hepatic nuclei.[234] The results indicated that the addition of valproic acid to hepatic nuclei or nuclear envelopes *in vitro* had little influence on their L-(5-³H)tryptophan binding. On the other hand, when valproic acid (80 mg per 100 g body weight) was tube-fed 2 h before killing, the isolated nuclei show decreased specific L-tryptophan binding (total binding minus nonspecific binding using unlabeled L-tryptophan (10^{-4} M), at 200-fold excess) compared with controls. Other fatty acids (oleic, palmitic, or linoleic acid at 10^{-4} M) when added with excess, unlabeled L-tryptophan (10^{-4} M) *in vitro* to hepatic nuclei revealed some decreased specific binding (but less than with valproic acid) compared with controls. At high doses, valproic acid (80 mg per 100 g body weight) appeared to decrease tryptophan-induced stimulation of hepatic protein synthesis, probably in a hepatotoxic manner.

Of interest is the ability of valproic acid to bind to albumin-binding sites[235] similar to the albumin binding of L-tryptophan[236] and of free fatty acids to displace the drug from binding sites in plasma proteins.[237] Also, the metabolism of valproic acid occurs primarily in the liver.[238] Currently, more than ten different metabolites have been identified and classified according to their routes of metabolism. The metabolic pathways identified include conjugation with glucuronic acid, β-oxidation, and W-1/W-2 oxidation via the cytochrome P-450 system.[239] Fisher et al.[240] reported that valproic acid or metabolites (2-en-valproic acid and 4-en-valproic acid, 300 mg/ml) inhibited hepatic protein synthesis of rat and human liver slices and, therefore, considered these levels as hepatotoxic. Also, they described that the co-administration of an antiepileptic drug, such as phenytoin and phenobarbital which themselves induced cytochrome P-450 enzymes, and of valproic acid have been linked to the formation of the more pronounced hepatotoxic metabolite 4-en-valproic acid.[241] In earlier studies,[219,242,243] it was reported that L-tryptophan enhanced hepatic cytochrome P-450 activity. Thus, it is possible that the combination of valproic acid and tryptophan *in vivo* led to the enhanced formation of the hepatotoxic metabolite 4-en-valproic acid, which adversely affected the hepatic protein synthesis mechanism and, therefore, accounted for less enhancement in hepatic protein synthesis due to L-tryptophan than when L-tryptophan was administered alone.

6.6.4   Concluding Remarks

In the previous sections, a number of chemicals that cause acute toxic liver injury have been reviewed in relation to their biochemical actions with or without tryptophan administration. It is of special interest that tryptophan was able to improve hepatic protein metabolism when administered before, simultaneously, or after administering the toxic compound (Table 6.2). Like-wise, the effects of tryptophan on altered liver function due to the acute administration of selected drugs are reviewed. Overall, the experimental findings demonstrate that many of the regulatory effects of tryptophan on hepatic protein metabolism can occur even during acute liver injury. This raises many questions as to whether L-tryptophan may possibly have therapeutic applications under certain states of liver injury. Further experimental studies should establish whether this consideration is valid or not.

6.7   Cancer

6.7.1   Introduction

Relationships between nutrition and cancer have been of concern for many years and continue to be of great interest. A number of nutrients have been thought to play a role in the induction of certain tumors. On the basis of animal experimentation, L-tryptophan has been implicated dating back to 1950.[244] Since that time, a number of important developments have occurred that serve to highlight how L-tryptophan may be related to carcinogenesis. In 1977, it was first reported that the pyrolysis of tryptophan leads to highly mutagenic and carcinogenic compounds.[245] In 1978, it was reported that some indole-containing compounds (of which L-tryptophan may be a precursor) can act under certain circumstances to inhibit chemical carcinogenesis in animals;[246] the action of such compounds was attributed mainly to their ability to increase the activity of the microsomal mixed-function oxidase system, leading to inactivation of the carcinogen. The possible significance of these important developments in relation to L-tryptophan and carcinogenesis merits consideration.

6.7.2   Experimental Studies on Tryptophan and Carcinogenesis

Attention was initially focused on the possible relationship between the ingestion of L-tryptophan and the development of tumors of the bladder. Thus, it may be appropriate to focus attention first on the experimental findings relating to L-tryptophan and the bladder. Subsequently, interest has extended to L-tryptophan and tumorigenesis in the liver and on other organs.

6.7.2.1 Bladder

6.7.2.1.1 Tryptophan and Tumorigenesis

Table 6.3 summarizes the experimental studies dealing with tryptophan and bladder tumors in experimental animals (rats, mice, and dogs). In 1950, Dunning and co-workers[244] reported that Fischer female rats fed a purified diet supplemented with 1.4 or 4.3% DL-tryptophan and 0.06% 2-acetylaminofluorene, a potent carcinogen, exhibited a high incidence of bladder carcinomas; however, carcinomas did not develop when 2-acetylaminofluorene was administered without tryptophan. In 1954, Boyland and colleagues[247] confirmed these findings, reporting that 2% DL-tryptophan plus 0.045% 2-acetylaminofluorene induced bladder cancers in Wistar female rats, but bladder tumors did not develop when DL-tryptophan plus 0.067% 2-naphthylamine or 0.017% benzidine were used.

Based upon the report by Dunning and co-workers[244] and also on the knowledge that several primary aromatic amino metabolites, structurally similar to known environmental human bladder carcinogens, are derived from tryptophan and are present in human urine,[248] it was then hypothesized that bladder cancer may result from metabolic alterations manifested by increased urinary concentrations of certain tryptophan metabolites.[249] From 1966 to 1969, investigators directed their attention to assaying urinary tryptophan metabolite excretion patterns of patients with bladder cancer[249] and also to inducting bladder tumors in experimental animals by the administration of tryptophan or its metabolites.

In 1971, Radomski and colleagues[250] fed female beagle dogs a dog meal supplemented with DL-tryptophan (6 g/d) for 0.3 to 7 years and reported marked focal hyperplasia of the transitional cell epithelium of the bladder but no evidence of cancer. In 1973, Miyakawa and Yoshida[251] fed Wistar male rats a pyridoxine-deficient diet containing 1.4% DL-tryptophan for 56 weeks and found no bladder tumors or hyperplasia, but autoradiograms of the bladder revealed increased labeling of [³H]thymidine in bladder epithelia in comparison to controls fed a regular pellet diet. Subsequently, in 1977, Radomski and colleagues[252] reported that one of four female beagle dogs administered a single dose of 4-aminobiphenyl (50 mg/kg) and then fed the diet described earlier[250] for 4.5 years developed bladder tumors, although no tumors occurred in six dogs given 4-aminobiphenyl without supplemental DL-tryptophan in the diet. Using the same tryptophan-supplemented diet for 3 years after the administration of 2-naphthylamine (5 mg/kg/d) for 30 days, the authors noted bladder tumors in two of four dogs, although no tumors occurred in four dogs given 2-naphthylamine alone. Because dogs fed DL-tryptophan alone developed focal hyperplasia of the bladder epithelium, the authors considered that DL-tryptophan might be a co-carcinogen or promoter in the induction of bladder cancer.

TABLE 6.3

Experiments with Tryptophan and Induction of Bladder Tumors

Animals Studied			Experimental Conditions		
Species	Strain	Sex	Treatment[a]	Duration, Yrs	Bladder Tumor Incidence[b]
Dogs	Beagle	F	DL-Trp (6 g/d)	0.25–7	Hyperplasia 7/8 (88%)
Dogs	Beagle	F	4-Aminobiphenyl (50 mg/kg; 1×) + DL-Trp (6 g/d)	4.5	1/4 (25%)
			2-Naphthylamine (5 mg/kg; 30×) + DL-Trp (6 g/d)	3	2/4 (50%)
					Controls (0%)
Rats	Fischer	F	2-AAF (0.06%) + DL-Trp (1.4 or 4.3%)	1	11/11 (100%)
					11/12 (92%)
Rats	Wistar	F	2-AAF (0.045%) + DL-Trp (2%)	0.33–2	8/10 (80%)
					Controls 1/10 (10%)
Rats	Wistar	M	B-6-deficient diet + DL-Trp (1.4%)	1	↑[³H]thymidine labeling of epithelium
Rats	Fischer	M	FANFT (0.2%; 6 wks) + DL-Trp (2%)	2	10/19 (53%)
			Chow diet (6 wks between 2)		10/20 (50%)
					Controls (0–20%)
Rats	Fischer	M	FANFT (0.2%; 4 wks) + L-Trp (2%)	2	5/26 (19%)
					Controls (0–4%)
Rats	Fischer	M	FANFT (0.02%; 4 wks) + L-Trp (2%)	1.5	22/38 (29%)
			+ B-6-deficient diet		10/36 (28%)
			+ B-6-adequate diet alone		Controls 16/40 (40%)
			+ B-6-deficient diet alone		Controls 5/39 (13%)
Rats	Fischer	M	BBN (0.05%; 4 wks) + saccharin (5%) + DL-Trp (2%) + ascorbate (5%) (each 10 wks sequentially)	0.7	7/25 (28%)
			+ saccharin (5%) + DL-Trp (2%)		2/24 (8%)
			+ saccharin (5%)		2/25 (8%)
					Controls 0/25 (0%)
Mice	D-D	F	FANFT (0.1%; 4 wks) + L-Trp (0.2%)	1.2	2/30 (7%)
					Controls (0%)

[a] Abbreviations are as follows: 2-AAF, 2-acetylaminofluorene; Trp, tryptophan; FANFT, N-[4-(5-nitro-2-furyl)-2-thiazolyl]formamide; BBN, N-butyl-N-(4-hydroxybutyl)nitrosamine.

[b] Ratio of animals with tumors to animals in experimental group.

From 1977 to 1987, studies were concerned with two stages in the process of bladder carcinogenesis using N-[4-(5-nitro-2-furyl)-2-thiazolyl]formamide (FANFT). Matsushima[253] fed female mice (D-D strain) a diet containing 0.1% FANFT for 4 weeks and then divided the mice into two groups and fed for 56 weeks: one was placed on the basal diet with an additional 0.2% L-tryptophan and the other received the basal diet alone. In the first group, 2 of 30 mice developed bladder tumors; no tumors developed in the second group. Epithelial hyperplasia and labeling index were evaluated in both groups and revealed a significant increase in the bladders of the first group compared with the second group. Cohen and associates[254] fed Fischer male rats a chow diet containing 0.2% FANFT for 6 weeks and then switched to the chow diet containing 2% DL-tryptophan for 98 weeks; 10 of 19 rats developed bladder tumors. In another experiment, the FANFT chow diet was fed for 6 weeks, followed by the chow diet alone for 6 weeks, and then the high DL-tryptophan diet was fed for 92 weeks; 10 of 20 rats developed bladder tumors. Fukushima and others[255] fed Fischer male weanling rats a chow diet containing 0.2% FANFT for 4 weeks and then the chow diet alone containing 2% L-tryptophan for 100 weeks; 5 of 26 rats had bladder tumors and 7 had epithelial hyperplasia. Among the 25 rats fed the FANFT diet for 4 weeks followed by the chow diet alone for 100 weeks, 1 had a papilloma and 2 had hyperplasia. Birt and co-workers[256] fed Fischer male rats a semipurified diet containing 0.2% FANFT for 4 weeks and then the semipurified diet alone or altered (supplemented and/or deficient) for 80 weeks as follows: (1) control (basal semipurified diet), (2) 2% L-tryptophan, (3) vitamin B-6 deficient, or (4) 2% L-tryptophan plus vitamin B-6 deficient. Bladder tumors developed in rats of each group as follows: (1) 16 of 40 (40%), (2) 11 of 38 (29%), (3) 5 of 39 (13%), and (4) 10 of 36 (28%). Their findings suggested that L-tryptophan promoted tumor formation only when vitamin B-6 intake was deficient but not when vitamin B-6 intake was adequate.

Sakata and colleagues,[257] using N-butyl-N-(4-hydroxybutyl)nitrosamine (BBN) as an initiating agent, reported that 4 weeks of BBN (0.05%) treatment of Fischer male rats followed by sequential administration of promoting agents, 5% sodium saccharin, 2% DL-tryptophan, and 5% sodium L-ascorbate in the diet, each for 10 weeks, induced a higher incidence of bladder tumors than that observed after using saccharin alone or saccharin followed by DL-tryptophan. Thus, certain combinations of promoters, including DL-tryptophan, appear to be capable of working in an additive fashion.

6.7.2.1.2 *Tryptophan Metabolites or Related Compounds and Tumorigenesis*

In similar studies to those reported earlier,[244] Dunning and Curtis[258] reported that indole or indoleacetic acid could be substituted for tryptophan, without significantly lowering the incidence of bladder carcinoma. Adding indole[259] or tryptophan[247] to the purified diets containing 2-acetylaminofluorene prolonged the lives of the rats, modified liver injury, and increased the incidence of bladder tumors. After treatment with 2-acetylaminofluorene plus indole, neonatal rats were more susceptible than weanling or postweanling rats to bladder cancer.[260]

Since urinary bladder tumor induction in experimental animals by tryptophan or tryptophan metabolites alone, administered orally or subcutaneously, was generally unsuccessful, direct application of the test agent to the urinary bladder was investigated. A small pellet containing the test compound was suspended in a suitable vehicle and then surgically implanted into the lumen of the mouse bladder. The urine bathed the pellet, thereby eluding the test chemical, which then came in contact with the bladder mucosa. This approach was utilized by several laboratories in evaluating the carcinogenicity of test compounds.[249,261,262] Bryan[263] summarized their findings as follows: of 15 compounds adequately tested, 9 (L-kynurenine, acetyl-L-kynurenine, 3-hydroxy-L-kynurenine, 3-hydroxyanthranilic acid, 3-ethoxyanthranilic acid, 8-methyl ether of xanthurenic acid, xanthurenic acid, 8-hydroxyquinaldic acid, and quinaldic acid) were active and 6 (indican, 0-aminohippuric acid, anthranilic acid, 4,8-quinolinediol, kynurenic acid, and L-tryptophan) were inactive. The active compounds have been investigated in a number of studies.[249,263] Some, 3-hydroxykynurenine and 3-hydroxyanthranilic acid, have been demonstrated to be mutagenic for mammalian cells. The major role of urine, including pH and urinary tract calculi, in bladder carcinogenesis has been stressed as being a direct as well as an indirect influence.[264]

6.7.2.1.3   Tryptophan Pyrolysis Compounds and Bladder Tumors

In 1977, Sugimura and associates[245] reported that the charred material on the surface of broiled fish and meat contained a product that was highly mutagenic. This product was subsequently found to be the result of the pyrolysis of DL-tryptophan, which yields the pyrolysis products Trp-P-1 [3-amino-1,4-dimethyl-5*H*-pyrido-(4,3-b)indole and Trp-P-2 [3-amino-1-methyl-5*H*-pyrido(4,3-b)indole]. Although mutagenic compounds have been isolated from pyrolysates of other amino acids, glutamic acid, phenylalanine, and lysine, the pyrolysis products of tryptophan were found to be the most mutagenic of the other amino acid pyrolysates.[265]

Using the implantation technique described previously, Hashida and others[266] reported a high incidence of transitional cell carcinomas in the bladders of female mice with inserted pellets containing crude tryptophan pyrolysate (47.8%), Trp-P-1 (22.7%), or Trp-P-2 (3.7%) and controls (2.7%) for 40 weeks. Because the crude tryptophan pyrolysate as well as Trp-P-1 and Trp-P-2 were potent mutagens (which required metabolic activation by liver microsomes) to *Salmonella typhimurium* TA98 and TA100 in the Ames test,[245,267] Hashida and others[266] concluded that Trp-P-1 and Trp-P-2 from the implanted pellets were released and then absorbed by the bladder epithelium, where they were metabolized to carcinogenic metabolites by the epithelial cells. De Waziers and Decloitre[268] demonstrated that mutagenic derivatives of these compounds could be formed by rat intestinal enzymes (S9 fraction). Also, Mita and colleagues[269] reported that Trp-P-2 was metabolized by the same type of monooxygenase system in nuclei (nuclear membranes) as reported earlier in microsomes[270] of rat liver to the N-hydroxylated form of Trp-P-2 that was nonenzymatically bound to DNA.[271] This suggested that the conversion of Trp-P-2 to N-hydroxy-Trp-P-2 by monooxygenase systems was an obligatory step for the mutagenicity of Trp-P-2.

6.7.2.2   Liver

6.7.2.2.1   Tryptophan and Tumorigenesis

The early experimental studies (1950–1977) dealing with tryptophan and liver tumors in experimental animals (rats) are summarized in Table 6.4. In 1950, Dunning and co-workers[244] reported a high incidence of liver cancers in Fischer female rats fed for 1 year a purified diet containing 0.06% 2-acetylaminofluorene and 1.4 or 4.3% DL-tryptophan (73 and 75%, respectively) compared with the lower incidence (37%) in rats fed 2-acetylaminofluorene without added tryptophan. Also, using Wistar female rats, Boyland and colleagues[247] reported a higher incidence (36%) of liver cancers in rats fed an acid-hydrolyzed casein diet containing 0.07% β-naphthylamine plus 2% DL-tryptophan than in rats fed the carcinogen-containing diet without added tryptophan (11%). Subsequently, Kawachi and associates[272] demonstrated that Wistar male rats fed a laboratory meal diet containing 1% L-tryptophan and receiving water containing diethylnitrosamine (DEN, 20 mg/l) for 6.5 months developed a greater incidence (62%) of liver tumors than rats that did not receive the added tryptophan (17%).

On the other hand, Okajima and co-workers[273] reported that Wistar male rats receiving N-nitrosodibutylamine (0.05%) in their drinking water and fed a purified basal diet containing 1.4% DL-tryptophan developed no (0 of 12) liver tumors after 7 months, but the control rats receiving the carcinogen with the basal diet without added tryptophan had liver tumors (4 of 12, 33%). Also, in contrast to the findings by Kawachi and associates,[272] Evarts and Brown[274] demonstrated that Wistar male rats fed a commercial laboratory diet supplemented with 1% L-tryptophan and receiving DEN (0.002% wt/vol) in the drinking water for 5.5 months developed fewer liver tumors (59%) than rats not receiving the tryptophan-supplemented diet (88%). The discrepancy between the results of Kawachi and associates and those of Evarts and Brown has not been explained. Possibly it may be attributed to differences in the commercial laboratory diets used, because the liver tumor incidences in the control rats differed in the two studies, from 17% after 6.5 months in the study by Kawachi and associates to 88% after 5.5 months in the study by Evarts and Brown. Also, Evarts and Brown found that Wistar male rats fed a commercial laboratory diet supplemented with 0.05% 3′-methyl-4-N-dimethyl-aminoazobenzeone and 1.0% L-tryptophan for 5.5 months developed fewer liver tumors (40%) than those fed the carcinogen-containing diet without added tryptophan (83%).

Sidransky et al.[275] investigated whether the ingestion of an elevated level of L-tryptophan (2%) in a purified diet would influence the induction of γ-glutamyltranspeptidase(GGT)-positive foci in livers of rats exposed to the

TABLE 6.4

Experiments with Tryptophan and Liver Carcinogenesis

Animals Studied		Experimental Conditions		
Strain of Rats	Sex	Treatment[a]	Duration (Years)	Liver Tumor Incidence[b]
Fischer	F	2-AAF (0.06%) + DL-Trp (1.4 or 4.3%)	1	1.4% 8/11 (73%)
				4.3% 9/12 (75%)
				Controls 6/16 (37%)
Wistar	F	β-Naphthylamine (0.067%) + DL-Trp (2%)	1.3–3.5	4/11 (36%)
				Controls 1/9 (11%)
Wistar	M	DEN (0.002% in water; 140 d) + L-Trp (1%)	0.5	15/21 (62%)
				Controls 4/23 (17%)
Wistar	M	DBN (0.05% in water) + DL-Trp (1.4%)	0.6	0/12 (0%)
				Controls 4/12 (33%)
Wistar	M	DEN (0.02% in water; 128 d) + L-Trp (1%)	0.6	17/29 (59%)
				Controls 22/25 (88%)
Wistar	M	3′-Me-DAB (0.05%; 96 d) + L-Trp (1%)	0.6	12/30 (40%)
				Controls 24/29 (83%)
Sprague-Dawley	M	DEN (30 mg/kg) x 1 after partial hepatectomy L-Trp (2%) + CS or + CD diet	0.2	GGT + foci (% liver)[c]
				CS 0.06
				CS + Trp 0.24
				CD 0.42
				CD + Trp 0.28

[a] Abbreviations are as follows: 2-AAF, 2-acetylaminofluorene; DEN, dimethylnitrosamine; DBN, dibutylnitrosamine; CD, choline-deficient diet; CS, choline-supplemented diet; GGT, γ-glutamyltranspetidase; 3′-Me-DAB, 3′-dimethy-lamino-azobenzene.

[b] Ratio of animals with tumors over animals in experimental or control group. Percentage in parenthesis.

[c] Presence of GGT + foci as percent of total livers (means) of test groups.

hepatocarcinogen DEN. The enzyme-altered foci that develop in the livers of rats treated with a hepatocarcinogen are considered to be precursor lesions to neoplastic nodules and hepatomas.[276] Using the model established by others,[276,277] Sprague-Dawley male rats were subjected to subtotal hepatectomy, and, after 18 h, were injected intraperitoneally with DEN (30 mg/kg). Ten days later, groups of rats were placed on one of four diets: (1) control (CS) diet,[276] (2) CS + tryptophan diet, (3) choline-deficient (CD) diet, and (4) CD + tryptophan diet. Rats were then followed for 10 weeks. Rats fed the CS + tryptophan diet or the CD diet developed more and larger GGT-positive foci than rats fed the CS diet. Rats fed the CD + tryptophan diet revealed changes similar to those in rats fed the CD diet (Table 6.4). The findings based upon the induction of GGT-positive foci in livers of rats exposed to DEN suggested that increased dietary tryptophan had a promoting effect on liver carcinogenesis. A potentiating effect of tryptophan on the livers of rats fed the CD + tryptophan diet over that on the livers of rats fed the CD diet was not observed, probably because the CD diet itself had a marked promoting effect. In further studies, the levels of dietary fat[278] or dietary protein[279] in the above diets were not observed to influence or vary the increased induction of GGT-positive foci in livers of rats exposed to DEN and dietary tryptophan.

6.7.2.2.2 *Tryptophan Pyrolysis Compounds and Tumorigenesis*

Matsukura and associates[280] examined the carcinogenicity of crude pyrolysis products of tryptophan (the basic fraction of tryptophan pyrolysate) using Wistar rats of both sexes. They observed neoplastic liver nodules in 2 of 22 males and 5 of 18 females fed the basal diet containing 0.2% tryptophan pyrolysate. Also, they reported that mice fed a pellet diet containing the purified mutagens from tryptophan pyrolysis, Trp-P-1 and Trp-P-2 (0.02%), for up to 621 days developed hepatocellular carcinomas.[281] The incidence for Trp-P-1 was 21% for males and 62% for females; for Trp-P-2, the incidence was 16% for males and 92% for females. Subsequently, Hosaka and others[282] reported that ACI rats fed a diet containing 0.01% Trp-P-2 developed neoplastic nodules of the liver in 6 of 9 female rats, but no tumors developed in 10 males or in 60 controls fed for 666 to 870 days. Thus, Trp-P-1 and Trp-P-2 have been demonstrated to induce cancers in the liver as well as in the urinary bladder.[266] Ishikawa and associates[283] reported that Trp-P-1 induced fibrosarcomas locally when injected subcutaneously into rats and hamsters.

Several groups of investigators have described the induction of enzyme-altered foci in the livers of rats fed diets containing tryptophan pyrolysis products. Ishikawa and associates[284] reported that Sprague-Dawley male weanling rats injected with Trp-P-1 alone or together with phenobarbital compared with controls developed an increased incidence of adenosintriphosphatase-deficient foci in the livers after 18 weeks. Also, Tamano and co-workers[285] found that Trp-P-1 administered at the initiation or the promotion stage significantly increased the induction of GGT-positive foci in the livers of Fischer male rats that had received partial hepatectomies or CCl_4 treatment to potentiate the effects.

In a long-term assay (about 500 d), an intake of 2 g of pyrolysates of tryptophan or arginine–tryptophan per kg of diet containing 12% of protein appeared to induce a sex-dependent decrease in the growth of rats. Pyrolysate withdrawal in accustomed rats (second and third generations) demonstrated an acquired inurement to these products. Indeed, their removal caused increased food consumption and growth.[286]

The level of these potential carcinogens in some broiled or roasted foods, such as broiled sardines, is about 10 ng/g. This amount is much lower than those used in the carcinogenicity assays. The long-term cumulative effect of the carboline intake may be of great concern. In some experimental studies, tryptophan itself appears to promote the formation of tumors.[287–289] Also, a tryptophan–riboflavin photoinduced adduct may have a role in the pathogenesis of hepatic dysfunction observed during parenteral nutrition.[290]

In view of the extremely high mutagenic activity of the heterocyclic amines derived from browning reactions toward both bacteria (Ames test) and mammalian cell lines, the question arises whether such short-term tests of genotoxicity are good predictors of carcinogenicity. According to some investigators,[291–293] this is indeed the case. The heterocyclic amines tested induce multiple tumors in rats and mice. Target organs include breast, colon, and pancreas, major sites of human cancer throughout the world. The heterocyclic amines derived from tryptophan induced liver cancer.

Sugimura[291] estimates that the average person consumes about 100 μg of heterocyclic amines per day. These compounds have extremely high mutagenic activities; the possibility exists that the effects in animals and humans could be cumulative, and the need is stressed to develop new approaches and strategies to prevent the formation of heterocyclic amines and other browning products during food processing.[291,292,294,295]

It is worth noting that a form of cytochrome P-450 responsible for activation of Trp-1 and Trp-2 *in vivo* to active carcinogens is inducible by dietary treatment of mice or rats with these compounds.[296] These workers reported that the amount of both native and inducible cytochrome P-450 is related to the species, sex, and organ differences in their carcinogenic susceptibility to the tryptophan derivatives.

6.7.2.3 Breast

6.7.2.3.1 Tryptophan and Tumorigenesis

Dunning and colleagues[244] reported that AXC female rats fed a purified diet containing 25% tryptophan-free casein hydrolysate plus 1.4% DL-tryptophan compared to those fed a 26% casein diet had an increase in the number (79 vs. 51) and percentage (100 vs. 75%) of induced mammary cancers, as well as a reduction in the average latent period (316 vs. 363 days). Tumors were induced by the implantation of cholesterol pellets containing 4 to 6 mg of diethylstilbestrol subcutaneously in the scapular region. However, rats fed the purified diet with 4.3% DL-tryptophan revealed the smallest number and percentage (60%) of mammary cancers with an increased average latent period (399 days). The consequent inanition and decrease in body weight were thought to account for the latter finding.

6.7.2.4 Tryptophan Alone and Tumorigenesis

In addition to the previously cited studies in which dogs were fed elevated levels of tryptophan alone for long durations and only bladder hyperplasia developed,[250,252] in long-term studies, large groups of rats and mice given elevated amounts of tryptophan without carcinogens in their diets for most of their lives were reported to have no increased incidence of cancer.[297]

6.7.2.5 Consideration of Mechanisms by which Tryptophan Acts as a Stimulatory or Inhibitory Agent in Chemical Carcinogenesis

In reviewing experimental studies dealing with L-tryptophan and carcinogenesis, it becomes apparent that L-tryptophan acts in most cases as a stimulatory agent in chemical carcinogenesis. However, in some cases, it appears to act in an inhibitory manner. In attempting to possibly explain each of the above actions of L-tryptophan, the following considerations should be reviewed.

6.7.2.5.1 Tryptophan as a Stimulatory Agent

In searching for an explanation for how the ingestion of L-tryptophan may be involved in the process of chemical carcinogenesis in experimental studies, several studies have concluded that L-tryptophan acts as a co-carcinogen or promoter.[250,252,275] Some of the following effects or actions of L-tryptophan may influence such processes in carcinogenesis.

Tryptophan's effects on enzymes — L-tryptophan administration has been demonstrated to elevate the activity of many enzyme systems.[101,220,222,298–301] The mechanisms by which tryptophan acts to affect hepatic enzyme levels are variable and have been reviewed.[219,220,301] In most studies, the effect of L-tryptophan on the overall enhancement of specific enzyme activity was measured. In some cases, it was shown to be due to a decrease in enzyme degradation [tryptophan dioxygenase[300,301]]. However, in other cases, it was shown that L-tryptophan stimulates hepatic protein synthesis (including enzyme protein synthesis) by acting to influence transcriptional, posttranscriptional, and translational controls.[220] Although some of the enzymes investigated play a role in detoxifying or deactivating chemical carcinogens, others activate them into ultimate carcinogens. Conceivably, in some cases the balance may become tilted toward greater levels of ultimate carcinogens that induce tumors.

Tryptophan's effect on cell proliferation and ornithine decarboxylase activity — The role of increased cell proliferation in the process of carcinogenesis has merited much attention.[302] However, whether the presence of cell proliferation by itself or by stimulation of cell proliferation in a quiescent tissue or organ with low mitotic activity is a risk factor for the process of cancer development has been questioned.[303] On the other hand, many have stressed the overall importance of cell proliferation during the process of carcinogenesis. Increased cell proliferation has been described in transitional cell epithelium of bladder of animals fed diets supplemented with tryptophan.[250–253] In liver, nodular hyperplasia is observed frequently in the course of hepatocarcinogenesis.[276] In one experimental study, elevated dietary tryptophan induced an increase in hyperplastic foci containing GGT-positive hepatocytes of DEN-pretreated rats.[275] In a study with adult rat hepatocyte cultures, it has been reported that the addition of L-tryptophan stimulates [³H]thymidine incorporation into DNA.[304] Conceptionally, this proliferative action by L-tryptophan in conjunction with exposure to carcinogen may be of great importance.

In proliferating tissues, ornithine decarboxylase (ODC) activity is markedly elevated.[305] Many investigators have attempted to correlate elevated ODC activity with the process of promotion in experimental skin[306,307] or bladder[308] carcinogenesis. L-tryptophan administration stimulated rat hepatic ODC activity.[309] ODC is the rate-controlling enzyme in the biosynthesis of polyamines, and its increased activity correlates with cell growth.[305–308,310] Also, increased ODC activity has been found in proliferating tissues,[305] in L1210 leukemia cells,[311] and in experimental hepatomas.[312] ODC activity is increased in the livers of rats treated with chemical carcinogens[310–312] or fed a choline-deficient diet.[313] Conceptionally, tryptophan's ability to stimulate hepatic ODC activity may be related to promotion in hepatocarcinogenesis.

6.7.2.5.2 Tryptophan as an Inhibitory Agent

Findings in some experimental studies concerned with increased dietary tryptophan and carcinogenesis related to chemical carcinogenesis indicated that tryptophan appeared to be protective[273,274] rather than stimulatory[244,247,272,275] in the induction of liver tumors. A rational explanation for the differences in the results is not apparent. However, in searching for a possible explanation, the following findings may be helpful. A number of indole-containing compounds present in the diet, such as indole-3-acetonitrile, indole-3-carbinol, and 3,3'-diindolylmethane, have been reported to increase the activity of the microsomal mixed-function oxidase system and thereby inhibit chemical carcinogenesis in animals.[246] Indole itself has been reported to have a suppressive effect on 2-acetylaminofluorene-induced hepatocarcinogenesis in animals.[259,314] Indole-3-carbinol, a naturally occurring component of cruciferous vegetables, has been shown to be an effective cancer chemopreventive agent in a number of animal models, and its proposed mechanism of action involves binding of indole-3-carbinol acid condensation products (formed in the stomach) to the aryl hydrocarbon (Ah) receptor, with resultant induction of phase I and phase II enzymes.[315] Indeed, bacteria in the gastrointestinal tract are capable of metabolizing tryptophan to compounds that are able to bind the Ah receptor.[316] L-tryptophan, an important indole-containing indispensable amino acid, has been reported to have a suppressive effect on dibutylnitrosomine-, DEN-, and 3'-methyl-4-*N*-dimethylamino-azobenzene-induced hepatocarcinogenesis.[273,274] L-tryptophan enhances the activities of many hepatic enzymes,[222,298–301,318] and examples can be cited. A diet containing 1% L-tryptophan or L-tryptophan administered alone significantly increased hepatic cytochrome P-450 concentrations[219,242] and also increased dimethylnitrosamine demethylase[318] and aniline hydroxylase activities[242] in rat livers. Such findings suggest that tryptophan may stimulate enzymes to inactivate certain chemical carcinogens, thereby negating their carcinogenic effects. Whether L-tryptophan itself may interact with the Ah receptor as a ligand has not been determined. Yet tryptophan metabolites and related compounds clearly do interact with the Ah receptor.

A number of reports have stressed the importance of antioxidants in protecting cells from free radical damage, the kind that can lead to an array of degenerative diseases, including cancer.[319,320] Therefore, it is appropriate to mention that a number of tryptophan metabolites have been reported to have antioxidant activities.[321] Under certain conditions, such effects may play a role in relation to tryptophan and its preventative effect in carcinogenesis.

6.7.2.6   Effects of Tryptophan upon Cancer Tissue

6.7.2.6.1   Liver Cancer

Although the end stage of carcinogenesis, the cancer itself, is probably not good material to search for clues about the pathogenesis of carcinogenesis, it has been used in many studies with the hope that it may offer leads regarding the process as well as possible clues for therapy. Experimental studies designed to determine whether the response of hepatocellular carcinoma to tryptophan administration would be similar to or different from that of host liver or normal liver have been conducted. Utilizing intrahepatically transplanted hepatomas (H5123 and 19) in Buffalo rats, the response to administration of L-tryptophan was determined in the host liver as well as in the hepatoma. The results revealed that the transplantable hepatoma showed little or no change relative to protein synthesis after tryptophan administration.[322] On the other hand, host livers of the tumor-bearing rats revealed mild or moderate stimulatory changes (less than that of livers of normal rats) in protein synthesis. Table 6.5 summarizes these findings. Also, *in vitro* tryptophan-binding affinity to nuclei of rat liver, host liver, and hepatoma 5123 was investigated.[323] The results, summarized in Table 6.5, indicate that the binding affinities (total and specific) of L-tryptophan to nuclei of hepatoma were appreciably less than to nuclei of normal liver or host liver, and this was attributed mainly to a decrease in the number of binding sites (B_{max}). Protein-free tryptophan levels were appreciably higher in hepatoma than in host or normal livers. Whether the latter finding had an effect on the binding affinity in hepatoma is not known.

Another study[324] investigated whether tryptophan would influence the polyribosomes and protein synthesis of host liver and of intrahepatically transplanted hepatomas of rats that were treated with two hepatotoxic agents, hypertonic NaCl and CCl_4, that had been reported to affect these parameters adversely in the tumor-bearing rats.[325] Although treatment with hypertonic NaCl or CCl_4 caused disaggregation of polyribosomes and inhibition of protein synthesis in host liver and in hepatoma, the subsequent administration of tryptophan caused some improvement in both parameters in host liver but not in hepatoma. Thus, even after toxic injury to the hepatoma, it was not able to respond to tryptophan, as were the livers of normal rats or host livers of tumor-bearing rats.

TABLE 6.5

Effects of Tryptophan on Livers of Normal Rats and on Host Livers and Hepatomas of Tumor-Bearing Rats[a]

Parameters Assayed	Normal Rat Liver	Transplantable Hepatomas in Rats	
		Host Liver	Hepatoma
Normal State[b]			
[³H]Trp binding to nuclei *in vitro*			
Total binding, %	100	99	25
Specific binding, %	64.4	66.3	57.3
K_D, nM	15.7	18.1	13.3
B_{max} fmol/mg protein	2911	1803	281
Protein-free Trp			
Tissue, µg/g		3.8	8.2
Nuclei, µg/mg RNA		11.9	21.2
Response to Tryptophan Administration[c,d]			
Aggregation of polyribosomes	1+	0	1–
Protein synthesis (*in vitro*)	4+	1+	0
Poly(A)mRNA synthesis	3+	3+	1+
Nuclear efflux of RNA			
Nuclear effect	4+	3+	1–
Cytosol effect	4+	0	0
Nuclear enzyme activity changes			
Nucleoside triphosphatase	4+	2+	0
RNA polymerase I	3+	2+	2–
RNA polymerase II	3+	1+	0

[a] Abbreviations are as follows: K_D, dissociation constant; B_{max}, binding capacity.
[b] Normal state indicates that rats, normal or tumor bearing, were fasted overnight and tube-fed water in the morning before they were killed (control group).
[c] Experimental groups were the same as controls, except they were tube-fed L-tryptophan in the morning before they were killed.
[d] Changes as increases (+), decreases (-), or little or no change (0): 4+ or 4–, >60%; 3+ or 3–, 40–59%; 2+ or 2–, 20–30%; 1+ or 1–, 10–19%; 0, 0–9%.

Since hepatoma, because of its rapid cell division and growth, may become resistant to the effects of tryptophan, investigations of whether regenerating livers, after partial hepatectomy (1 or 2 days), would respond to the administration of tryptophan were conducted. The regenerating livers responded to tryptophan with a shift toward heavier aggregation of polyribosomes and an increase in protein synthesis,[322] similar to that observed in livers of normal animals. Thus, the inhibitory or resistant effect found in the hepatoma probably rests in the anaplasia of the cells rather than merely in the rapid division or growth of the cells. Another study dealing with rapidly growing liver cells under different physiologic conditions, as in fetuses or in pups of rats, failed to reveal responses to tryptophan as did maternal livers or normal livers.[15] However, the failure to respond under the latter circumstances may be related to environmental factors (e.g., maternal and lactating amino acid supplies, hormonal effects) rather than rapid cell growth, as occurs in the regenerating livers of adult rats.[322]

6.7.2.6.2 Relating Tryptophan's Effects on Cellular Regulatory Controls to Carcinogenesis

Under normal conditions, the administration of L-tryptophan affects the transcriptional and translational controls involving hepatic protein synthesis.[220] Earlier studies have reported enhanced outflow of mRNA from hepatic nuclei in rats treated with chemical carcinogens,[326] similar to that described with the administration of L-tryptophan to normal controls.[298] Altered or uncontrolled release of nuclear RNA has been considered as a potential basis for the phenotypic expression of chemically induced neoplasms.[327] Possibly the stimulation of nuclear mRNA efflux induced by L-tryptophan in conjunction with that induced by the chemical carcinogen may in some cases potentiate the overall process involved in carcinogenesis.

Information relating to a specific receptor for L-tryptophan in the nuclear envelope of hepatocytes[78,79] adds a new dimension to the consideration of how L-tryptophan may act in the process of carcinogenesis. Since L-tryptophan has a specific nuclear receptor in liver,[78,79] it was important to investigate whether its receptor was similar or related to other hepatic nuclear receptors. Much is known about the steroid hormone nuclear receptors, such as those for glucocorticoids and triiodothyronine, and the complexity of their actions on a vast number of physiologic and pathologic processes.[83] Recently, the hepatic nuclear receptor has been found to be affected by the administration of certain hormones.[84,328-330] Since steroid and thyroid hormones may exert their effects through fundamentally similar mechanisms,[82,331] it was especially important to determine whether L-tryptophan may possibly act similarly. It has long been established that hormones are vitally linked to or involved in the process of chemical carcinogenesis.[332] Whether L-tryptophan acts in some cases in a similar manner needs to be determined.

Searches for possible hepatic nuclear and nuclear membrane alterations during the process of carcinogenesis are ongoing. It is of interest that such

alterations have been described in studies with animals fed a choline-deficient (CD) diet.[333] Although the mechanism(s) by which a CD diet exerts
its carcinogenic[334] and/or promotional[335] effects are not known, it is conceivable that alterations in hepatic nuclear membranes may play some role.
Hepatic nuclei of rats fed a CD diet revealed a decreased affinity for
[³H]tryptophan binding *in vitro*. However, the affinity is increased in hepatic
nuclei of rats fed the CD + 2% L-tryptophan diet.[174] Also, some of the
functional responses of hepatic nuclei to tryptophan are different in rats
fed the CD diet than in control rats.[174] Whether these alterations were related
in any way to the increased or potentiated induction of GGT-positive foci
(precancerous foci) due to tryptophan in DEN-treated rats after partial
hepatectomy[275] is conjectural.

Interesting coincidences have been observed recently. The affinity for
L-tryptophan binding to hepatic nuclei is markedly less in $NZBWF_1$ mice
than in Swiss and other strains of mice.[91] Likewise, Kurl (personal communication) reported a diminished affinity for hepatic specific binding for
³H-labeled 2,3,7,8-tetrachlorodilenzo-*p*-dioxin (TCDD) in $NZBWF_1$ mice
compared with C57B/6 mice. Also, because guinea pigs were susceptible to
TCDD and hamsters were resistant to TCDD in relation to TCDD lethality,[336]
the binding affinities for L-tryptophan to hepatic nuclei of guinea pigs and
hamsters were studied, and it was revealed that the binding affinity was low
in the hamsters (as in $NZBWF_1$ mice) and high in guinea pigs (as in rats and
other mouse strains).[93] Using an acryl hydrocarbon receptor (AHR)-deficient
mouse, Fernandez-Salguerao and co-workers[337] reported that such mice were
relatively unaffected by high doses of TCDD that induced severe toxic and
pathologic effects in littermates expressing a functional AHR. The AHR is a
ligand-activated transcription factor that is required in laboratory animals
to mediate the toxic effects of chemicals such as TCDD. Recent data indicate
that genetic differences do exist in relation to L-tryptophan binding and
subsequent metabolic responses. Whether these genetic differences in
response to tryptophan binding and effects may be related to the actions of
TCDD, including the tumor promotion effects mediated through the Ah
receptor, is not known.

6.7.2.7 Concluding Remarks

A literature review of animal experimental studies with tryptophan and
carcinogenesis, particularly involving bladder and liver, indicates that tryptophan alone does not induce tumors but is capable of acting in many cases
as a promoting agent in chemical carcinogenesis. Whether this effect is due
to tryptophan alone or to tryptophan metabolites is not clear. In the induction
of bladder cancer, tryptophan metabolites are clearly implicated.

In some experimental studies, L-tryptophan has been observed to have
a protective or inhibitory effect against chemically induced cancers. A
possible explanation appears to rely on the ability of tryptophan or its
metabolite to enhance the activities of many enzymes, some of which are

capable of deactivating (detoxifying) the chemical carcinogen. Also, because L-tryptophan and some metabolites are considered to be antioxidant agents, they may serve as scavengers against chemical carcinogens that act via free radical injury, speculated events considered to be essential in chemical carcinogenesis.

Explanations for the promotional (stimulatory) effects or actions of L-tryptophan on carcinogenesis are more complex. In consideration of the process of enhancing enzyme activities, some enzymes affected by tryptophan may play a role in activating chemical carcinogens into ultimate carcinogens, thereby potentiating their effects. Also, tryptophan appears to stimulate ODC activity and cellular proliferation, a process vital in promotion. Last, L-tryptophan's action via nuclear receptor binding and its transduction effects relating to enhanced protein synthesis (in some ways analogous to the effects of some hormones) suggest that it, along with induced disturbances in nuclear regulatory mechanism by chemical carcinogens, may contribute by enhancing the process of carcinogenesis. Genetic alterations in nuclear receptor binding affinity for L-tryptophan have been described in animal studies and may relate to tryptophan's ability to affect the process of promotion in carcinogenesis. Further investigative studies are needed to explore whether such alterations affecting the transduction effects of L-tryptophan may be involved in the process of carcinogenesis.

Reports that the pyrolysate of L-tryptophan forms products that are potent carcinogens in animals merit caution and raise important questions. With regard to humans, the recent occurrence of a new human disease, eosinophilia-myalgia syndrome, related to L-tryptophan and contaminants/impurities from a Japanese manufacturer, clearly demonstrates that tryptophan together with other agents can induce chronic disease in some susceptible individuals. A better understanding of the pathogenesis of this disease and its consequences is needed. Such information may offer clues as to the actions of L-tryptophan and contaminants in the process of carcinogenesis.

6.8   Immunomodular Effects: Interferon and Tryptophan

Interferons represent a class of proteins with various biological properties.[338,339] These include the ability to inhibit intracellular replication of viruses and certain parasites,[340] the ability to inhibit replication of certain types of tumor cells *in vitro*,[341] and the ability to modulate immune responses *in vitro* and *in vivo* in a positive or negative manner.[339] Of the interferons, interferon-γ (IFN-γ) is thought to be a more effective immunomodulary agent and a more effective inhibitor of division of certain tumor cells *in vitro* than other interferons.[339] One mechanism of IFN-γ–mediated growth inhibition is the stimulation of cellular oxidation of tryptophan by indoleamine 2,3-dioxygenase.[342,343]

Aune and Pogue[344] presented data indicating that at least two distinct mechanisms, (1) stimulation of cellular catabolism of tryptophan and (2) stimulation of cellular catabolism of nicotinamide adenine dinucleotide (NAD) by adenosine diphosphate-ritosyl transferase (ADP-RT), can account for IFN-γ–mediated inhibition of tumor cell growth. Both mechanisms appear to be sensitive to oxygen tension and to changes in intracellular glutathione concentrations, and both mechanisms lead to loss of intracellular NAD.

Werner-Felmayer et al.[345] studied IFN-γ–induced tryptophan metabolism of human macrophage and compared this to 10 human neoplastic cell lines of various tissue origin. Tryptophan and metabolites were determined. Most (8 out of 10) cell lines revealed that tryptophan degradation was induced by IFN-γ. Five of the ten formed only kynurenine, and three formed kynurenine and anthranilic acid. Only one line showed the same pattern of metabolites as macrophages (kynurenine, anthranilic acid, and 3-hydroxyanthranilic acid). IFN-γ regulated only the activity of indoleamine 2,3-dioxygenase, and other enzyme activities were independent of IFN-γ. Increasing the extracellular L-tryptophan concentration resulted in a marked induction of tryptophan degradation by macrophages but a significant decrease of tryptophan degrading activity with tumor cell lines. Their study demonstrated that the induction of indoleamine 2,3-dioxygenase was a common feature of IFN-γ action and that the extent of this induction was influenced by extracellular L-tryptophan concentration.

Rubin et al.[346] reported the cloning and characterization of a cDNA, representing a gene where expression is upregulated in INF-treated cells. This gene encodes a protein that has sequence homology with and the biological activity of a tryptophanyl-tRNA synthetase.

Feng and Taylor[347] reported that the human cell line ME 180 undergoes cell death very rapidly following treatment with IFN-γ. This cell death appears to be the result of starvation for tryptophan due to the induction of IDO.[343,344] In ME 180 mutants resistant to the antiproliferative effects of IFN-γ, there was no induction of IDO.[347] Moreover, the antiproliferative response to IFN-γ could be reversed by addition of tryptophan back to the medium.[347,348] More recently, Taylor et al.[349] and Konan and Taylor[350] reported that the antiproliferative response to IFN-γ results in apoptosis of treated cells and tryptophan starvation by itself appears to be sufficient to drive the cell to apoptosis through the same or similar mechanisms. Also, apoptosis was prevented on adding back tryptophan to IFN-γ–treated cells or those induced by removing tryptophan from the medium in the absence of IFN-γ.

The influence of IFN-γ on tryptophan metabolism of cells (macrophages and tumor cell lines) via stimulation of IDO appears to be an important process. It may affect cell proliferation as well as apoptosis. The preceding cited findings that the levels of L-tryptophan in a medium containing cultured cells is important in inducing apoptosis deserve further investigation. *In vivo* experimental studies directed toward similar effects are needed. This important field should be pursued to clarify a possibly important feature of cellular tryptophan levels as influenced by IFN-γ.

In Chapter 5, the relationship of tryptophan and IFN-γ in a few disease states was reviewed. These diseases involve disturbances in the patient's immune system.

6.9 Concluding Comments

This chapter reviewed the possible involvement of L-tryptophan in a number of conditions or diseases. It reviewed the state-of-the-art developments pertaining to L-tryptophan and its possible relationship with each of a number of important conditions or disease states.

Since most of the diseases are chronic, it is important to consider certain aspects relating to chronic diseases themselves. First, it is generally thought that most or all chronic diseases have a genetic component. Genes are considered to define susceptibility to disease with nutrition considered an environmental factor that may influence which susceptible individuals may develop disease. L-tryptophan, a vital and unique amino acid, is a nutritional component that may play an important role in influencing the development of certain chronic diseases in susceptible individuals.

Using the tools of molecular biology and genetics, research should define the mechanisms by which genes influence nutrient (L-tryptophan) absorption, metabolism, excretion, and other actions and also the mechanisms by which the nutrient (L-tryptophan) influences gene expression. Such studies should be productive and will clarify whether and how L-tryptophan may be primarily or secondarily involved in and during the pathogenesis of a variety of important chronic diseases.

References

1. Schrocksnadel, H., Baier-Bitterlich, G., Dapunt, O., Wachter, H., and Fuchs, D., Decreased plasma tryptophan in pregnancy, *Obstet. Gynecol.,* 88, 47, 1996.
2. Zamenhof, S., Hall, S. M., Grauel, L., Van Marthens, E., and Donahue, M. J., Deprivation of amino acids and prenatal brain development in rats, *J. Nutr,* 104, 1002, 1974.
3. Zamenhof, S., Van Marthens, E., and Grauel, L., DNA (cell number) and protein in neonatal rat brain: Alteration by timing of maternal dietary protein restriction, *J. Nutr.,* 101, 1265, 1971.
4. Sanfilippo, S., Imbesi, R. M., and Sanfilippo, S., Jr., Pre- and postnatal sexual morphogenesis and maturation in tryptophan deprived rats during ontogeny. Postulated control in the male by serotonin-prolactin system, *Biogenic Amines,* 11, 87, 1995.

5. Matsueda, S. and Niiyama, Y., The effects of excess amino acids on maintenance of pregnancy and fetal growth in rats, *J. Nutr. Sci. Vitaminol.*, 28, 557, 1982.
6. Meier, A. H. and Wilson, J. .M., Tryptophan feeding adversely influences pregnancy, *Life Sci.*, 32, 1193, 1983.
7. Waugh, D. and Pearl, M. J., Serotonin-induced acute nephrosis and renal cortical necrosis in rats. A morphologic study with pregnancy correlation, *Am. J. Pathol.*, 36, 431, 1960.
8. Paulson, E., Robson, J. M., and Sullivan, F. M., Teratogenic effect of 5-hydroxy-tryptamine in mice, *Science*, 141, 717, 1963.
9. Hammar, R., Embryotoxic effects of serotonin during early pregnancy in the rat, 196, 71A, 1980.
10. Fernstrom, J. D. and Wurtman, R. J., Brain serotonin content: Physiological dependence on plasma tryptophan levels, *Science*, 173, 149, 1971.
11. Green, H., Greenberg, S. M., Erickson, R. W., Sawyer, J. L., and Ellison, T., Effect of dietary phenylalanine and tryptophan upon rat brain amine levels, *J. Pharmacol. Exp. Ther.*, 136, 174, 1962.
12. Biggio, G., Fadda, F., Fanni, P., Tagliamonte, A., and Gessa, G. L., Rapid depletion of serum tryptophan, brain tryptophan, serotonin and 5-hydroxyindoleacetic acid by a tryptophan-free diet, *Life Sci.*, 14, 1321, 1974.
13. Blundell, J. E., Serotonin and skin diseases, in *Serotonin in Health and Disease*, Vol. 5, Essman, W. B., Ed., S.P. Medical and Scientific Books, New York, 1979, 403–450.
14. Hartmann, E. and Spinweber, C. L., Sleep induced by L-tryptophan. Effect of dosages within the normal dietary intake, *J. Nerv. Ment. Dis.*, 167, 497, 1979.
15. Sidransky, H. and Verney, E., Effect of tryptophan on livers of pregnant and lactating rats and their fetuses and pups, *Exp. Biol. Med.*, 187, 309, 1988.
16. van Heyningen, R., Experimental studies on cataract, *Invest. Ophthalmol. Vis. Sci.*, 15, 685, 1976.
17. Albanese, A. A., Holt, L. E., Jr., Kajdi, C. N., and Frankston, J. E., Observations on tryptophane deficiency in rats. Chemical and morphological changes in the blood, *J. Biol. Chem.*, 148, 299, 1943.
18. Cole, A. S. and Scott, P. P., Tissue changes in the adult tryptophan-deficient rat, *Br. J. Nutr.*, 8, 125, 1954.
19. Scott, E. B., Histopathology of amino acid deficiencies. IV. Tryptophan, *Am. J. Pathol.*, 31, 1111, 1955.
20. Adamstone, F. B. and Spector, H., Tryptophan deficiency in the rat. Histologic changes induced by forced feeding of an acid hydrolyzed casein diet, *Arch. Pathol.*, 49, 173, 1950.
21. Samuels, L. T., Goldthorpe, H. C., and Dougherty, T. F., Metabolic effects of specific amino acid deficiencies, *Fed. Proc.*, 10, 393, 1951.
22. Mertz, E. T., Beeson, W. M., and Jackson, H. D., Classification of essential amino acids for the weanling pig, *Arch. Biochem. Biophys.*, 38, 121, 1952.
23. Van Pilsum, J. F., Speyer, J. F., and Samuels, L. T., Essential amino acid deficiency and enzyme activity, *Arch. Biochem.*, 68, 42, 1957.
24. Bauer, C. D. and Berg, C. P., The amino acids required for growth in mice and the availability of their optical isomer, *J. Nutr.*, 26, 51, 1943.
25. Spector, H. and Adamstone, F. B., Tryptophan deficiency in the rat induced by forced feeding of an acid hydrolyzed casein diet, *J. Nutr.*, 40, 213, 1950.

26. Arevalo, R., Afonso, D., Castro, R., and Rodriguez, M., Fetal brain serotonin synthesis and catabolism is under control by mother intake of tryptophan, *Life Sci.*, 49, 53, 1991.

27. Martin, L., Rodriguez, D. M., Santana-Herrera, C., Milena, A., and Santana, C., Tryptophan ingestion by gestant mothers alters prolactin and luteinizing hormone release in the adult male offspring, *Brain Res.*, 774, 265, 1997.

28. Hernandez-Rodriguez, J. and Chagoya, G., Brain serotonin synthesis and Na+,K+-ATPase activity are increased postnatally after prenatal administration of L-tryptophan, *Brain Res.*, 390, 221, 1986.

29. Henderson, M. and Kitos, P. A., Do organophosphate insecticides inhibit the conversion of tryptophan to NAD+ in ovo? *Teratology*, 26, 173, 1982.

30. Snawder, J. E. and Chambers, J. E., Critical time periods and the effect of tryptophan in malathion-induced developmental defects in *Xenopus* embryos, *Life Sci.*, 46, 1635, 1990.

31. Miller, M., Leahy, J. P., Stern, W. C., Morgane, P. J., and Resnick, O., Tryptophan availability: Relation to elevated brain serotonin in developmentally protein-malnourished rats, *Exp. Neurol.*, 57, 142, 1977.

32. Miller, M. and Resnick, O., Tryptophan availability: The importance of prepartum and postpartum dietary protein on brain indoleamine metabolism in rats, *Exp. Neurol.*, 67, 298, 1980.

33. Aoki, K. and Siegel, F. L., Hyperphenylalaninemia: Disaggregation of brain polyribosomes in young rats, *Science*, 168, 129, 1970.

34. Blazek, R. and Shaw, D. M., Tryptophan availability and brain protein synthesis, *Neuropharmacology*, 17, 1065, 1978.

35. Sobotka, T. J., Cook, M. P., and Brodie, R. E., Neonatal malnutrition: Neurochemical, hormonal and behavioral manifestations, *Brain Res.*, 65, 443, 1974.

36. Hamon, M. and Bourgoin, S., Ontogenesis of tryptophan transport in the rat brain, *J. Neural Transm.* (Suppl.), 93, 1979.

37. Bourgoin, B., Faivre-Bauman, A., Hery, F., Ternaux, J. P., and Hamon, M., Characteristics of tryptophan binding in the serum of the newborn rat, *Biol. Neonate*, 31, 141, 1977.

38. Jaeger, W., Kafer, O. Schmidt, H., and Lutz, P., Bilateral optic atrophy in childhood caused by tryptophan deficiency, *Metab. Pediatr. Ophthal.*, 3, 167, 1979.

39. De Antoni, A., Allegri, G., Costa, C., Vanzan, S., Bertolin, A., Carretti, N., and Zanardo, V., Total and free tryptophan levels in serum of newborn infants. Relationships with the serotonin and nicotinic acid pathways, *Acta Vitaminol. Enzymol.*, 2, 17, 1980.

40. Tricklebank, M.D., Pickard, F. J., and de Souza, S. W., Free and bound tryptophan in human plasma during the perinatal period, *Acta Paediatr. Scand.*, 68, 199, 1979.

41. Hernandez, J., Manjarrez, G. G., and Chagoya, G., Newborn humans and rats malnourished *in utero*: Free plasma L-tryptophan, neutral amino acids and brain serotonin synthesis, *Brain Res.*, 488, 1, 1989.

42. Manjarrez, G., Contreras, J. L., Chagoya, G., and Hernandez, R., Free tryptophan as an indicator of brain serotonin synthesis in infants, *Pediatr. Neurol.*, 18, 57, 1998.

43. Zammarchi, E., La Rosa, S., Pierro, U., Lenzi, G., Bartolini, P., and Falorni, S., Free tryptophan decrease in jaundiced newborn infants during phototherapy, *Biol. Neonate*, 55, 224, 1989.

44. Cortamira, N. O., Seve, B., Lebreton, Y. and Ganier, P., Effect of dietary tryptophan on muscle, liver and whole-body protein synthesis in weaned piglets: Relationship to plasma insulin, *Br. J. Nutr.*, 66, 423–435, 1991.

45. Ponter, A. A., Cortamira, N. O., Seve, B., Salter, D. N., and Morgan, L. M., The effects of energy source and tryptophan on the rate of protein synthesis and on hormones of the entero-insular axis in the piglet, *Br. J. Nutr.*, 71, 661, 1994.

46. Lin, F. D., Smith, T. K., and Bayley, H. S., A role for tryptophan in regulation of protein synthesis in porcine muscle, *J. Nutr.*, 118, 445, 1988.

47. Seve, B., Impact of dietary tryptophan and behavioral type on growth performance and plasma amino acids of young pigs, *J. Anim. Sci.*, 69, 3679, 1991.

48. Montgomery, G. W., Flux, D. S., and Greenway, R. M., Tryptophan deficiency in pigs: Changes in food intake and plasma levels of glucose, amino acids, insulin and growth hormone, *Hormone Metab. Res.*, 12, 304, 1980.

49. McCay, C. M., Chemical aspects of aging and the effect of diet upon aging, in *Cowdry's Problems of Aging*, 3rd ed., Liansing, A. I., Ed., Williams & Wilkins, Baltimore, 1952, 139.

50. Berg, B. N., Nutrition and longevity in the rat. I. Food intake in relation to size, health and fertility, *J. Nutr.*, 71, 242, 1960.

51. Berg, B. N., Nutrition and longevity in the rat. II. Longevity and onset of disease with different levels of food intake, *J. Nutr.*, 71, 255, 1960.

52. Ross, M. H., Length of life and caloric intake, *Am. J. Clin. Nutr.*, 25, 834, 1972.

53. Yu, B. P., How diet influences the aging process of the rat, *Exp. Biol. Med.*, 205, 97, 1994.

54. Roth, G. S., Ingram, D. K., and Lane, M. A., Calorie restriction in primates: Will it work and how will we know? *J. Am. Geriatr. Soc.*, 47, 896, 1999.

55. Segall, P. E. and Timiras, P. S., Patho-physiologic findings after chronic tryptophan deficiency in rats: A model for delayed growth and aging, *Mech. Ageing Dev.*, 5, 109, 1976.

56. Ooka, H., Segall, P. E., and Timiras, P. S., Histology and survival in age-delayed low-tryptophan-fed rats, *Mech. Ageing Dev.*, 43, 79, 1988.

57. De Marte, M. L. and Enesco, H. E., Influence of low tryptophan diet on survival and organ growth in mice, *Mech. Ageing Dev.*, 36, 161, 1986.

58. Segall, P. E., Interrelations of dietary and hormonal effects in aging, *Mech. Ageing Dev.*, 9, 515, 1979.

59. Sidransky, H., Chemical and cellular pathology of experimental acute amino acid deficiency, in *Methods of Achievment in Experimental Pathology*, Vol. 6, Bajusz, E. and Jasmin, G., Eds., Basel, Kargeer, 1972, 1–24.

60. Felig, P., Amino acid metabolism in man, *Annu. Rev. Biochem.*, 44, 933, 1975.

61. Demling, J., Langer, K., and Mehr, M. Q., Age dependence of large neutral amino acid levels in plasma. Focus on tryptophan, *Adv. Exp. Med. Biol.*, 398, 579, 1996.

62. Fuchs, D., Forsman, A., Hagberg, L., Larsson, M., Norkrans, G., Reibnegger, G., Werner, E. R., and Wachter, H. Immune activation and decreased tryptophan in patients with HIV-1 infection, *J. Interferon Res,*, 10, 599, 1990.

63. Sainio, E. L., Pulkki, K., and Young, S. N., L-tryptophan: Biochemical, nutrition and pharmacological aspects, *Amino Acids*, 10, 21, 1996.

64. Tang, J. P. and Melethil, S., Effect of aging on the kinetics of blood–brain barrier uptake of tryptophan in rats, *Pharm. Res.*, 12, 1085, 1995.

65. Yeung, J. M. and Friedman, E., Effect of aging and diet restriction on monoamines and amino acids in cerebral cortex of Fischer-344 rats, *Growth Dev. Aging*, 55, 275, 1991.
66. Navab, F. and Winter, C. G., Effect of aging on intestinal absorption of aromatic amino acids *in vitro* in the rat, *Am. J. Physiol.*, 254, G631, 1988.
67. Fleck, C., Renal transport of endogenous amino acids. I. Comparison between immature and adult rats, *Renal Physiol. Biochem.*, 15, 257, 1992.
68. Patnaik, S. K. and Patnaik, R., Age-related differential induction of tryptophan pyrrolase by hydrocortisone in the liver of male rats, *Biochem. Int.*, 18, 1221, 1989.
69. Kanungo, M. S., *Biochemistry of Ageing: Changes in Enzymes during Ageing*, Academic Press, London, 1980, 79–126.
70. Kalimi, M., Glucocorticoid receptors: From development to aging. A review, *Mech. Ageing Dev.*, 24, 129, 1984.
71. Sharma, R. and Timiras, P. S., Age-dependent regulation of glucocorticoid receptors in the liver of male rats, *Biochim. Biophys. Acta*, 930, 237, 1987.
72. Roth, G. S., Age-related changes in specific glucocorticoid binding by steroid-responsive tissues of rats, *Endocrinology*, 94, 82, 1974.
73. Kalimi, M., Beato, M., and Feigelson, P., Interaction of glucocorticoids with rat liver nuclei. I. Role of the cytosol proteins, *Biochemistry*, 12, 3365, 1973.
74. Cole, G. M., Segall, P. E., and Timiras, P. S., Hormones during aging, in *Hormones in Development and Aging*, Vernadaker, A. and Timiras, P. S., Eds., SP Medica and Scientific Books, New York, 1982, 477–550.
75. Valcana, T., The role of triiodothyronine in brain development, in *Neural Growth and Differentiation*, Meisami, E. and Brazier, M. A. B., Eds., Raven Press, New York, 1979, 39–58.
76. Valcana, T. and Timiras, P. S., Nuclear triiodothyronine receptors in the developing rat brain, *Mol. Cell. Endocrinol.*, 11, 31, 1978.
77. Margarity, M., Valcana, T., and Timiras, P. S., Thyroxine deiodination, cytoplasmic distribution and nuclear binding of thyroxine and triiodothyronine in liver and brain of young and aged rats, *Mech. Ageing Dev.*, 29, 181, 1985.
78. Kurl, R. N., Verney, E., and Sidransky, H., Tryptophan binding sites on nuclear envelopes of rat liver, *Nutr. Rep. Int..*, 36, 669, 1987.
79. Kurl, R. N., Verney, E., and Sidransky, H., Identification and immunohistochemical localization of a tryptophan binding protein in nuclear envelopes of rat liver, *Arch. Biochem. Biophys.*, 265, 286, 1988.
80. Kurl, R. N., Verney, E., and Sidransky, H., Mechanism of action of tryptophan: new insights in *Regulatory Processes in Biology: A Festschrift*, W. B. Saunders, Philadelphia, 1990, 93–108.
81. Sap, J., Munoz, A., Damm, K., Goldberg, Y., Ghysdael, J., Leutz, A., Beug, H., and Vennstrom, B., The c-erb-A protein is a high-affinity receptor for thyroid hormone, 324, 635, 1986.
82. Weinberger, C., Thompson, C. C., Ong, E. S., Lebo, R., Gruol, D. J., and Evans, R. M., The c-erb-A gene encodes a thyroid hormone receptor, *Nature*, 324, 641, 1986.
83. Beato, M., Herrlich, P., and Schutz, G., Steroid hormone receptors: Many actors in search of a plot, *Cell*, 83, 851, 1995.
84. Sidransky, H. and Verney, E., Hormonal influences on tryptophan binding to rat hepatic nuclei, *Metab. Clin. Exp.*, 48, 144, 1999.

85. Sidransky, H. and Verney, E., Hormonal influences on tryptophan binding to rat hepatic nuclei, *Adv. Exp. Med. Biol.*, 467, 369, 1999.

86. Touitou, Y., Bogdan, A., Auzeby, A., and Selmaoui, B., Melatonin and aging, *Therapie*, 53, 473, 1998.

87. Kilberg, M. S., Hutson, R. G., and Laine, R. O., Amino acid-regulated gene expression in eukaryotic cells, *FASEB J.*, 8, 13, 1994.

88. Lefebvre, Y. A. and Novosad, Z., Binding of androgens to a nuclear-envelope fraction from the rat ventral prostate, *Biochemical J.*, 186, 641, 1980.

89. Simmer, R. C. M., Means, A. R., and Clark, J. H., Estrogen modulation of nuclear-associated steroid hormone binding, *Endocrinology*, 115, 1197, 1984.

90. Kaufmann, S. H., Okret, S., Wikstrom, A. C., Gustafsson, J. A., and Shaper, J. H., Binding of the glucocorticoid receptor to the rat liver nuclear matrix. The role of disulfide bond formation, *J. Biol. Chem.*, 261, 11962, 1986.

91. Sidransky, H. and Verney, E., Differences in tryptophan binding to hepatic nuclei of NZBWF1 and Swiss mice: Insight into mechanism of tryptophan's effects, *J. Nutr.*, 127, 270, 1997.

92. Yunis, E. J., Teague, P. O., Stutman, O., and Good, R. A., The thymus, autoimmunity and the involution of the lymphoid system, in *Tolerance Autoimmunity, and Aging*, Sigel, M. M., Ed., Charles C Thomas, Springfield, IL, 1972, 62–119.

93. Sidransky, H. and Verney E., L-tryptophan binding to hepatic nuclei: Age and species differences, *Amino Acids*, 12, 77, 1997.

94. Sidransky, H., Ethanol and liver injury: Aspects relating to hepatic protein synthesis, *Rev. Environ. Health*, 7, 81, 1987.

95. Preedy, V. R., Duane, P., and Peters, T. J., Comparison of the acute effects of ethanol on liver and skeletal muscle protein synthesis in the rat, *Alcohol & Alcoholism*, 23, 155, 1988.

96. Sellers, E. M., Higgins, G. A., and Sobel, M. B., 5-HT and alcohol abuse, *Trends Pharmacol. Sci.*, 13, 69, 1992.

97. LeMarquand, D., Phil, R. O., and Benkelfat, C., Serotonin and alcohol intake, abuse, and dependence: Clinical evidence, *Biol. Psychiatr.*, 36, 326, 1994.

98. LeMarquand, D., Phil, R. O., and Benkelfat, C., Serotonin and alcohol intake, abuse and dependence: Findings in animal studies, *Biol. Psychiatr.*, 36, 395, 1994.

99. Lucas, C. C., Ridout, J. H., and Lumchick, G. L., Dietary protein and chronic intoxication with ethanol, *Can. J. Physiol. Pharmacol.*, 46, 475, 1968.

100. Sidransky, H., Nutritional disturbances of protein metabolism in the liver, *Am. J. Pathol.*, 84, 649, 1976.

101. Murty, C. N., Hornseth, R., Verney, E., and Sidransky, H., Effect of tryptophan on enzymes and proteins of hepatic nuclear envelopes of rats, *Lab. Invest.*, 48, 256, 1983.

102. Jarowski, C. I. and Ward, C. O., Effect of tryptophan on toxicity and depressant effects of barbiturates and ethanol in rats, *Toxicol. Appl. Pharmacol.*, 18, 603–606, 1971.

103. Jarowski, C. I., Puccini, A. V., Winitz, M., and Otey, M. C., Utility of fasting essential amino acid plasma levels in formulation of nutritionally adequate diets. 1. Sprague-Dawley rats, *Agric. Biol. Chem.*, 35, 1007, 1971.

104. Ward, C. O., Lau, C. C., Tang, A. S., Breglia, R. J., and Jarowski, C. I., Effects of lysine on toxicity and depressant effects of ethanol in rats, *Toxicol. Appl. Pharmacol.*, 22, 422, 1972.

105. Breglia, R. J., Ward, C. O., and Jarowski, C. I., Effect of selected amino acids on ethanol toxicity in rats, *J. Pharm. Sci.*, 62, 49, 1973.
106. Dubroff, L. S., Ward, C. O., and Jarowski, C. I., Effect of dietary lysine and tryptophan supplementation on growth rate and toxicity of barbiturates and ethanol in rats, *J. Pharm. Sci.*, 68, 1554, 1979.
107. Jeejeebhoy, K. N., Phillips, M. J., Bruce-Robertson, A., Ho, J., and Sodtke, U., The acute effect of ethanol on albumin, fibrinogen and transferrin synthesis in the rat, *Biochemical J.*, 126, 1111, 1972.
108. Rothschild, M. A., Oratz, M., Mongelli, J., and Schreiber, S. S., Alcohol-induced depression of albumin synthesis: Reversal by tryptophan, *J. Clin. Invest.*, 50, 1812, 1971.
109. Rothschild, M. A., Oratz, M., and Schreiber, S. S., Effect of tryptophan on the hepatotoxic effects of alcohol and carbon tetrachloride, *Trans. Assoc. Am. Phys.*, 84, 313, 1971.
110. Gullino, P., Winitz, M., Birnbaum, S. M., Cornfield, J., Otey, M. C., and Greenstein, J. P., Studies on the metabolism of amino acids and related compounds *in vivo*. I. Toxicity of essential amino acids individually, in mixtures and the protective effect of L-arginine, *Arch. Biochem. Biophys.*, 319, 332, 1956.
111. Badawy, A. A. B. and Evans, M., The regulation of rat liver tryptophan pyrrolase activity by reduced nicotinamide-adenine dinucleotide (phosphate). Experiments with glucose and nicotinamide, *Biochemical J.*, 156, 381, 1976.
112. Stowell, L. and Morland, J., Ethanol-induced increase in liver tryptophan oxygenase activity in the starved rat: Evidence against tryptophan mediation, *Biochem. Pharmacol.*, 33, 2397, 1984.
113. Eriksson, T., Carlsson, A., Liljequist, S., Hagman, M., and Jagenburg, R., Decrease in plasma amino acids in rat after acute administration of ethanol, *J. Pharm. Pharmacol.*, 32, 512, 1980.
114. Eriksson, T., Magnusson, T., Carlsson, A., Hagman, M., Jagenburg, R., and Eden, S., Effects of hypophysectomy, adrenalectomy and (-)-propranolol on ethanol-induced decrease in plasma amino acids, *Naunyn-Schmiedebergs Arch. Pharmacol.*, 317, 214, 1981.
115. Cobb, C. F. and Van Thiel, D. H., Mechanism of ethanol-induced adrenal stimulation, *Alcoholism Clin. Exp. Res.*, 6, 202, 1982.
116. Khawaja, J. A., Effect of ethanol ingestion on the nucleocytoplasmic transport of hepatic RNA, *Toxicol. Lett.*, 15, 199, 1983.
117. Murty, C. N., Verney, E., and Sidransky, H., The effect of tryptrophan on nucleocytoplasmic translocation of RNA in rat liver, *Biochim. Biophys. Acta*, 474, 117, 1977.
118. Hazan, N. and McCauley, R., Effect of phenobarbitone on the nucleocytoplasmic transport of ribonucleic acid *in vitro*, *Biochemical J.*, 156, 665, 1976.
119. Murty, C. N. and Sidransky, H., The effect of tryptophan on messenger RNA of the liver of fasted mice, *Biochim. Biophys. Acta*, 262, 328, 1972.
120. Murty, C. N., Verney, E., and Sidransky, H., Effect of tryptophan on polyriboadenylic acid and polyadenylic acid-messenger ribonucleic acid in rat liver, *Lab. Invest.*, 34, 77, 1976.
121. Sidransky, H., Murty, C. N., and Verney, E., Nutritional control of protein synthesis. Studies relating to tryptophan-induced stimulation of nucleocytoplasmic translocation of mRNA in rat liver, *Am. J. Pathol.*, 117, 298, 1984.
122. Harris, R. A. and Schroeder, F., Ethanol and the physical properties of brain membranes: Fluorescence studies, *Mol. Pharmacol.*, 20, 128, 1981.

123. Gordon, L. M., Sauerheber, R. D., Esgate, J. A., Dipple, I., Marchmont, R. J., and Houslay, M. D., The increase in bilayer fluidity of rat liver plasma membranes achieved by the local anesthetic benzyl alcohol affects the activity of intrinsic membrane enzymes, *J. Biol. Chem.*, 255, 4519, 1980.

124. Harris, R. A., Defining the membrane pathology produced by chronic alcohol consumption [editorial], *Lab. Invest.*, 50, 113, 1984.

125. Rubin, E. and Rottenberg, H., Ethanol-induced injury and adaptation in biological membranes, *Fed. Proc.*, 41, 2465, 1982.

126. Badawy, A. A., Tryptophan metabolism in alcoholism, *Adv. Exp. Med. Biol.*, 467, 265, 1999.

127. Badawy, A. A. B. and Evans M., Tryptophan pyrrolase in ethanol administration and withdrawal, *Adv. Exp. Med. Biol.*, 35, 105, 1973.

128. Badawy, A. A. and Evans, M., The effects of ethanol on tryptophan pyrolase activity and their comparison with those of phenobarbitone and morphine, *Adv. Exp. Med. Biol.*, 59, 229, 1975.

129. Davis, V. E., Brown, H., Huff, J. A., and Cashaw, J. L., The alteration of serotonin metabolism to 5-hydroxytryptophan by ethanol ingestion in man, *J. Lab. Clin. Med,.* 69, 132, 1967.

130. Badawy, A. A., Morgan, C. J., Lovett, J. W., Bradley, D. M., and Thomas, R., Decrease in circulating tryptophan availability to the brain after acute ethanol consumption by normal volunteers: Implications for alcohol-induced aggressive behaviour and depression, *Pharmacopsychiatry*, 28 (Suppl. 2), 93, 1995.

131. Badawy, A. A., Punjani, N. F., and Evans, M., Enhancement of rat brain tryptophan metabolism by chronic ethanol administration and possible involvement of decreased liver tryptophan pyrrolase activity, *Biochem. J.*, 178, 575, 1979.

132. Walsh, M. P., Howart, P. J. N., and Marks, V., Pyridoxine deficiency and tryptophan metabolism in chronic alcoholics, *Am. J. Clin. Nutr.*, 19, 379, 1966.

133. Friedman, M. J., Krstulovic, A. M., Severinghaus, J. M., and Brown, S. J., Altered conversion of tryptophan to kynurenine in newly abstinent alcoholics, *Biol. Psychiatr.*, 23, 89, 1988.

134. Sved, A. F., Van Itallie, C. M., and Fernstrom, J. D., Studies on the antihypertensive action of L-tryptophan, *J. Pharmacol. Exp. Ther.*, 221, 329, 1982.

135. Wolf, W. A. and Kuhn, D. M., Effects of L-tryptophan on blood pressure in normotensive and hypertensive rats, *J. Pharmacol. Exp. Ther.*, 230, 324, 1984.

136. Fregly, M. J. and Fater, D. C., Prevention of DOCA-induced hypertension in rats by chronic treatment with tryptophan, *Clin. Exp. Pharmacol. Physiol.*, 13, 767, 1986.

137. Fregly, M. J., Lockley, O. E., and Cade, J. R., Effect of chronic dietary treatment with L-tryptophan on the development of renal hypertension in rats, *Pharmacology*, 36, 91, 1988.

138. Lark, L. A., Witt, P. A., Becker, K. B., Studzinski, W. M., and Weyhenmeyer, J. A., Effect of dietary tryptophan on the development of hypertension in the Dahl salt-sensitive rat, *Clin. Exp. Hypertension Pt. A, Theory Pract.*, 12, 1, 1990.

139. Riesselmann, A., Baron, A., Fregly, M. J., and Cade, J. R., Effect of chronic dietary treatment with L-tryptophan on the development of cold-induced hypertension in rats, *Pharmacology*, 42, 349, 1991.

140. Fregly, M. J., Effects of tryptophan on the development of deoxycorticosterone acetate (DOCA)-induced hypertension in rats, *Adv. Exp. Med. Biol.*, 294, 619, 1991.

141. Squadrito, F., Sturniolo, R., Trimarchi, G. R., Campo, G. M., De Luca, G., Gorini, A., and Caputi, A. P. , Antihypertensive activity of indolepyruvic acid: A keto analogue of tryptophan, *J. Cardiovasc. Pharmacol.*, 15, 102, 1990.

142. Tang, J. P., Xu, Z. Q., Douglas, F. L., Rakhit, A., and Melethil, S. Increased blood-brain barrier permeability of amino acids in chronic hypertension, *Life Sci.*, 53, L417, 1993.

143. Dawson, R. J., Nagahama, S., and Oparil, S., Yohimbine-induced alterations of monoamine metabolism in the spontaneously hypertensive rat of the Okamoto strain (SHR). II. The central nervous system (CNS), *Brain Res. Bull.*, 19, 525, 1987.

144. Dawson, R., Jr., Nagamhama, S., and Oparil, S., Central serotonergic alterations in deoxycorticosterone acetate/NaCl(DOCA/NaCl)-induced hypertension, *Neuropharmacology*, 27, 417, 1988.

145. Dawson, R. and Oparil, S., Genetic and salt-related alterations in monoamine neurotransmitters in Dahl-salt-sensitive and salt-resistant rats, *Pharmacology*, 33, 322, 1986.

146. Baron, A., Riesselmann, A., and Fregly, M. J., Reduction in the elevated blood pressure of Dahl salt-sensitive rats treated chronically with L-5-hydroxytryptophan, *Pharmacology*, 42, 15, 1991.

147. Patterson, T. S. A., Dawson, R., Jr., Iyer, S. N., and Katovich, M. J., Plasma tryptophan is altered in the Dahl rat model of hypertension, *Biogenic Amines*, 11, 109, 1995.

148. Fregly, M. J., Lockley, O. E., Van, D. V., Sumners, C., and Henley, W. N., Chronic dietary administration of tryptophan prevents the development of deoxycorticosterone acetate salt induced hypertension in rats, *Can. J. Physiol. Pharmacol.*, 65, 753, 1987.

149. Fregly, M. J. and Cade, J. R., Effect of pyridoxine and tryptophan, alone and combined, on the development of deoxycorticosterone acetate-induced hypertension in rats, *Pharmacology*, 50, 298, 1995.

150. Fregly, M. J., Lockley, O. E., Torres, J. L., and Cade, J. R., Effect of chronic dietary treatment with nicotinic acid on the development and maintenance of deoxy-corticosterone-acetate-salt-induced hypertension, *Pharmacology*, 37, 50, 1988.

151. Fregly, M. J., Sumners C., and Cade, J. R., Effect of chronic dietary treatment with L-tryptophan on the maintenance of hypertension in spontaneously hypertensive rats, *Can. J. Physiol. Pharmacol.*, 67, 656, 1989.

152. Sidransky, H., Sarma, D. S., Bongiorno, M., and Verney, E., Effect of dietary tryptophan on hepatic polyribosomes and protein synthesis in fasted mice, *J. Biol. Chem.*, 243, 1123, 1968.

153. Sidransky, H., Verney, E., and Sarma, D. S., Effect of tryptophan on polyribosomes and protein synthesis in liver, *Am. J. Clin. Nutr.*, 24, 779, 1971.

154. Cade, J. R., Fregley, M. J., and Privette, M., Effect of L-tryptophan on the blood pressure of patients with mild to moderate essential hypertension, in *Amino Acids, Chemistry, Biology and Medicine*, Lubec, G. and Rosenthal, G. A., Eds., ESCOM Science, Leiden, 1990, 738–744.

155. Feltkamp, H., Meurer, K. A., and Godehardt, E., Tryptophan-induced lowering of blood pressure and changes of serotonin uptake by platelets in patients with essential hypertension, *Klin. Wochenschrift*, 62, 1115, 1984.

156. Wolf, W. A. and Kuhn, D. M., Antihypertensive effects of L-tryptophan are not mediated by brain serotonin, *Brain Res.*, 295, 356, 1984.

157. Tomoda, F., Takata, M., Oh-Hashi, S., Ueno, H., Yasumoto, K., Iida, H., and Sasayama, S., Altered renal response to enhanced endogenous 5-hydroxy-tryptamine after tryptophan administration in essential hypertension, *Clin. Sci.*, 82, 551, 1992.

158. Kuhn, D. M., Wolf, W. A., and Lovenberg, W., Review of the role of the central serotonergic neuronal system in blood pressure regulation, *Hypertension*, 2, 243, 1980.

159. Chandra, M. and Chandra, N., Serotonergic mechanisms in hypertension, *Int. J. Cardiol.*, 42, 189, 1993.

160. Wolf, W. A., Kuhn, D. M., and Lovenberg, W., Serotonin and central regulation of arterial blood pressure, in *Serotonin and the Cardiovascular System*, VanHoutte, P. M., Ed., Raven Press, New York, 1985, 63–73.

161. Frazer, A., Maayani, S., and Wolfe, B. B., Subtypes of receptors for serotonin, *Annu. Rev. Pharmacol. Toxicol.*, 30, 307, 1990.

162. Peters, J. C., Tryptophan nutrition and metabolism: An overview, *Adv. Exp. Med. Biol.*, 294, 345, 1991.

163. Rudrzite, V., Sileniece, G., Jirgensons, J., Schlossberger, H. G., Kochen, W., Linzen, B., and Sternhart, H., Eds., *Progress in Tryptophan and Serotonin Research*, Walter de Gruyter, Berlin, 1984, 365–381.

164. During, M. J., Heyes, M. P., Freese, A., Markey, S. P., Martin, J. B., and Roth, R. H., Quinolinic acid concentrations in striatal extracellur fluid reach potentially neurotoxic levels following systemic L-tryptophan loading, *Brain Res.*, 476, 384, 1989.

165. Herken, H. and Weber, H. J., L-tryptophan-induced increase of renal sodium reabsorption, *Naunyn-Schmiedebergs Arch. Pharmakol.*, 271, 206, 1971.

166. Reuter, E., Weber, H.-J., and Herken, H., Studies of sodium ion retention and antidiuretic effects after administration of L-tryptophan to rats, *Naunyn-Schmiedebergs Arch. Pharmakol.*, 297, 213, 1977.

167. Sidransky, H., Verney, E., and Orenstein, J., Effects of altered tonicity by sodium chloride on L-tryptophan binding to hepatic nuclei, *Am. J. Physiol. Cell Physiol.*, 278, C1237, 2000.

168. Sidransky, H., Verney, E., and Murty, C. .N., Effect of tryptophan on hepatic polyribosomal disaggregation due to hypertonic sodium chloride, *Lab. Invest.*, 34, 291, 1976.

169. Sidransky, H., Possible role of dietary proteins and amino acids in atherosclerosis, *Ann. N.Y. Acad. Sci.*, 598, 464, 1990.

170. Raja, P. K. and Jarowski, C. I., Utility of fasting essential amino acid plasma levels in formulation of nutritionally adequate diets. IV. Lowering of human plasma cholesterol and triglyceride levels by lysine and tryptophan supplementation, *J. Pharm. Sci.*, 64, 691, 1975.

171. Hartroft, W. S., Ridout, J. H., Sellers, E. A., and Best, C. H., Atheromatous changes in aorta, carotid and coronary arteries of choline-deficient rats, *Proc. Soc. Exp. Biol. Med.*, 81, 384, 1952.

172. Wilgram, G. F., Best, C. H., and Blumenstein, J., Aggravating effect of cholesterol on cardiovascular changes in choline-deficient rats, *Proc. Soc. Exp. Biol. Med.*, 89, 476, 1955.

173. Salman, W. D. and Newberne, P. M., Cardiovascular disease in choline-deficient rats, *J. Nutr.*, 73, 26, 1962.

174. Sidransky, H., Verney, E., and Kurl, R. N., Effect of feeding a choline-deficient diet on the hepatic nuclear response to tryptophan in the rat, *Exp. Mol. Pathol.*, 51, 68, 1989.

175. Aviram, M., Cogan, U., and Mokady, S., Excessive dietary tryptophan enhances plasma lipid peroxidation in rats, 88, 29, 1991.

176. Heron, D. S., Shinitzky, M., Hershkowitz, M., and Samuel, D., Lipid fluidity markedly modulates the binding of serotonin to mouse brain membranes, *Proc. Natl. Acad. Sci. U.S.A.*, 77, 7463, 1980.

177. Engelberg, H., Low serum cholesterol and suicide, *Lancet*, 339, 727, 1992.

178. Baldo-Enzi, G., Baiocchi, M. R., Bertazzo, A., Costa, C. V., and Allegri, G., Tryptophan and atherosclerosis, *Adv. Exp. Med. Biol.*, 398, 429, 1996.

179. McMenamy, R. M. and Oncley, J. L., The specific binding of L-tryptophan to serum albumin, *J. Biol. Chem.*, 233, 1436, 1958.

180. Thomas, S. R. and Stocker R., Antioxidant activities and redox regulation of interferon-gamma-induced tryptophan metabolism in human monocytes and macrophages, *Adv. Exp. Med. Biol.*, 467, 541, 1999.

181. Christen, S., Thomas, S. R., Garner, B., and Stocker, R., Inhibition by interferon-gamma of human mononuclear cell-mediated low density lipoprotein oxidation. Participation of tryptophan metabolism along the kynurenine pathway, *J. Clin. Invest.*, 93, 2149, 1994.

182. Slater, T. F., Necrogenic action of carbon tetrachloride in the rat: A speculative mechanism based on activation, *Nature*, 209, 36, 1966.

183. Recknagel, R. O., Carbon tetrachloride hepatotoxicity, *Pharmacol. Rev.*, 19, 145, 1967.

184. Smuckler, E. A. and Koplitz, M., The effects of carbon tetrachloride and ethionine on RNA synthesis *in vivo* and in isolated rat liver nuclei, *Arch. Biochem. Biophys.*, 132, 62, 1969.

185. Farber, E., Biochemical pathology, *Annu. Rev. Pharmacol.*, 11, 71, 1971.

186. Sarma, D. S., Reid, I. M., Verney, E., and Sidransky, H., Studies on the nature of attachment of ribosomes to membranes in liver. I. Influence of ethionine, sparsomycin, CCl₄, and puromycin on membrane-bound polyribosomal disaggregation and on detachment of membrane-bound ribosomes from membranes, *Lab. Invest.*, 27, 39, 1972.

187. Sidransky, H., Verney, E., and Murty, C. N., Effect of tryptophan on hepatic polyribosomes and protein synthesis in rats treated with carbon tetrachloride, *Toxicol. Appl. Pharmacol.*, 39, 295, 1977.

188. Sidransky, H., Murty, C. N., and Verney, E., Effect of tryptophan on the inhibitory action of selected hepatotoxic agents on hepatic protein synthesis, *Exp. Mol. Pathol.*, 37, 305, 1982.

189. De Ferreyra, E. C., De Fenos, O. M., Bernacchi, A. S., de Castro, C. R., and Castro, J. A., Treatment of carbon tetrachloride-induced liver necrosis with chemical compounds, *Toxicol. Appl. Pharmacol.*, 42, 513, 1977.

190. De Ferreyra, E. C., De Fenos, O. M., and Castro, J. A., Tryptophan potentiation of the late cysteine preventive effects in carbon tetrachloride-induced necrosis, *Res. Commun. Chem. Pathol. Pharmacol.*, 40, 515, 1983.

191. De Toranzo, E. G., De Ferreyra, E. C., De Fenos, O. M., and Castro, J. A., Prevention of carbon tetrachloride-induced liver necrosis by several amino acids, *Br. J. Nutr.*, 64, 166, 1983.

192. Meister, A., Metabolism and functions of glutathione, *Trends Biochem. Sci.*, 6, 231, 1981.

193. Reed, D. J. and Beatty, P. W., Biosynthesis and regulation of glutathione: Toxicological implications, *Rev. Biochem. Toxicol.*, 2, 213, 1980.
194. Wang, D., Verney, E., and Sidransky, H., Protective effect of tryptophan and cysteine against carbon tetrachloride-induced liver injury, *Exp. Mol. Pathol.*, 43, 364, 1985.
195. De Ferreyra, E. C., De Fenos, O. M., and Castro, J. A., Modulation of galactosamine-induced liver injury by some amino acids or Triton WR1339, *Toxicol. Lett.*, 16, 63, 1983.
196. Ohta, Y., Kongo, M., Sasaki, E., Nishida, K., and Ishiguro, I., Therapeutic effect of melatonin on carbon tetrachloride-induced acute liver injury in rats, *J. Pineal Res.*, 28, 119, 2000.
197. Sidransky, H., Verney, E., and Sarma, D. S., Effect of tryptophan on hepatic polyribosomal disaggregation due to ethionine, *Exp. Biol. Med.*, 140, 633, 1972.
198. Sidransky, H. and Verney, E., Effect of diet and tryptophan on hepatic polyribosomal disaggregation due to actinomycin D, *Exp. Mol. Pathol.*, 17, 233, 1972.
199. Sarma, D. S., Bongiorno, M., Verney, E., and Sidransky, H., Effect of oral administration of tryptophan or water on hepatic polyribosomal disaggregation due to puromycin, *Exp. Mol. Pathol.*, 19, 23, 1973.
200. Sidransky, H. and Verney, E., Effect of cycloheximide on tryptophan binding to rat hepatic nuclei, *Amino Acids*, 18, 103, 2000.
201. Haussinger, D., Lang, F., and Gerok, W., Regulation of cell function by the cellular hydration state, *Am. J. Physiol.*, 267, E343, 1994.
202. Haussinger, D. and Schliess, F., Cell volume and hepatocellular function, *J. Hepatol.*, 22, 94, 1995.
203. Lynn, J. K., Murty, C. N., and Sidransky, H., Osmoregulation of ribosomal function in mouse liver, *Biochim. Biophys. Acta*, 299, 444, 1973.
204. Lynn, J. K., Sarma, D. S., and Sidransky, H., Response of hepatic polyribosomes of the mouse to the administration of anisotonic solutions, *Life Sci. Pt. 2 Biochem. Gen. Mol. Bio.*, 10, 385, 1971.
205. Lynn, J. K. and Sidransky, H., Effect of changes of osmotic pressure of portal blood on hepatic protein synthesis, *Lab. Invest.*, 31, 332, 1974.
206. Roeder, R. G. and Rutter, W. J., Multiple ribonucleic acid polymerases and ribonucleic acid synthesis during sea urchin development, *Biochemistry*, 9, 2543, 1970.
207. Sidransky, H., Verney, E., Murty, C. N., and Sarma, D. S., Sparsomycin-induced disaggregation but not detachment of hepatic membrane-bound polyribosomes, *Exp. Biol. Med.*, 157, 660, 1978.
208. Simons, S. S., Jr., Chakraborti, P. K., and Cavanaugh, A. H., Arsenite and cadmium(II) as probes of glucocorticoid receptor structure and function, *J. Biol. Chem.*, 265, 1938, 1990.
209. Tashima, Y., Terui, M., Itoh, H., Mizunuma, H., Kobayashi, R., and Marumo, F., Effect of selenite on glucocorticoid receptor, *J. Biochem.*, 105, 358, 1989.
210. Telford, W. G. and Fraker, P. J., Zinc reversibly inhibits steroid binding to murine glucocorticoid receptor, 238, 86, 1997.
211. Tonner, L. E., Katz, D. I., and Heiman, A. S., The acute effect of lead acetate on glucocorticoid receptor binding in C6 glioma cells, *Toxicology*, 116, 109, 1997.
212. Sidransky, H. and Verney, E., Influence of lead acetate and selected metal salts on tryptophan binding to rat hepatic nuclei, *Toxicol. Pathol.*, 27, 441, 1999.
213. Sidransky, H. and Verney, E., Influence of L-leucine on L-tryptophan binding to rat hepatic nuclei, *J. Nutr. Biochem.*, 8, 592, 1997.

214. Chen, S.-H., Estes, L. W., and Lombardi, B., Lecitin depletion in hepatic microsomal membranes of rats fed a choline-deficient diet, *Exp. Mol. Pathol.*, 17, 176, 1972.

215. Filipowicz, C. M. and McCauley, R. B., The effect of choline deficiency on the outer membranes of rat liver mitochondria, *Biochim. Biophys. Acta*, 734, 373, 1983.

216. Rushmore, T. H., Lim, Y. P., Farber, E., and Ghoshal, A. K., Rapid lipid peroxidation in the nuclear fraction of rat liver induced by a diet deficient in choline and methionine, *Cancer Lett.*, 24, 251, 1984.

217. Gupta, C., Hattori, A., Betschart, J. M., Virji, M. S., and Shinozuka, H., Modulation of epidermal growth factor receptors in rat hepatocytes by two liver tumor-promoting regimens, a choline-deficient diet and a phenobarbital diet, *Cancer Res.*, 48, 1162, 1988.

218. Betschart, J. M., Virji, M. A., Perera, M. I., and Shinozuka, H., Alterations in hepatocyte insulin receptors in rats fed a choline-deficient diet, *Cancer Res.*, 46, 4425, 1986.

219. Sidransky, H., Verney, E., and Murty, C. N., Effect of elevated dietary tryptophan on protein synthesis in rat liver, *J. Nutr.*, 111, 1942, 1981.

220. Sidransky, H., Tryptophan. Unique action by an essential amino acid, in *Nutritional Pathology: Pathobiochemistry of Dietary Imbalances*, Sidransky, H., Ed., Marcel Dekker, New York, 1985, 1–62.

221. Agutter, P. S., McArdle, H. J., and McCaldin, B., Evidence for involvement of nuclear envelope nucleoside triphosphatase in nucleocytoplasmic translocation of ribonucleoprotein, *Nature*, 263, 165, 1976.

222. Kurl, R. N., Verney, E., and Sidransky, H., Effect of tryptophan on rat hepatic nuclear poly(A)polymerase activity, *Amino Acids*, 5, 263, 1993.

223. Kroger, H., Gratz, R., Museteanu, C., and Haase, J., The influence of nicotinamide, tryptophan, and methionine upon galactosamine-induced effects in the liver, *Arzneimittel-Forschung*, 31, 987, 1981.

224. Franke, W. W., Structure, biochemistry, and functions of the nuclear envelope, *Int. Rev. Cytol.*, Suppl. 4, 71, 1974.

225. Oravec, M. and Korner, A., Stimulation of ribosomal and DNA-like RNA synthesis by tryptophan, *Biochim. Biophys. Acta*, 247, 404, 1971.

226. Sarma, D. S. R., Verney, E., Bongiorno, M., and Sidransky, H., Influence of tryptophan on hepatic polyribosomes and protein synthesis in non-fasted mice, *Nutr. Rep. Int.*, 4, 1, 1971.

227. Sidransky, H., Verney, E., Kurl, R. N., and Razavi, T., Effect of tryptophan on toxic cirrhosis induced by intermittent carbon tetrachloride intoxication in the rat, *Exp. Mol. Pathol.*, 49, 102, 1988.

228. Ohta, Y., Sahashi, D., Sasaki, E., and Ishiguro, I., Alleviation of carbon tetrachloride-induced chronic liver injury and related dysfunction by L-tryptophan in rats, *Ann. Clin. Biochem.*, 36, 504, 1999.

229. Sidransky, H., Verney, E., Cosgrove, J. W., and Schwartz, A. M., Inhibitory effect of demoxepam on tryptophan binding to rat hepatic nuclei, *Biochem. Med. Metab. Biol.*, 47, 270, 1992.

230. Braestrep, C. and Nielsen M., Benzodiazepine receptors, in *Handbook of Psychopharmacology. Biochemical Studies of CNS Receptors*, Iverson, L. L., Iverson, S. D., and Snyder, S. H., Eds. Plenum Press, New York, 1983, 285–384.

231. Ronnelspacher, H., Nanz, C., Borbe, H. O., Fehske, K. J., Muller, W. E., and Wollert, U., 1-Methyl-beta-carboline(harmane), a potent endogenous inhibitor of benzodiazepine receptor binding., *Naunyn-Schmiedebergs Arch. Pharmakol.*, 314, 97, 1980.

232. Sidransky, H., Verney, E., Cosgrove, J. W., and Schwartz, A.M., Effect of benzodiazepines on tryptophan binding to rat hepatic nuclei, *Toxicol. Pathol.*, 20, 350, 1992.

233. Verney, E. and Sidransky, H., Effect of metyrapone on tryptophan binding to rat hepatic nuclei, *Metab. Clin. Exp.*, 43, 79, 1994.

234. Sidransky, H. and Verney, E., Toxic effect of valproic acid on tryptophan binding to rat hepatic nuclei, *Toxicology*, 109, 39, 1996.

235. Bowdle, A. T., Patel, I. H., Levy, R. H., and Wilensky, A. J., Valproic acid dosage and plasma protein binding and clearance, *Clin. Pharmacol. Ther.*, 28, 486, 1980.

236. McMenemy, R. M., Lund, C. C., and Oncley, J. L., Unbound amino acid concentrations in human blood plasmas, *J. Clin. Invest.*, 36, 1672, 1957.

237. Gatti, G., Crema, F., Attardo-Parrinello, G., Fratino, P., Aguzzi, F., and Perucca, E., Serum protein binding of phenytoin and valproic acid in insulin-dependent diabetes mellitus, *Ther. Drug Monitor.*, 9, 389, 1987.

238. Nurge, M. E., Anderson, C. R., and Bates, E. B., Metabolic and nutritional implications of valproic acid, *Nutr. Res.*, 11, 949, 1991.

239. Prickett, K. S. and Baillie, T. A., Metabolism of valproic acid by hepatic microsomal cytochrome P-450, *Biochem. Biophys. Res. Commun.*, 122, 1166, 1984.

240. Fisher, R. L., Sanuik, J. T., Nau, H., Gandolfi, A. J., and Brendel, K., Comparative toxicity of valproic acid and its metabolites in liver slices from adult rats, weanling rats and humans, *Toxicol. in Vitro*, 8, 371, 1994.

241. Rettie, A. E., Rettenmeier, A. W., Howald, W.N., and Baillie, T. A., Cytochrome P-450-catalyzed formation of delta 4-VPA, a toxic metabolite of valproic acid, *Science*, 235, 890, 1987.

242. Jorgensen, A. J. and Majumdar, A. P., Influence of tryptophan on the level of hepatic microsomal cytochrome P-450 in well-fed normal, adrenalectomized, and phenobarbital-treated rats, *Biochim. Biophys. Acta*, 444, 453, 1976.

243. Evarts, R. P. and Mostafa, M. H., Effects of indole and tryptophan on cytochrome P-450, dimethylnitrosamine demethylase, and arylhydrocarbon hydroxylase activities, *Biochem. Pharmacol.*, 30, 517, 1981.

244. Dunning, W. F., Curtis, M. R., and Maun, M. E., The effect of added dietary tryptophane on the occurrence of 2-acetylaminofluorene-induced liver and bladder cancer in rats, *Cancer Res.*, 10, 454, 1950.

245. Sugimura, T., Kawachi, T., Nagao, M., et al., Mutagenic principle(s) in tryptophan and phenylalanine pyrolysis products, *Proc. Jpn. Acad.*, 53, 58, 1977.

246. Wattenberg, L W., Inhibitors of chemical carcinogenesis, in *Environmental Carcinogenesis*, Emmelot, P. and Kriek, E., Eds., Elsevier/North Holland Biomedical, Amsterdam, 1979, 241–264.

247. Boyland, E., Harris, J., and Horning, E. S., The induction of carcinoma of the bladder in rats with acetaminofluorene, *Br. J. Cancer*, 8, 647, 1954.

248. Brown, R. and Price, J. M., Quantitative studies on metabolism of tryptophan in the urine of the dog, cat, and man, *J. Biol. Chem.*, 219, 985, 1956.

249. Bryan, T., Role of tryptophan metabolites in urinary bladder cancer, *Am. Ind. Hyg. Assoc. J.*, 30, 27, 1969.

250. Radomski, J. L., Glass, E. M., and Deichmann, W. B., Transitional cell hyperplasia in the bladders of dogs fed DL-tryptophan, *Cancer Res.*, 31, 1690, 1971.

251. Miyakawa, M. and Yoshida, O., DNA synthesis of the urinary bladder epithelium in rats with long-term feeding of dl-tryptophan-added and pyridoxine-deficient diet, *Gann*, 64, 411, 1973.
252. Radomski, J. L., Radomski, T., and MacDonald, W. E., Cocarcinogenic interaction between D,L-tryptophan and 4-aminobiphenyl or 2-naphthylamine in dogs, *J. Natl. Cancer Inst.*, 58, 1831, 1977.
253. Matsushima, M., The role of L-tryptophan's promoting factor on tumorgenesis in the urinary bladder. 2. Urinary bladder carcinogenicity of FANFT (initiating factor) and L-tryptophan (promoting factor) in mice (author's transl., Japanese), *Jpn. J. Urol.*, 68, 731, 1977.
254. Cohen, S. M., Arai, M., Jacobs, J. B., and Friedell, G. H., Promoting effect of saccharin and DL-tryptophan in urinary bladder carcinogenesis, *Cancer Res.*, 39, 1207, 1979.
255. Fukushima, S., Friedell, G. H., Jacobs, J. B., and Cohen, S. M., Effect of L-tryptophan and sodium saccharin on urinary tract carcinogenesis initiated by N-[4-(5-nitro-2-furyl)-2-thiazolyl]formamide, *Cancer Res.*, 41, 3100, 1981.
256. Birt, D. F., Julius, A. D., Hasegawa, R., St. John, M., and Cohen, S. M., Effect of L-tryptophan excess and vitamin B6 deficiency on rat urinary bladder cancer promotion, *Cancer Res.*, 47, 1244, 1987.
257. Sakata, T., Shirai, T., Fukushima, S., Hasegawa, R., and Ito, N., Summation and synergism in the promotion of urinary bladder carcinogenesis initiated by N-butyl-N-(4-hydroxybutyl)-nitrosamine in F344 rats, *Gann*, 75, 950, 1984.
258. Dunning, W. F. and Curtis, M. R., The role of indole in incidence of 2-acetylaminofluorene-induced bladder cancer in rats, *Proc. Soc. Exp. Biol. Med.*, 99, 91, 1958.
259. Oyasu, R., Miller, D. A., McDonald, J. H., and Hass, G. M., Neoplasms of rat urinary bladder and liver: Rat fed 2-acetylaminofluorene and indole, *Arch. Pathol.*, 75, 184, 1963.
260. Oyasu, R., Battifora, H. A., Eisenstein, R., McDonald, J. H., and Hass, G. M., Enhancement of tumorigenesis in the urinary bladder of rats by neonatal administration of 2-acetylaminofluorene, *J. Natl. Cancer Inst.*, 40, 377, 1968.
261. Allen, M. J., Boyland, E., Dukes, C. E., Horning, E. S., and Watson, J. G., Cancer of the urinary bladder induced in mice with metabolites of aromatic amines and trptophan, *Br. J. Cancer*, 11, 212, 1957.
262. Clayson, D. B., Jull, J. W., and Bonser, G. M., The testing of ortho hydroxyamines and related compounds by bladder implantation and a discussion of their structural requirements for carcinogenic activity, *Br. J. Cancer*, 12, 222, 1958.
263. Bryan, G. T., The role of urinary tryptophan metabolites in the etiology of bladder cancer, *Am. J. Clin. Nutr.* 24, 841, 1971.
264. Cohen, S. M., Masui, T., Garland, E. M., and Arnold, L. L., Effects of diet on urinary bladder carcinogenesis and cancer prevention, *J. Nutr*, 127, 826S, 1997.
265. Nagao, M., Yahagi, T., Kawachi, T., et al., Mutagens in foods, especially pyrolysis products of protein, in *Progress in Genetic Toxicology*, Scott, D., Bridges, B. A., and Sobels, F. H., Eds., Elsevier/North Holland Biomedical, Amsterdam, 1977, 259–264.
266. Hashida, C., Nagayama, K., and Takemura, N., Induction of bladder cancer in mice by implanting pellets containing tryptophan pyrolysis products, *Cancer Lett.*, 17, 101, 1982.

267. Ames, B. N., Mccann, J., and Yamasaki, E., Methods for detecting carcinogens and mutagens with the *Salmonella*/mammalian-microsome mutagenicity test, *Mutation Res.*, 31, 347, 1975.

268. de Waziers, I. and Decloitre, F., Formation of mutagenic derivatives from tryptophan pyrolysis products (Trp P1 and Trp P2) by rat intestinal S9 fraction, *Mutation Res.*, 119, 103, 1983.

269. Mita, S., Yamazoe, Y., Kamataki, T., and Kato, R., Metabolic activation of a tryptophan pyrolysis product, 3-amino-1-methyl-5H-pyrido[4,3-b]indole (TRP-P-2) by isolated rat liver nuclei, *Cancer Lett.*, 14, 261, 1981.

270. Yamazoe, Y., Ishii, K., Kamataki, T., Kato, R., and Sugimura, T., Isolation and characterization of active metabolites of tryptophan-pyrolysate mutagen, TRP-P-2, formed by rat liver microsomes, *Chemico-Biol. Interact.*, 30, 125, 1980.

271. Mita, S., Ishii, K., Yamazoe, Y., Kamataki, T., Kato, R., and Sugimura, T., Evidence for the involvement of N-hydroxylation of 3-amino-1-methyl-5H-pyrido[4,3-b]indole by cytochrome P-450 in the covalent binding to DNA, *Cancer Res.*, 41, 3610, 1981.

272. Kawachi, T., Hirata, Y., and Sugimura, T., Enhancement of N-nitrosodiethylamine hepato-carcinogenesis by L-tryptophan in rats, *Gann*, 59, 523, 1968.

273. Okajima, E., Hiramatsu, T., Motomiya, Y., Iriya, K., and Ijuin, M., Effect of DL-tryptophan on tumorigenesis in the urinary bladder and liver of rats treated with N-nitrosodibutylamine, *Gann*, 62, 163, 1971.

274. Evarts, R. P. and Brown, C. A., Effect of L-tryptophan on diethylnitrosamine and 3'-methyl-4-n-dimethylaminoazobenzene hepatocarcinogenesis, *Food & Cosmetics Toxicol.*, 15, 431, 1977.

275. Sidransky, H., Garrett, C. T., Murty, C. N., Verney, E., and Robinson, E. S., Influence of dietary tryptophan on the induction of gamma-glutamyltranspeptidase-positive foci in the livers of rats treated with hepatocarcinogen, *Cancer Res.*, 45, 4844, 1985.

276. Takahashi, S., Lombardi, B., and Shinozuka, H., Progression of carcinogen-induced foci of gamma-glutamyltranspeptidase-positive hepatocytes to hepatomas in rats fed a choline-deficient diet, *Int. J. Cancer*, 29, 445, 1982.

277. Shinozuka, H. and Lombardi, B., Synergistic effect of a choline-devoid diet and phenobarbital in promoting the emergence of foci of gamma-glutamyl-transpeptidase-positive hepatocytes in the liver of carcinogen-treated rats, *Cancer Res.*, 40, 3846, 1980.

278. Sidransky, H., Verney, E., and Wang, D., Effects of varying fat content of a high tryptophan diet on the induction of gamma-glutamyltranspeptidase positive foci in the livers of rats treated with hepatocarcinogen, *Cancer Lett.*, 31, 235, 1986.

279. Verney, E., Wang, D., and Sidransky, H., Influence of level of dietary protein on tryptophan-induced promotional activity in induction of gamma-glutamyl transpeptidase-positive foci of rat liver, *Exp. Mol. Pathol.*, 47, 279, 1987.

280. Matsukura, N., Kawachi, T., Wakabayashi, K., Ohgaki, H., Morino, K., Sugimura, T., Nukaya, H., and Kosuge, T., Liver cancer and precancerous changes in rats induced by the basic fraction of tryptophan pyrolysate, *Cancer Lett.*, 13, 181, 1981.

281. Matsukura, N., Kawachi, T., Morino, K., Ohgaki, H., Sugimura, T., and Takayama, S., Carcinogenicity in mice of mutagenic compounds from a tryptophan pyrolyzate, *Science*, 213, 346, 1981.

282. Hosaka, S., Matsushima, T., Hirono, I., and Sugimura, T., Carcinogenic activity of 3-amino-1-methyl-5H-pyrido [4,3-b]indole (Trp-P-2), a pyrolysis product of tryptophan, *Cancer Lett.*, 13, 23, 1981.

283. Ishikawa, T., Takayama, S., Kitagawa, T., et al., *In vivo* experiments of trptophan pyrolysis products, in *Naturally Occurring Carcinogens-Mutagens and Modulators of Carcinogenesis*, Miller, E. C., Miller, I., Hirono, T., et al., Eds., University Park, Baltimore, MD, 1979, 159–167.

284. Ishikawa, T., Takayama, S., Kitagawa, T., Kawachi, T., and Sugimura, T., Induction of enzyme-altered islands in rat liver by tryptophan pyrolysis products, *J. Cancer Res. Clin. Oncol.*, 95, 221, 1979.

285. Tamano, S., Tsuda, H., Tatematsu, M., Hasegawa, R., Imaida, K., and Ito, N., Induction of gamma-glutamyl transpeptidase positive foci in rat liver by pyrolysis products of amino acids, *Gann*, 72, 747, 1981.

286. Rabache, M. and Adian J., Effects des Pyrolysate de Tryptophan et D'arginine-tryptophan Sue L'ingere, la Croissance et l'Effecacite Alimentaire Chez le Rat, *Sci. Aliments*, 4, 299, 1984.

287. Berry, D. L. and Helmes, C. T., Role of epigenetic factors in dietary carcinogenesis, in *Nutritional and Toxicological Aspects of Food Safety*, Friedman, M., Ed., Plenum Press, New York, 1984, 91.

288. Sidransky, H., Role of tryptophan in carcinogenesis, *Adv. Exp. Med. Biol.*, 72, 187, 1986.

289. Williams, D. J., Tryptophan, urinary quinolines, and bladder cancer, *Nutr. Cancer*, 11, 81, 1988.

290. Donoso, M. L. N., Valenzuela, A., and Silva, E., Tryptophan-riboflavin photoinduced adduct and hepatic dysfunction in rats, *Nutr. Rep. Int.*, 37, 599, 1988.

291. Sugimura, T., Studies on environmental chemical carcinogenesis in Japan, *Science*, 233, 312, 1986.

292. Weisburger, J. H., On the mechanisms relevant to nutritional carcinogenesis, *Prev. Med.*, 16, 586, 1987.

293. Krone, C. A., Yeh, S. M., and Iwaoka, W. T., Mutagen formation during commercial processing of foods, *Environ. Health Persp.*, 67, 75, 1986.

294. Ohgaki, H., Hasegawa, H., Kato, T., Suenaga, M., Ubukata, M., Sato, S., Takayama, S., and Sugimura, T. Carcinogenicity in mice and rats of heterocyclic amines in cooked foods, *Environ. Health Persp.*, 67, 129, 1986.

295. Hatch, T. F. and Felton J. S., Toxicologic strategy for mutagens in foods during cooking, *Genetic Toxicology of the Diet*, Knudsen, I., Ed., Alan R. Liss, New York, 109, 1986.

296. Degawa, M., Hishinuma, T., Yoshida, H., and Hashimoto, Y., Species, sex and organ differences in induction of a cytochrome P-450 isozyme responsible for carcinogen activation: Effects of dietary hepatocarcinogenic tryptophan pyrolysate components in mice and rats, *Carcinogenesis*, 8, 1913, 1987.

297. National Cancer Institute, Bioassay of L-tryptophan for Possible Carcinogenicity, DHEW Publ. (NIH) 78-1321, U. S. Government Printing Office, Washington, D.C., 1978.

298. Kurl, R. N., Barsoum, A. L., and Sidransky, H., Association of poly(A)polymerase with tryptophan receptor in rat hepatic nuclei, *J. Nutr. Biochem.*, 3, 366, 1992.

299. Schimke, R. T., Sweeney, E. W., and Berlin, C. M., The roles of synthesis and degradation in the control of rat liver tryptophan pyrrolase, *J. Biol. Chem.*, 240, 322, 1965.

300. Cihak, A. L., Tryptophan action on hepatic RNA synthesis and enzyme induction, *Mol. Cell. Biochem.*, 24, 131, 1979.

301. Smith, S. A., Marston, F. A., Dickson, A. J., and Pogson, C. I., Control of enzyme activities in rat liver by tryptophan and its metabolites, *Biochem. Pharmacol.*, 28, 1645, 1979.

302. Farber, E., Hepatocyte proliferation in stepwise development of experimental liver cell cancer, *Dig. Dis. Sci.*, 36, 973, 1991.

303. Farber, E., Cell proliferation as a major risk factor for cancer: A concept of doubtful validity, *Cancer Res.*, 55, 3759, 1995.

304. Wang, D., Verney, E., Kurl, R. N., and Sidransky, H., Effect of tryptophan on isolated hepatocytes of rats, *Virchows Archiv B, Cell Pathol. Mol. Pathol.*, 53, 125, 1987.

305. Janne, J., Holtta, E., and Guha, S. K., Polyamines in mammalian liver during growth and development, in *Progress in Liver Disease*, Popper, H. and Schaffner, F., Eds., Grune & Stratton, New York, 1976, 5, 100–124.

306. Boutwell, R. K., Biochemical mechanism of tumor promotion, in *Carcinogenesis*, 2nd ed., Slaga, J. J., Swak, A., and Boutwell, R. K., Eds., Raven Press, New York, 1978, 49–58.

307. O'Brien, T. G., The induction of ornithine decarboxylase as an early, possibly obligatory, event in mouse skin carcinogenesis, *Cancer Res.*, 36, 2644, 1976.

308. Matsuschima, M., Takano, S., Erturk, E., and Bryan, G. T., Induction of ornithine decarboxylase activity in mouse urinary bladder by L-tryptophan and some of its metabolites, *Cancer Res.*, 42, 3587, 1982.

309. Sidransky, H., Murty, C. N., Myers, E., and Verney, E., Tryptophan-induced stimulation of hepatic ornithine decarboxylase activity in the rat, *Exp. Mol. Pathol.*, 38, 346, 1983.

310. Byus, C. V., Costa, M., Sipes, I. G., Brodie, B. B., and Russell, D. H., Activation of 3':5'-cyclic AMP-dependent protein kinase and induction of ornithine decarboxylase as early events in induction of mixed-function oxygenases, *Proc. Natl. Acad. Sci. U.S.A.*, 73, 1241, 1976.

311. Russell, D. H. and Levy, C. C., Polyamine accumulation and biosynthesis in a mouse L1210 leukemia, *Cancer Res.*, 31, 248, 1971.

312. Cavia, E. and Webb, T. E., The polyamine content in two slow-growing rat hepatomas, *Biochemical J.*, 129, 223, 1972.

313. Mikol, Y. B. and Poirier, L. A., An inverse correlation between hepatic ornithine decarboxylase and S-adenosylmethionine in rats, *Cancer Lett.*, 13, 195, 1981.

314. Miller, J. A. and Miller, E. C., The metabolic activation of carcinogenic aromatic amines and amides, *Progr. Exp. Tumor Res.*, 11, 273, 1969.

315. Larsen-Su, S. and Williams, D. E., Dietary indole-3-carbinol inhibits FMO activity and the expression of flavin-containing monooxygenase form 1 in rat liver and intestine, *Drug Metab. Disposition*, 24, 927, 1996.

316. Perdew, G. H. and Babbs, C. F., Production of Ah receptor ligands in rat fecal suspensions containing tryptophan or indole-3-carbinol, *Nutr. Cancer*, 16, 209, 1991.

317. Vesley, J. and Cihak, A., Enhanced DNA-dependent RNA polymerase and RNA synthesis in rat liver nuclei after administration of L-tryptophan, *Biochim. Biophys. Acta*, 204, 614, 1970.

318. Evarts, R. P. and Mostafa, M.H., The effect of L-tryptophan and certain other amino acids on liver nitrosodimethylamine demethylase activity, *Food & Cosmetics Toxicol.*, 16, 585, 1978.

319. Ames, B. N., Gold, L. S., and Willett, W. C., The causes and prevention of cancer, *Proc. Natl. Acad. Sci. U.S.A.*, 92, 5258, 1995.
320. Weisburger, J. H., Nutritional approach to cancer prevention with emphasis on vitamins, antioxidants, and carotenoids, *Am. J. Clin. Nutr.*, 53, 226S, 1991.
321. Christen, S., Peterhans, E., and Stocker, R., Antioxidant activities of some tryptophan metabolites: Possible implication for inflammatory diseases, *Proc. Natl. Acad. Sci. U.S.A.*, 87, 2506, 1990.
322. Sidransky, H. and Verney, E., Effect of nutritional alterations on protein synthesis in transplantable hepatomas and host livers of rats, *Cancer Res.*, 39, 1995, 1979.
323. Sidransky, H., Kurl, R. N., Holmes, S. C., and Verney, E., Tryptophan binding to nuclei of rat liver and hepatoma, *J. Nutr. Biochem.*, 6, 73, 1995.
324. Sidransky, H., Verney, E., and Murty, C. N., Effect of tryptophan on hepatoma and host liver of rats. Influence after treatment with hypertonic sodium chloride and carbon tetrachloride, *Exp. Mol. Pathol.*, 35, 124, 1981.
325. Sidransky, H. and Verney, E., Effect of inhibitory and stimulatory agents on protein synthesis in hepatomas and host livers of rats, *J. Natl. Cancer Inst.*, 63, 81, 1979.
326. Patel, N. T., Yoshida, M., and Holoubek, V., *In vitro* incorporation of 3'-methyl-4-dimethylaminoazobenzene into liver nuclei and release of RNA from the nuclei, *Cancer Res.*, 41, 743, 1981.
327. Shearer, R. W. and Smuckler, E. A., A search for gene derepression in RNA of primary rat hepatomas, *Cancer Res.*, 31, 2104, 1971.
328. Brtko, J., Knopp, J. and Baker, M. E., Inhibition of 3,5,3'-triiodothyronine binding to its receptor by protease inhibitors and substrates, *Mol. Cell Endocrinol.*, 93, 811, 1993.
329. Brtko, J. and Filipcik, P., Effect of selenite and selenate on rat liver nuclear 3,5,3'-triiodothyronine (T3) receptor, *Biol. Trace Element Res.*, 41, 191, 1994.
330. Sidransky, H. and Verney, E., The presence of thiols in the hepatic nuclear binding site for L-tryptophan: Studies with selenite, *Nutr. Res.*, 16, 1023, 1996.
331. Thompson, C. C. and Evans, R. M., Trans-activation by thyroid hormone receptors: Functional parallels with steroid hormone receptors, *Proc. Natl. Acad. Sci. U.S.A.*, 86, 3494, 1989.
332. Sidransky, H., Wagner, B. P., and Morris, H. P., Sex differences in liver tumorigenesis in rats ingesting N-2-fluorenylacetamide, *J. Natl. Cancer Inst.*, 26, 151, 1987.
333. Kapoor, R. K., Kuksis, A., Farber, E., and Ghoshal, A. K., Alterations in hepatic nuclear membranes during hepatocarcinogenesis induced by a diet devoid of choline, *Proc. Am. Assoc. Cancer Res.*, 29, 150, 1988.
334. Ghoshal, A. K. and Farber, E., The induction of liver cancer by dietary deficiency of choline and methionine without added carcinogens, *Carcinogenesis*, 5, 1367, 1984.
335. Sidransky, H., Tryptophan and carcinogenesis: Review and update on how tryptophan may act, *Nutr. Cancer*, 29, 181, 1997.
336. Unkila, M., Ruotsalainen, M., Pohjanvirta, R., Viluksela, M., MacDonald, E., Tuomisto, J. T., Rozman, K., and Tuomisto, J., Effect of 2,3,7,8-tetrachlorodibenzo-p-dioxin (TCDD) on tryptophan and glucose homeostasis in the most TCDD-susceptible and the most TCDD-resistant species, guinea pigs and hamsters, *Arch. Toxicol.*, 69, 677, 1995.

337. Fernandez-Salguero, P., Pineau, T., Hilbert, D. M., McPhail, T., Lee, S. S., Kimura, S., Nebert, D. W., Rudikoff, S., Ward, J. M., and Gonzalez, F. J., Immune system impairment and hepatic fibrosis in mice lacking the dioxin-binding Ah receptor, *Science*, 268, 722, 1995.
338. Stewart, W. E., II., *The Interferon System*, Springer-Verlag, New York, 2001.
339. Villllcek, J. P. W., Grey, E., Rinderknrcht, E., and Sevastopoulos, C. G., Interferon-V: A lymphokine for all seasons, *Lymphokines*, 11, 1, 1985.
340. Pfefferkorn, E. R., Interferon gamma blocks the growth of *Toxoplasma gondii* in human fibroblasts by inducing the host cells to degrade tryptophan, *Proc. Natl. Acad. Sci. U.S.A.*, 81, 908, 1984.
341. Denz, H., Lechleitner, M., Marth, C., Daxenbichler, G., Gastl, G., and Braunsteiner, H., Effect of human recombinant alpha-2- and gamma-interferon on the growth of human cell lines from solid tumors and hematologic malignancies, *J. Interferon Res*, 5, 147, 1985.
342. de la Maza, L. M. and Peterson, E. M., Dependence of the *in vitro* antiproliferative activity of recombinant human gamma-interferon on the concentration of tryptophan in culture media, *Cancer Res.*, 48, 346, 1988.
343. Ozaki, Y., Edelstein, M. P., and Duch, D. S., Induction of indoleamine 2,3-dioxygenase: A mechanism of the antitumor activity of interferon gamma, *Proc. Natl. Acad. Sci. U.S.A.*, 85, 1242, 1988.
344. Aune, T.M. and Pogue, S. L., Inhibition of tumor cell growth by interferon-gamma is mediated by two distinct mechanisms dependent upon oxygen tension: Induction of tryptophan degradation and depletion of intracellular nicotinamide adenine dinucleotide, *J. Clin. Invest.*, 84, 863, 1989.
345. Werner-Felmayer, G., Werner, E. R., Fuchs, D., Hausen, A., Reibnegger, G., and Wachter, H., Characteristics of interferon induced tryptophan metabolism in human cells in vitro, *Biochim. Biophys. Acta*, 1012, 140, 1989.
346. Rubin, B. Y., Anderson, S. L., Xing, L., Powell, R. J., and Tate, W. P., Interferon induces tryptophanyl-tRNA synthetase expression in human fibroblasts, *J. Biol. Chem.*, 266, 24245, 1991.
347. Feng, G.S. and Taylor, M.W., Interferon gamma-resistant mutants are defective in the induction of indoleamine 2,3-dioxygenase, *Proc. Natl. Acad. Sci. U.S.A.*, 86, 7144, 1989.
348. Ozes, O. N. and Taylor, M. W., Reversal of an interferon-gamma-resistant phenotype by poly(I:C): Possible role of double-stranded RNA-activated kinase in interferon-gamma signaling, *J. Interferon Res.*, 13, 283, 1993.
349. Taylor, M. W., Konan, V. K., and Yu, D., Tryptophan starvation is involved in human interferon-gamma mediated apoptosis, *Adv. Exp. Med. Biol.*, 398, 155, 1996.
350. Konan, K. V. and Taylor, M. W., Treatment of ME180 cells with interferon-gamma causes apoptosis as a result of tryptophan starvation, *J. Interferon Cytokine Res.*, 16, 751, 1996.

7

Effects or Influences on Organ Systems

CONTENTS

7.1 Central Nervous System

The effects of L-tryptophan on the central nervous system have been investigated mainly in studies with acute tryptophan depletion. This approach has been utilized on a wide variety of neuropsychiatric conditions in humans and also in experimental models in animals. The rationale is that the rapid decrease in L-tryptophan levels in the circulation leads to a decrease in brain serotonin levels.

This section describes the rationale for the utilization of dietary tryptophan depletion. Also, it reviews a number of studies designed to determine the consequences of acute tryptophan depletion upon a variety of disorders in humans and conditions in animals. The literature contains a plethora of reports utilizing acute tryptophan depletion. Selected examples have been chosen to illustrate the effects or influences of L-tryptophan levels on a variety of behavioral and psychiatric states.

7.1.1 Rationale for Utilization of Acute Tryptophan Depletion to Decrease Circulating Tryptophan Levels

Gessa et al.[1] were the first to demonstrate that the acute administration of an amino acid mixture containing all of the essential amino acids, except tryptophan, caused a rapid fall in plasma free and total tryptophan in rats. Furthermore, this effect was associated with a parallel depletion in brain tryptophan, serotonin, and 5-hydroxyindole acetic acid in rats.[2] These early studies opened the way for subsequent studies, using acute tryptophan depletion by feeding a tryptophan-free amino acid mixture, a simple, specific, and nontoxic method, to delete brain serotonin and thus provide a tool for clarifying the physiological role of serotonin in the central nervous system.

In considering the mechanism for the observed fall in serum tryptophan in acute tryptophan depletion studies, Gessa et al.,[3] as well as others,[4] have attributed the fall to a rapid renewal of endogenous tryptophan from the circulation, secondary to an increased incorporation of tryptophan into proteins in liver and other organs. Support for this hypothesis came from studies on the effect of the ingestion of the tryptophan-free diet in rats that had been treated with cycloheximide, a protein synthesis inhibitor, 1 or 2 h prior to food ingestion.[3,4] Under these conditions, the tryptophan-free diet failed to decrease the tryptophan concentrations in serum and in the central nervous system. However, Moja et al.[4] reported that the control (saline) group that received cycloheximide alone showed an elevation of plasma and brain tryptophan levels. This suggests that cycloheximide alone, probably via inhibition of protein synthesis, may cause a rise in plasma tryptophan by a protein catabolism.

The interpretation of the data based upon the administration of cycloheximide merits caution in regard to identifying its principal effect as the inhibition of protein synthesis. For example, it may have other actions.

Sidransky and Verney[5] reported that cycloheximide added *in vitro* diminished ^{3}H-tryptophan binding to hepatic nuclei, probably related to its structural effect on the nuclear receptor. This effect may also occur *in vivo*, in addition to cycloheximide's action in inhibiting tissue and organ protein synthesis, and may possibly contribute in a minor way to the alteration in tryptophan level in serum.

A number of experimental studies have revealed that responses relating to hepatic protein synthesis are variable depending upon the experimental conditions. For example, the acute administration of one feeding of a complete amino acid mixture or of L-tryptophan alone has a stimulatory effect on hepatic protein synthesis compared to that of a tryptophan-free amino acid mixture which does not.[6] This occurs in fasted[6] or fed rats.[7] On the other hand, multiple tube feedings of a complete diet devoid of tryptophan compared to that of a complete diet for 1 day stimulated hepatic protein synthesis.[8] Also, in other experiments where rats were tube-fed for 1 to 7 days complete diets devoid of other single essential amino acids compared to those of rats tube-fed complete diets, they revealed enhanced hepatic protein synthesis.[9–13] Thus, experimental conditions relating to route of feeding, dosage, timing, and other variable-controlled conditions may influence the response of hepatic protein synthesis. Such may be the case in studies with cycloheximide.

Many studies have described how L-tryptophan itself may be an important regulator of hepatic protein synthesis under normal or abnormal conditions.[14–16] Based upon these reports, the hypothesis of Gessa et al.[3] that the primary effect of administering a tryptophan-free amino acid mixture that lowers endogenous tryptophan serum levels via increased incorporation of tryptophan into hepatic and other proteins must be viewed with caution. Possibly, the overall decrease in serum tryptophan that occurs is due to decreased ingestion of tryptophan along with adequate intake of other amino acids which may stimulate muscle protein catabolism. This may liberate tryptophan and other amino acids into the circulation, which may rapidly enhance hepatic protein synthesis and thereby deplete plasma tryptophan levels. This mechanism was proposed earlier in studies with dietary tryptophan deficiency.[17]

7.1.2 Experimental Studies with Acute Tryptophan Depletion

Acute tryptophan depletion has been a research strategy that rapidly reduces the availability of tryptophan, especially as it relates to being the precursor to serotonin, and thus provides a useful tool for studying the behavioral consequences of low brain serotonin.

7.1.2.1 Human Studies

Subjects were given a mixture of amino acids devoid of tryptophan. This led to a rapid (5 h) and substantial (80 to 90%) lowering of tryptophan in plasma and tissues.[18-21] This decline in tryptophan is considered to reduce the rate of brain serotonin synthesis. Resulting changes in mood or behavior are believed to be a consequence of the effects of the tryptophan-deficient amino acid mixture and, thereby, to result from a lowering of central nervous system serotonin. Also, the behavioral effects may be related in part to alterations in brain levels of other potentially psychoactive metabolites of tryptophan, such as tryptamine, melatonin, quinolinic acid, or kynurenic acid, and even to alterations in brain protein synthesis.

A unique aspect of acute tryptophan depletion is that it reduces brain serotonin with a specificity that most pharmacological probes are unable to achieve due to their simultaneous effects on multiple synaptic systems. For example, in healthy subjects, tryptophan depletion causes an acute, but brief, lowering of mood.[19,21-23]

In attempting to evaluate mood changes, studies of normal male volunteers on acute tryptophan depletion have resulted in significant lowering of mood in some subject groups[19,22,24] but not in others.[21,25,26] This discrepancy was considered to be due to differences in the baseline mood state among studies. Also, in depressed patients taking antidepressant medications, tryptophan depletion caused a return of depressive symptoms, with peak effects at 5 to 7 h after the tryptophan-free amino acid drink had been ingested.[20,27,28]

The literature contains many studies relating to tryptophan depletion and various psychiatric diseases. Before beginning a discussion of human conditions in which decreased availability of L-tryptophan may play a role in the symptomatology of the disorder, one must mention pellagra, which is caused by a deficiency of niacin. Pellagra was described as being associated with poverty and diets that relied heavily on corn, which is low in both niacin and its precursor, tryptophan.[29,30] Nonetheless, since it is not due per se to tryptophan deficiency itself, this condition is not included in the diseases reviewed in this chapter.

7.1.2.1.1 *Mood Disorders (General)*

Young et al.[19] reported that normal male human subjects who ingested an amino acid mixture that was tryptophan-free revealed a marked depletion of plasma tryptophan at 5 h and revealed a rapid mood-lowering effect. These subjects had significantly elevated scores on the depression scale of the Multiple Affect Adjective Checklist and performed scores in a proofreading task carried out while listening to a tape with themes of hopelessness and helplessness (dysphoric distractor) compared with controls (fed a balanced amino acid mixture or one with excess tryptophan).

Ellenbogen et al.[31] studied the mood response to acute tryptophan depletion in healthy euthymic women devoid of any personal or familial history of psychiatric illness. Like the males, the women exhibited a significant lowering of mood.

Leyton et al.[32] fed a tryptophan-free amino acid mixture to fully remitted, medication-free, former patients with major depression and observed no significant effect on mood. These results suggested that a previous report[20] that acute tryptophan depletion substantially lowered mood in pharmacologically treated patients probably reflected a mechanism involved in the therapeutic effects of antidepressants.

The involvement of the central nervous system serotonin function in the pathogenesis and treatment of affective disorders has been a subject of intensive research during the past 30 years.[33-36] Studies using serotonin precursors and agonists as pharmacologic probes and measurements of cerebrospinal fluid monoamine metabolite levels indicated that alterations in central nervous system serotonin function may be involved in the pathophysiology of depression. Since the synthesis of serotonin depends on dietary intake of the precursor tryptophan, many studies have utilized tryptophan depletion techniques by which patients were fed a tryptophan-free diet for various time intervals.

Delgado et al.[20] studied the behavioral effects of rapid (24 h) tryptophan depletion in patients in antidepressant-induced remission. Patients receiving antidepressants leading to remission were then given a tryptophan-free amino acid drink, and they experienced a depressive relapse. Free plasma tryptophan level was negatively correlated with the depression score during acute tryptophan depletion. A number of other studies on the effects of tryptophan depletion on relapse of depression after treatment confirmed the previous findings.[37-41]

In view of the interest in low serotonin levels in the etiology of depression, several groups have looked at tryptophan levels or the plasma ratio of tryptophan to other large neutral amino acids in depressed patients. Values are often found to be low in depression.[42-46] However, the magnitude of the decline is too small to cause an appreciable decline in brain serotonin, and it is unlikely that reduced tryptophan availability is involved in the etiology of most cases of depression. Nonetheless, the low plasma tryptophan ratio is capable of predicting the response to a variety of different antidepressant drugs.[47]

The consensus of the antidepressant effect of tryptophan is that it is not as effective as a standard antidepressant in severely depressed inpatients.[48-50] However, one clinical trial of tryptophan in depression conducted on mild to moderately depressed outpatients concluded that tryptophan (3 g/d) was more effective than placebo and was as effective as amitriptyline.[51] Tryptophan produced no more side effects than placebo and significantly fewer side effects than amitriptyline.

Several early studies suggest that tryptophan can potentiate the antidepressant effect of monoamine oxidase inhibitors. However, since it also tends to potentiate the side effects of these drugs, the combination is usually used only in treatment-resistant patients. Even though tryptophan potentiates the action of monoamine oxidase inhibitors, it does not seem to potentiate the action of other antidepressant treatments such as tricyclic antidepressant and electroconvulsive therapy.[52]

Seasonal affective disorder (SAD), or winter depression, is a subtype of mood disorder characterized by recurrent major depressive episodes that occur regularly in the fall and winter months, with spontaneous remission in the spring and summer. It appears to respond to exposure to bright light, termed light therapy. However, the mechanism of action of light therapy, as well as the pathophysiology of SAD, is still poorly understood. Several lines of research suggest that the serotonin mechanisms may be important. Lam et al.[53] examined the effects of rapid tryptophan depletion using a low tryptophan diet in patients with SAD who were in remission with light therapy. Indeed, this rapid tryptophan depletion appeared to reverse the antidepressant effect of bright light therapy in patients with SAD. They interpreted their findings to suggest that the therapeutic effect of bright light in SAD may involve a serotonergic mechanism. These findings were substantiated by Neumeister et al.,[54] who found that short-term tryptophan depletion, which induced a significant decrease in plasma free and total tryptophan levels, led to a transient depressive relapse.

In 1990, McGrath et al.[55] in a small study used tryptophan treatment of seasonal affective disorder and reported that the response was significantly better than with placebo.

7.1.2.1.2 Specific Conditions

7.1.2.1.2.1 Aggression — The putative role of serotonin in aggressive behavior has been the subject of much varied research. Using tryptophan depletion or enhancement as a mechanism for altering brain levels of serotonin acutely, selected studies have been conducted. Cleare and Bond[24] reported on a study that used an amino acid mixture drink without or with tryptophan on patients with high trait aggression or with low trait aggression. The former group on the tryptophan-free mixture became more angry, aggressive, annoyed, hostile, and quarrelsome, whereas those given the tryptophan-containing mixture responded in the opposite way. In the latter group, no consistent effects were found. In other studies using healthy male subjects given a tryptophan-free amino acid mixture, the findings indicated that such subjects demonstrated increased aggressive responses.[56,57]

Reilly et al.[58] reviewed the literature for the period from 1980 through 1996 which covered 44 double-blind studies in humans and 3 clinical case reports, covering a range of psychiatric disorders including mood disorders and aggression. They suggested that the mood change induced by tryptophan depletion might predict those likely to respond to serotonin-specific drugs. Rapid tryptophan depletion has been reported by many studies to exacerbate aggression in vulnerable individuals.

Dougherty and co-workers[59,60] reported in 1999 that, in male subjects following the ingestion of a tryptophan-depleted beverage, laboratory aggression increased but not after ingestion of a tryptophan-containing beverage. The increases in aggression under tryptophan-depleted conditions were specific to men who scored the highest on the Buss-Perry Aggressive Questionnaire. They concluded that hostile men, compared to nonhostile men, might be more prone to behavior change induced by the perturbation of the serotonin neurotransmitter system. In another report,[61] they concluded from their studies with males that (1) subsets of individuals (e.g., persons self-rating high on aggressive or hostility scales) may differ in their susceptibility to aggression produced through plasma tryptophan depletion, and (2) alcohol in combination with tryptophan depletion has an addictive effect on aggression.

In a recent report, Bjork et al.[62] measured laboratory aggression in men selected for presence or absence of aggressive histories. Testing occurred before and after tryptophan depletion, tryptophan loading, and under a food-restricted control condition. Subjects were provoked by subtractions of money, and aggression was measured as the responses the subject made to ostensibly subtract money from the instigator of the subtractions. When subjects were highly provoked, there was a significant tryptophan condition to aggression history interaction effect on aggressive responding. In particular, laboratory aggression in aggressive men was elevated under tryptophan-depleted conditions relative to tryptophan-loaded conditions, whereas the opposite occurred in nonaggressive men. Moreover, plasma total tryptophan levels after tryptophan loading were significantly higher in nonaggressive men, and plasma-free (but not total) tryptophan levels after tryptophan loading correlated negatively with aggressive responses in the aggressive men. These data corroborated earlier findings that aggressive men may be more prone to aggression induced by reductions in plasma tryptophan.

In view of clinical studies that suggested that aggressive patients have low levels of the serotonin metabolite 5-hydroxyindoleacetic acid in their cerebrospinal fluid,[63,64] two studies investigated the possible effect of tryptophan in pathologically aggressive patients. In the first, Morand et al.,[65] using aggressive schizophrenics, reported that tryptophan caused a significant reduction in uncontrolled behavior relative to placebo. In the second study, Volavka et al.,[66] using aggressive psychiatric inpatients, reported that tryptophan did not decrease aggressive acts relative to placebo. However, the patients required significantly less neuroleptic medication to control their aggression when they were on tryptophan.

7.1.2.1.2.2 Schizophrenia — In 1958, Lauer et al.[67] reported the first study using tryptophan to affect mood. Using seven schizophrenic patients receiving a monoamine oxidase inhibitor, they treated them with L-tryptophan (20 mg/kg/d for 6 weeks). They reported "the patients exhibited an increase in energy level and motor activity and improvement in the ability to accept interpersonal relationships, and displayed more affect."

Rosse et al.,[68] in an open-labeled treatment trial, utilized a low tryptophan diet as an adjunctive approach to conventional antipsychotic pharmacotherapy over several days in patients with schizophrenia. They found statistically (but not clinically) significant improvement in behavioral ratings and emphasized that the low tryptophan diet enhanced performance on the Stroop Color and Word test.

Sharma et al.[69] utilized the acute tryptophan depletion paradigm to evaluate patients with schizophrenia under controlled conditions. They observed no clinical or statistically significant improvement in symptoms compared to baseline when tryptophan depletion was imposed. The authors considered that their findings with schizophrenic or schizoaffective patients (treated but still symptomatic) may differ from those in untreated symptomatic patients. Other studies with the effects of tryptophan depletion differ markedly in treated remitted vs. untreated symptomatic depressed patients.[20,70]

7.1.2.1.2.3   Obsessive-Compulsive Disorder — Barr et al.[71] investigated the effects of short-term tryptophan depletion on patients with obsessive-compulsive disorder who demonstrated symptom reduction following treatments with serotonin reuptake inhibitors. Such low tryptophan diets did not significantly change mean ratings of obsessions and compulsions but, in contrast, mean depression ratings were significantly increased with tryptophan depletion compared with controls (tryptophan-supplemented diet).

Smeraldi et al.[72] likewise reported that mean ratings of obsessions and compulsions, measured by Visual Analogue Scales ratings, did not worsen with patients fed the tryptophan-devoid amino acid mixture. However, tryptophan depletion also failed to alter mood in contrast to findings by others.

Huwig-Poppe et al.[73] studied the effects of tryptophan depletion in 12 patients with obsessive-compulsive disorder and in 12 healthy subjects. They reported that tryptophan depletion led to more pronounced disturbances of sleep continuity in the patients than in healthy subjects, in terms of an increase of wake time and a decrease of total sleep time.

7.1.2.1.2.4   Autistic Disorder — Autistic disorder is characterized by a disturbance in social relatedness often accompanied by obsessive-compulsive symptoms and aggressive/impulsive behavior. A number of lines of evidence suggest that abnormalities in the serotonin system may contribute to the pathophysiology of autism. Since dietary tryptophan depletion may specifically reduce brain serotonin function,[74] investigations using this dietary regime (low-tryptophan diet or a tryptophan-free amino acid mixture) on autistic patients were undertaken.[75,76] The results of these studies revealed that such a dietary regime resulted in an acute worsening of some symptoms characteristic of autism.

D'Eufemia et al.[77] reported that there was a significantly lower serum tryptophan to large neutral amino acids ratio in children with idiopathic infantile autism than in control children. Their findings suggest that a low brain tryptophan availability due to a low serum tryptophan to large neutral amino acids ratio could be one of the possible mechanisms involved in the alteration of serotonergic function in autism.

Croonenberghs et al.[78] examined serotonergic and noradrenergic markers in a study group of 13 male, post-pubertal, Caucasian autistic patients (ages

12 to 28 years) and 13 matched volunteers. Plasma concentrations of tryptophan were significantly lower in autistic patients than in healthy volunteers. There were no significant differences between autistic and normal children in the serum concentrations of serotonin or the 24-h urinary excretion of 5-hydroxy-indoleacetic acid, adrenaline, noradrenaline, and dopamine. There were highly significantly positive correlations between age and 24-h urinary excretion of 5-hydroxy-indoleacetic acid and serum tryptophan. The results suggested that (1) serotonergic disturbances, such as defects in the serotonin transporter system and lower plasma tryptophan, may play a role in the pathophysiology of autism; (2) autism is not associated with alterations in the noradrenergic system; and (3) the metabolism of serotonin in humans undergoes significant changes between the ages of 12 and 18 years.

7.1.2.1.2.5 Tourette's Syndrome — Tourette's syndrome is a chronic, neuropsychiatric disorder of childhood onset characterized by motor and phonic ties that wax and wane in severity, as well as by symptoms of obsessive-compulsive disorder. Comings[79] measured blood tryptophan and serotonin levels in Tourette's syndrome patients The mean level of tryptophan in 315 patients was 1.48 mg/dl (1.93 mg/dl for controls) and mean level of serotonin in 359 patients was 71.6 ng/ml (98.1 ng/ml for controls). The author attributed the wide range of behavioral disorders in Tourette's syndrome to the low blood tryptophan and serotonin levels and suggested tryptophan oxygenase as a possible candidate gene. Rasmusson et al.[80] studied the effects of acute tryptophan depletion in a group of patients with Tourette's syndrome and found no worsening of tic, obsessive-compulsive, or mood symptoms. It is of interest that Chandler et al.[81] reported the successful treatment of stimulant-induced tics with oral tryptophan.

Richards et al.[82] measured fasting plasma levels of tryptophan, kynurenine and the pteridines, neopterin, and tetrahydrobiopterin in seven patients with Tourette's syndrome and ten healthy controls. Plasma kynurenine was significantly elevated in the patients. The lowest patient value was higher than the highest control value. Values for tryptophan, neopterin, and tetrahydrobiopterin were similar in patients and controls. However, in patients only, there was a significant negative correlation between tryptophan and neopterin and a significant positive correlation between kynurenine and neopterin when controlling for tryptophan. This finding suggested that activation of cellular immune processes is a possible explanation for the rise in plasma kynurenine.

7.1.2.1.2.6 Panic Disorder — Goddard et al.[83] conducted studies in which the effects of tryptophan depletion were evaluated in panic disorder patients. In this study, tryptophan depletion was not found to be anxiogenic in unmedicated panic disorder patients. They concluded that tryptophan depletion alone is not particularly panicogenic.

7.1.2.1.2.7   Miscellaneous Findings — In a review concerned with tryptophan in neuropsychiatric disorders, Sandyk[84] reviewed the evidence that abnormalities of serotonin functions are related to the pathophysiology of diverse neurological conditions, including Parkinson's disease, tardive dyskinesia, akathisia, dystonia, Huntington's disease, familial tremor, restless legs syndrome, myoclonus, Tourette's syndrome, multiple sclerosis, sleep disorders, and dementia. The psychiatric disorders of schizophrenia, mania, depression, aggressive and self-injurious behavior, obsessive-compulsive disorder, seasonal affective disorder, substance abuse, hypersexuality, anxiety disorders, bulimia, childhood hyperactivity, and behavioral disorders in geriatric patients have been linked to impaired central serotonin functions. Since tryptophan is a natural constituent of the diet and is the precursor of serotonin, dietary tryptophan supplementation has been used in the management of neuropsychiatric disorders with variable success. Clinical use of tryptophan supplementation in a variety of neuropsychiatric disorders has been described.

Park et al.[85] investigated the effect of tryptophan depletion during a single day upon learning and memory in normal subjects. This produced selective impairments in learning and memory in the normal volunteers.

7.1.2.2   Animal Studies

7.1.2.2.1   Grooming Chain Completion

Grooming behavior may be a useful model to study some of the motor disturbances associated with both obsessive-compulsive disorders and motor sterotypies. Serotonin has been implicated in the magnitude of novelty-induced grooming behavior. Therefore, del Angel-Meza et al.[86] investigated the effect of a tryptophan-deficient diet on grooming chain completion in rats. They found that the tryptophan-deficient diet produced fewer chain-associated face washings, more face washings alone, fewer number of chains as well as elementary units into chains. They concluded that an apparent lower threshold for emotional responsiveness also took place.

7.1.2.2.2   Spontaneous Alternation

Spontaneous alternation is controlled by septal cholinergic terminals in the hippocampus. Serotoninergic terminals end on cholinergic nerve endings in the hippocampus. Gonzalez-Burgos et al.[87] investigated the effects of a tryptophan-deficient diet on spontaneous alternation in rats (weaning to 60 days of age). Using a T-maze as the test, they observed that, at age 40 days, an increase in spontaneous alternation occurred in the rats fed the tryptophan-deficient diet, although this effect disappeared by 60 days of age.

7.1.2.2.3   Rat–Mouse Aggressive Behavior

Giammanco et al.[88] reported that alimentation of rats for 4 days with a diet composed of precooked cornmeal (tryptophan < 0.025%) induced the appearance of aggressive-cidal or aggressive noncidal behavior toward the mouse in more than half of the Wistar rats. They attributed this behavior to a decrease in brain serotonin.

7.1.2.2.4 Sexual Performance

Chronic dietary restriction of tryptophan has been reported to be associated with clear-cut changes in behavior, including increased sexual performance (mounting behavior) in male rats and rabbits,[89,90] presumably by attenuating serotonergic function.

Female rats, receiving estradiol valerate after ovariectomy, were given a tryptophan-free amino acid mixture, and sexual contact was followed. The tryptophan-free amino acid mixture in the female rats, unlike in male rats, failed to modify sexual motivation.[91]

7.1.3 Concluding Remarks

Experimental tryptophan depletion studies in humans and in animals have been utilized to determine the effects of reduced serotonin levels in the brain. Since acute tryptophan depletion leads to diminished serotonin levels, it has been considered a desirable and specific way to study effects or influences of serotonin. In general, it appears that alterations in serotonin levels influence a variety of mood disorders and neuropsychiatric conditions. This raises the question of whether the administration of tryptophan may prove to be beneficial in treating some patients. This aspect is considered further in Chapter 8.

7.2 Liver and Hepatic Coma

The many effects of L-tryptophan (deficiency or excess) on the liver have been considered in detail in earlier chapters (Chapters 2, 4, and 6). The liver is the organ that is intimately involved in the metabolism of ingested L-tryptophan and determines the pathways available and rates of formation of the various metabolites (see Chapter 4, Figure 4.1). Thus, alterations in the metabolism of L-tryptophan in the liver can have consequences throughout the body. Other than the brain, where the effects of L-tryptophan and its product, serotonin, have been extensively investigated, the liver is probably the second most investigated organ in regard to the effects or influence of L-tryptophan. How the liver in disease states is affected by L-tryptophan has been of much interest.

Chapter 6 reviewed tryptophan and toxic liver disease. This section deals with the effects or influences of tryptophan on chronic liver disease in association with hepatic coma. Chronic liver disease in humans is often association with hepatic encephalopathy, a neuropsychiatric syndrome usually beginning with changes in mood and signs of intellectual impairment, leading to confusion, slurred speech, drowsiness, hypersomnia, stupor, and coma as the condition worsens. Liver dysfunction is characterized by a known number of metabolic abnormalities, including increased concentrations of aromatic amino acids in plasma and cerebrospinal fluid.[92] These changes include an increase in plasma free tryptophan and are associated with raised CSF levels of tryptophan and 5-hydroxyindoleacetic acid, a precursor and the terminal metabolite of serotonin. Indeed, many workers[93-98] have considered tryptophan to be implicated in the pathogenesis of hepatic coma. However, overall, an elevation of plasma tryptophan is not generally considered to be pathognomonic of hepatic encephalopathy.[92]

A study by Rao et al.[99] measured the levels of amino acids using *in vivo* cerebral microdialysis in the frontal cortex of portacaval-shunted rats administered ammonium acetate to precipitate severe portal-systemic encephalopathy. In comparison to sham-operated control rats, tryptophan levels increased by 63% along with those of other amino acids. However, the experimental animals did not have a significant increase in extracellular fluid concentration of tryptophan, suggesting that increased spontaneous release of tryptophan in cerebral cortex is not implicated in the pathogenesis of hepatic coma.

The involvement of tryptophan in hepatic coma may be explained by the action of one of its metabolites, serotonin, which is known to exert profound effects on the central nervous system.[100] Although it is generally agreed that the turnover of brain serotonin is related directly to the concentration of brain tryptophan, questions remain regarding the regulation of brain tryptophan levels. The apparent increased turnover of brain serotonin in patients with hepatic encephalopathy and coma cannot be explained by corresponding increases in plasma total tryptophan levels because the reported values in these patients range from low, normal, to mildly elevated.[94,96,98,101] However, all reports seem to agree that plasma-free tryptophan levels become increased. The raised free tryptophan concentration is important because it is this fraction that is available for transport into the brain and that plays a key role in regulating the entry of tryptophan into the brain.[102,103] In attempting to explain the elevation in plasma-free tryptophan levels, there are a few probable mechanisms that operate singly or in combination: (1) a rise in plasma concentration of unesterified fatty acids occurs,[104] which releases tryptophan from plasma protein,[105] thus increasing its availability to the brain, and (2) the drop in plasma albumin in chronic liver disease may account for some of the increase in the free-to-bound tryptophan ratio. Also, brain tryptophan concentration is influenced by the ratio of its plasma concentration to the sum of the concentrations of five other amino acids (tyrosine, phenylalanine, leucine, isoleucine, and valine), which compete with tryptophan for uptake into the brain.[106,107]

An altered plasma amino acid pattern is observed in patients with liver cirrhosis and hepatic encephalopathy: low concentrations of the branched-chain amino acids (leucine, valine, and isoleucine) and high levels of the aromatic amino acids (tryptophan, tyrosine, and phenylalanine) and methionine.[108–110] These changes, together with an increased blood–brain barrier permeability,[111,112] may augment the influx of aromatic amino acids into the brain, causing an imbalance in the synthesis of neurotransmitters, which may in turn contribute to the disturbed brain function. An increased concentration of the branched-chain amino acids in the blood has been proposed to normalize these reactions.[113] Experimental studies have indeed demonstrated that the administration of branched-chain amino acids to patients with liver cirrhosis is accompanied by reduced arterial blood levels and diminished brain uptake of aromatic amino acids.[110] Although some case reports have suggested that intravenous or oral administration of branched-chain amino acids may be beneficial in patients with liver cirrhosis and hepatic encephalopathy,[108,114,115] a multicenter study with 50 patients reported that such therapy, while reducing the concentration of plasma aromatic amino acids, did not appear to improve cerebral function or decrease mortality in patients with hepatic encephalopathy.[116] Thus, the possible pathogenetic importance of the observed derangements of plasma amino acid levels is still in doubt. Kienzl et al.[117] reviewed changes in and modulation of receptor activity in hepatic encephalopathy. They reported that in hepatic encephalopathy brain, uptake of large neutral amino acids is impaired, with tryptophan crossing the blood–brain barrier to a much larger extent than all other competing amino acids. The disturbance in the steady-state of transmitter was paralleled to the change of their kinetic data. This was reflected by an increase in serotonin synthesis and turnover; while the number of postsynaptic serotonin 1-binding sites was decreased, serotonin 2-receptor activity was dropping to a much smaller extent. On the other hand, presynaptic dopaminergic activity remained unchanged, with no change in D2-receptor activity. Valine improved the postsynaptic serotonin function via modulating activity due to a regulatory mechanism at the membranal level *in vitro* and *ex vivo*. Furthermore, valine led to a significant reduction of serum ammonia (NH_4^+) and brain NH_4^+ concentration. Valine was able to antagonize the binding density, diminishing effects of NH_4^+ on 5-HT binding sites. In attempting to propose a unified hypothesis of hepatic encephalopathy, Fischer and Bower[118] have considered ammonia, plasma amino acid imbalance, deranged hormonal profile, and a deranged plasma amino acid pattern as all contributing to the deranged brain amino acid profile, resulting in distortion of the aminergic neurotransmitter profile within the central and peripheral nervous system.

Although there is much evidence relating to the association between changes in plasma and brain tryptophan levels with hepatic coma, the underlying cause of the coma is still not clear. In experimental animals, it has been established that tryptophan is a very toxic amino acid in terms of lethality.[119] In fact, the ingestion of high levels of tryptophan by humans is able to induce significant central nervous system signs and symptoms.[120] However, these manifestations are different from but have been confused with hepatic coma.[92] In humans, a tryptophan dose of 100 mg/kg body weight per os is usually well tolerated with the exception of some minor gastric disturbances

(vomiting, etc.).[121] A simple toxicity of tryptophan itself can hardly be responsible, as up to 15 g/d of DL-tryptophan has been given by mouth in the
treatment of depression,[122] and plasma free tryptophan of human subjects
has been raised almost 100-fold by tryptophan infusion without grossly
apparent effect.[123] In normal rats, injection of a lethal dose of tryptophan
(510 to 775 mg per 100-g body weight) produced dyspnea, dehydration,
prostration, and death, with an intervening phase of coma, while the plasma
and brain concentrations increased more than 300-fold.[92] However, it is conceivable that raised serotonin levels in the brain might enhance the toxicity
in the central nervous system of other substances accumulating in subjects
with liver disease. Moroni et al.[124] proposed that quinolinic acid, an excito-
toxic tryptophan metabolite, should be added to the list of compounds
possibly involved in the pathogenesis and symptomatology of brain disorders associated with liver failure. They based this on the increased concentration of quinolinic acid in the CSF in patients during coma compared to
controls as well as in the frontal cortex of patients who died after episodes
of hepatic encephalopathy. Thus, tryptophan may certainly be implicated in
hepatic coma, but the true extent of its effects or actions on the brain awaits
further clarification.

7.3 Protein Synthesis in Various Organs

In considering how L-tryptophan can affect various organs, it is appropriate
to review how it affects protein synthesis in specific organs. In addition to
reports that tryptophan stimulates hepatic and plasma protein synthesis as
described in Chapter 4, it has also been reported that tryptophan stimulates
protein synthesis in other organs. These studies, other than in liver, are cited
in this section.

7.3.1 Brain

Jorgensen and Majumdar[125] reported that a single tube-feeding of L-tryptophan to well-fed adrenalectomized rats stimulated *in vivo* incorporation
of [³H]leucine into brain proteins as well as liver proteins. Also, Nakhla
and Majumdar[126] reported that tube-feeding tryptophan to well-fed adrenalectomized rats induced an increase in the activity of cerebral acetylcholinesterase, which could be prevented when the animals were pretreated
with actinomycin D. Whether or not the enhanced protein synthesis in the
brain following tryptophan administration may be related to a rise in brain
serotonin level caused by increased plasma tryptophan concentration is
not known.

   Blazek and Shaw[127] studied the effects of tryptophan availability on brain
protein synthesis in male rats. Using α-methyltryptophan acutely (6 h) to

decrease plasma and brain tryptophan concentrations, they measured the rate of protein synthesis in plasma and brain and observed that the α-methyl-tryptophan-treated rats revealed a significant decrease (65 and 45%, respect-fully) in both, which they attributed to the tryptophan depletion.

Although the report by Cosgrove et al.[128] was not concerned per se with rat brain protein synthesis, it investigated tryptophan binding *in vitro* to whole rat brain nuclei. On Scatchard analysis, brain nuclei appeared to contain one binding site for ^{3}H-tryptophan and the K_D was 263 nM. This was similar to the liver nuclear binding for tryptophan reported earlier. Kurl et al.[129,130] suggested that the nuclear binding in liver may likewise be impli-cated in affecting protein synthesis in brain tissue.

7.3.2 Gastrointestinal Tract

Since starvation lowers protein synthesis in a number of organs or tissues and refeeding reverses the situation, Majumdar[131] investigated the impor-tance of tryptophan in regulating protein synthesis in one such tissue, the gastric mucosa. He reported that refeeding a nutritionally complete diet to fasted rats stimulated the ability of gastric mucosal polyribosomes to syn-thesize protein in a cell-free system. In contrast, a tryptophan-free diet (oth-erwise nutritionally complete) was ineffective. Also, Majumdar[132] demonstrated that tube-feeding tryptophan to well-fed adrenalectomized rats stimulated *in vivo* amino acid incorporation into gastric total proteins. Thinking that tryptophan may influence enzymes of the gastrointestinal tract, specifically the stomach and small intestine, Majumdar reported that tube feeding tryptophan to adrenalectomized rats increased the activities of gastric mucosal pepsin[132] and disaccharidases (lactase and maltase) in the jejunum and ileum.[133] Also, Majumdar reported that, using fasted (2 d) rats, refeeding of a complete diet, but not a tryptophan-free diet, increased the activities of small-intestinal alkaline phosphatase and disaccharidases (mal-tase and sucrase) to normal levels.[134]

Ponter et al.[135] reported that in piglets the fractional protein synthesis rates were generally not increased in duodenal or jejunal mucosa by adequate or excess tryptophan in high carbohydrate or high fat diets, although in stom-ach small increases occurred. Also, the fractional protein synthesis rate was increased with adequate or excess tryptophan diets compared to inadequate tryptophan diets (controls).

7.3.3 Kidney

Jorgensen and Majumdar[125] reported that a single tube-feeding of L-tryp-tophan to well-fed adrenalectomized rats stimulated *in vivo* incorporation of [^{3}H]leucine into kidney proteins.

7.3.4 Lungs

Gacad et al.[136] reported that tryptophan administration to food-deprived rabbits at 45 min before killing induced an increase in protein synthesis ([14C]leucine incorporation into protein) by lung slices.

7.3.5 Skin

Ponter et al.[135] reported an increase in fractional protein synthesis rate in the skin of piglets tube-fed adequate or excess tryptophan diets compared to controls (tryptophan-inadequate diet).

7.3.6 Bone (Femur)

Ponter et al.[135] reported that the fractional protein synthesis rate was increased with tryptophan-adequate or -excess diets high in fat compared to the control group (inadequate tryptophan, high fat diet).

7.3.7 Muscle

Lin et al.[137] reported that there was a depressive effect of tryptophan deficiency on the protein synthesis rate in pig muscle. Also, Cortamira et al.[138] reported that the fractional protein synthesis rates in piglet muscle (longissimus dorsi and semitendinosus) were increased in animals fed tryptophan-adequate diets compared to controls (tryptophan-inadequate diets). This was confirmed in a later study by Ponter et al.[135]

7.3.8 Conclusion

Based upon data of many experimental studies, it appears that L-tryptophan has the ability to stimulate protein synthesis in a number of organs. Many of the findings are based upon adding tryptophan to a diet inadequate in tryptophan. However, other studies indicate that intake of elevated levels of tryptophan can likewise stimulate protein synthesis in many organs. Speculation as to the mechanism of tryptophan's actions on stimulating protein synthesis is based mainly on studies with the liver (Chapter 4). However, it is likely that similar mechanisms may be involved in other organs. However, further investigative studies are needed to confirm whether other organs respond by similar mechanisms as occur in liver.

References

1. Gessa, G. L., Biggio, G., Fadda, F., Corsini, U., and Tagliamonte, A., Effect of the oral administration of tryptophan-free amino acid mixtures on serum tryptophan, brain tryptophan, and serotonin metabolism, *J. Neurochem.*, 22, 869, 1974.

2. Biggio, G., Fadda, F., Fanni, P., Tagliamonte, A., and Gessa, G. L., Rapid depletion of serum tryptophan, brain tryptophan, serotonin and 5-hydroxyindoleacetic acid by a tryptophan-free diet, *Life Sci.*, 14, 1321, 1974.

3. Gessa, G. L., Biggio, G., Fadda, F., Corsini, G. U., and Tagliamonte, A., Tryptophan-free diet: A new means for rapidly decreasing brain tryptophan content and serotonin synthesis, *Acta Vitaminol. Enzymol.*, 29, 72, 1975.

4. Moja, E. A., Restani, P., Corsini, E., Stacchezzini, M. C., Assereto, R., and Galli, C. L., Cycloheximide blocks the fall of plasma and tissue tryptophan levels after tryptophan-free amino acid mixtures, *Life Sci.*, 49, 1121, 1991.

5. Sidransky, H. and Verney, E., Effect of cycloheximide on tryptophan binding to rat hepatic nuclei, *Amino Acids*, 18, 103, 2000.

6. Sidransky, H., Sarma, D. S., Bongiorno, M., and Verney, E., Effect of dietary tryptophan on hepatic polyribosomes and protein synthesis in fasted mice, *J. Biol. Chem.*, 243, 1123, 1968.

7. Sarma, D. S. R., Verney, E., Bongiorno, M., and Sidransky, H., Influence of tryptophan on hepatic polyribosomes and protein synthesis in non-fasted mice, *Nutr. Rep. Int.*, 4, 1, 1971.

8. Sidransky, H. and Verney, E., Enhanced hepatic protein synthesis in rats force-fed a tryptophan-devoid diet, *Exp. Biol. Med.*, 135, 618, 1970.

9. Sidransky, H. and Farcer E., Chemical pathology of acute amino acid deficiencies. II. Biochemical changes in rats fed threonine- or methionine-devoid diets, *AMA Arch. Pathol.*, 66, 135, 1958.

10. Sidransky, H., Staehelin, T., and Verney E., Protein synthesis enhanced in the liver of rats force-fed a threonine-devoid diet, *Science*, 146, 766, 1964.

11. Sidransky, H. and Verney E., Chemical pathology of acute amino acid deficiencies. VIII. Influence of amino intake on the morphologic and biochemical changes in young rats force-fed a threonine-devoid diet, *J. Nutr.*, 86, 73, 1965.

12. Sidransky, H., Wagle, D. S., and Verney, E., Hepatic protein synthesis in rats force-fed a threonine-devoid diet and treated with cortisone acetate or threonine, *Lab. Invest.*, 20, 364, 1969.

13. Sidransky, H. and Verney, E., Studies on hepatic protein synthesis in rats force-fed a threonine-devoid diet, *Exp. Mol. Pathol.*, 13 12, 1970.

14. Sidransky, H., Tryptophan. Unique action by an essential amino acid, in *Nutritional Pathology: Pathobiochemistry of Dietary Imbalances*, Sidransky, H., Ed., Marcel Dekker, New York, 1985, 1–62.

15. Sidransky, H., Murty, C. N., and Verney, E., Evidence for the role of glycosylation of proteins in the tryptophan-induced stimulation of nucleocytoplasmic translocation of mRNA in rat liver, *Lab. Invest.*, 54, 93, 1986.

16. Sidransky, H., Verney, E., Latham, P., and Schwartz, A., Effects of tryptophan-related compounds on nuclear regulatory control. Possible role in the eosinophilia-myalgia syndrome, *Adv. Exp. Med. Biol.*, 398, 343, 1996.

17. Sidransky, H., Chemical and cellular pathology of experimental acute amino acid deficiency, Bajusz, E. and Jasmin, G., Eds., *Methods and Achievements in Experimental Pathology*, Vol. 6, Basel, Kargeer, 1972, 1–24.
18. Moja, E. A., Antinoro, E., Cesa-Bianchi, M., and Gessa, G. L., Increase in stage 4 sleep after ingestion of a tryptophan-free diet in humans, *Pharmacol. Res. Commun.*, 16, 909, 1984.
19. Young, S. N., Smith, S. E., Pihl, R. O., and Ervin, F. R., Tryptophan depletion causes a rapid lowering of mood in normal males, *Psychopharmacology*, 87, 173, 1985.
20. Delgado, P. L., Charney, D. S., Price, L. H., Aghajanian, G. K., Landis, H., and Heninger, G. R., Serotonin function and the mechanism of antidepressant action. Reversal of antidepressant-induced remission by rapid depletion of plasma tryptophan, *Arch. Gen. Psychiatr.*, 47, 411, 1990.
21. Benkelfat, C., Ellenbogen, M. A., Dean, P., Palmour, R. M., and Young, S. N., Mood-lowering effect of tryptophan depletion. Enhanced susceptibility in young men at genetic risk for major affective disorders, *Arch. Gen. Psychiatr.*, 51, 687, 1994.
22. Smith, S. E., Pihl, R. O., Young, S. N., and Ervin, F. R., A test of possible cognitive and environmental influences on the mood lowering effect of tryptophan depletion in normal males, *Psychopharmacology*, 91, 451, 1987.
23. Young, S. N., Pihl, R. O., and Ervin, F. R., The effect of altered tryptophan levels on mood and behavior in normal human males, *Clin. Neuropharmacol.*, 11 (Suppl. 1), S207, 1988.
24. Cleare, A. J. and Bond, A. J., The effect of tryptophan depletion and enhancement on subjective and behavioural aggression in normal male subjects, *Psychopharmacology*, 118, 72, 1995.
25. Danjou, P., Hamon, M., Lacomblez, L., Warot, D., Kreckemeti, S., and Puech, A., Psychomotor, subjective and neuroendocrine effects of acute tryptophan depletion in the healthy volunteer, *Psychiatr. Psychobiol.*, 5, 31, 1990.
26. Abbott, F. V., Etienne, P., Franklin, K. B., Morgan, M. J., Sewitch, M. J., and Young, S. N., Acute tryptophan depletion blocks morphine analgesia in the cold-pressor test in humans, *Psychopharmacology*, 108, 60, 1992.
27. Delgado, P. L., Price, L. H., Miller, H. L., Salomon, R. M., Licinio, J., Krystal, J. H., Heninger, G. R., and Charney, D. S., Rapid serotonin depletion as a provocative challenge test for patients with major depression: Relevance to antidepressant action and the neurobiology of depression, *Psychopharmacol. Bull.*, 27, 321, 1991.
28. Salomon, R. M., Miller H. L., Delgado P. L., and Charney D., The use of tryptophan depletion to evaluate central serotonin function in depression and other neuropsychiatric disorders, *Int. Clin. Psychopharmacol.*, 8 (Suppl. 2), 41, 1993.
29. Golberger, J. and Wheeler G. A., Experimental pellegra in the human subject brought about by a restricted diet, *Publ. Health Rep.*, 30, 3336, 1915.
30. Sebrell, W. H., History of pellagra, *Fed. Proc.*, 40, 1520, 1981.
31. Ellenbogen, M. A., Young, S. N., Dean, P., Palmour, R. M., and Benkelfat, C., Mood response to acute tryptophan depletion in healthy volunteers: Sex differences and temporal stability, *Neuropsychopharmacology*, 15, 465, 1996.

32. Leyton, M., Young, S. N., Blier, P., Ellenbogen, M. A., Palmour, R. M., Ghadirian, A. M., and Benkelfat, C., The effect of tryptophan depletion on mood in medication-free, former patients with major affective disorder, *Neuropsychopharmacology*, 16, 294, 1997.

33. Fernstrom, J. D. and Wurtman, R. J., Nutrition and the brain, *Sci. Am.*, 230, 84, 1974.

34. Wurtman, R. J. and Fernstrom, J. D., Control of brain neurotransmitter synthesis by precursor availability and nutritional state, *Biochem. Pharmacol.*, 25, 1691, 1976.

35. Wurtman, R. J., Nutrients that modify brain function, *Sci. Am.*, 246, 50, 1982.

36. Fernstrom, J. D., Can nutrient supplements modify brain function? *Am. J. Clin. Nutr.*, 71, 1669S, 2000.

37. Heninger, G. R., Delgado, P. L., Charney, D. S., Price, L. H., and Aghajanian, G. K., Tryptophan-deficient diet and amino acid drink deplete plasma tryptophan and induce a relapse of depression in susceptible patients, *J. Chem. Neuroanat.*, 5, 347, 1992.

38. Delgado, P. L., Price, L. H., Heninger, G. R., and Charney, D. S., Neurochemistry of affective disorders, in *Handbook of Affective Disorders*, Paytkel, E. S., Ed., Churchill Livingstone, New York, 1992, 219–253.

39. Smith, K. A., Fairburn, C. G., and Cowen, P. J., Relapse of depression after rapid depletion of tryptophan, *Lancet*, 349, 915, 1997.

40. Leyton, M., Young, S. N., and Benkelfat, C., Relapse of depression after rapid depletion of tryptophan, *Lancet*, 349, 1840, 1997.

41. Aberg-Wistedt, A., Hasselmark, L., Stain-Malmgren, R., Aperia, B., Kjellman, B. F., and Mathe, A. A., Serotonergic 'vulnerability' in affective disorder: A study of the tryptophan depletion test and relationships between peripheral and central serotonin indexes in citalopram-responders, *Acta Psychiatr. Scand.*, 97, 374, 1998.

42. Maes, M., Vandewoude, M., Schotte, C., Martin, M., D'Hondt, P., Scharpe, S., and Blockx, P., The decreased availability of L-tryptophan in depressed females: Clinical and biological correlates, *Progr. Neuro-Psychopharmacol. Biol. Psychiatr.*, 14, 903, 1990.

43. DeMeyer, M. K., Shea, P. A., Hendrie, H. C., and Yoshimura, N. N., Plasma tryptophan and five other amino acids in depressed and normal subjects, *Arch. Gen. Psychiatr.*, 38, 642, 1981.

44. Dunlop, S. R., Hendrie, H. C., Shea, P. A., and Brittain, H. M., Ratio of plasma tryptophan to five other amino acids in depressed subjects: A follow-up, *Arch. Gen. Psychiatr.*, 40, 1033, 1983.

45. Lucca, A., Lucini, V., Piatti, E., Ronchi, P., and Smeraldi, E., Plasma tryptophan levels and plasma tryptophan/neutral amino acids ratio in patients with mood disorder, patients with obsessive-compulsive disorder, and normal subjects, *Psychiatr. Res.*, 44, 85, 1992.

46. Joseph, M. S., Brewerton, T. D., Reus, V. I., and Stebbins, G. T., Plasma L-tryptophan/neutral amino acid ratio and dexamethasone suppression in depression, *Psychiatr. Res.*, 11, 185, 1984.

47. Moller, S. E., Plasma neutral amino acids associated with the efficacy of antidepressant treatment: A summary, in *Amino Acids in Psychiatric Disease*, Richardson, M. A., Ed., American Psychiatric Press, Bethesda, MD, 1990, 99–129.

48. Young, S. N., The clinical psychopharmacology of tryptophan, in *Nutrition and the Brain. Food Constituents Affecting Normal and Abnormal Behavior*, Vol. 7, Wurtman, R. J. and Wurtman, J. J., Eds., Raven Press, New York, 1986, 49–88.

49. Cole, J. O., Hartmann, E., and Brigham, P., L-tryptophan: Clinical studies, in *Psychopharmacology Update*, Cole, J. O., Ed., Collamore Press, Lexington, MA, 1980, 119–148.

50. Baldessarini, R. J., Treatment of depression by altering monoamine metabolism: Precursors and metabolic inhibitors, *Psychopharmacol. Bull.*, 20, 224, 1984.

51. Thomson, J., Rankin, H., Ashcroft, G. W., Yates, C. M., McQueen, J. K., and Cummings, S. W., The treatment of depression in general practice: A comparison of L-tryptophan, amitriptyline, and a combination of L-tryptophan and amitriptyline with placebo, *Psychol. Med.*, 12, 741, 1982.

52. Young, S. N., Use of tryptophan in combination with other antidepressant treatments: A review, *J. Psychiatr. Neurosci.*, 16, 241, 1991.

53. Lam, R. W., Zis, A. P., Grewal, A., Delgado, P. L., Charney, D. S., and Krystal, J. H., Effects of rapid tryptophan depletion in patients with seasonal affective disorder in remission after light therapy, *Arch. Gen. Psychiatr.*, 53, 41, 1996.

54. Neumeister, A., Praschak-Rieder, N., Besselmann, B., Rao, M. L., Gluck, J., and Kasper, S., Effects of tryptophan depletion on drug-free patients with seasonal affective disorder during a stable response to bright light therapy, *Arch. Gen. Psychiatr.*, 54, 133, 1997.

55. McGrath, R. E., Buckwald, B., and Resnick, E. V., The effect of L-tryptophan on seasonal affective disorder, *J. Clin. Psychiatr.*, 51, 162, 1990.

56. Pihl, R. O., Young, S. N., Harden, P., Plotnick, S., Chamberlain, B., and Ervin, F. R., Acute effect of altered tryptophan levels and alcohol on aggression in normal human males, *Psychopharmacology*, 119, 353, 1995.

57. Moeller, F. G., Dougherty, D. M., Swann, A. C., Collins, D., Davis, C. M., and Cherek, D. R., Tryptophan depletion and aggressive responding in healthy males, *Psychopharmacology*, 126, 97, 1996.

58. Reilly, J. G., McTavish, S. F., and Young, A. H., Rapid depletion of plasma tryptophan: A review of studies and experimental methodology, *J. Psychopharmacol.*, 11, 381, 1997.

59. Dougherty, D. M., Bjork, J. M., Marsh, D. M., and Moeller, F. G., Influence of trait hostility on tryptophan depletion-induced laboratory aggression, *Psychiatr. Res.*, 88, 227, 1999.

60. Bjork, J. M., Dougherty, D. M., Moeller, F. G., Cherek, D. R., and Swann, A. C., The effects of tryptophan depletion and loading on laboratory aggression in men: Time course and a food-restricted control, *Psychopharmacology*, 142, 24, 1999.

61. Dougherty, D. M., Moeller, F. G., Bjork, J. M., and Marsh, D. M., Plasma L-tryptophan depletion and aggression. *Adv. Exp. Med. Biol.*, 467, 57, 1999.

62. Bjork, J. M., Dougherty, D. M., Moeller, F. G., and Swann, A. C., Differential behavioral effects of plasma tryptophan depletion and loading in aggressive and nonaggressive men, *Neuropsychopharmacology*, 22, 357, 2000.

63. Virkkunen, M., De Jong, J., Bartko, J., Goodwin, F. K., and Linnoila, M., Relationship of psychobiological variables to recidivism in violent offenders and impulsive fire setters. A follow-up study (erratum appears in *Arch. Gen. Psychiatr.*, Oct 46(10), 913, 1989), *Arch. Gen. Psychiatr.*, 46, 600, 1989.

64. Coccaro, E. F., Impulsive aggression and central serotonergic system function in humans: An example of a dimensional brain-behavior relationship, *Int. Clin. Psychopharmacol.*, 7, 3, 1992.
65. Morand, C., Young, S. N., and Ervin, F. R., Clinical response of aggressive schizophrenics to oral tryptophan, *Biol. Psychiatr.*, 18, 575, 1983.
66. Volavka, J., Crowner, M., Brizer, D., Convit, A., Van Praag, H., and Suckow, R. F., Tryptophan treatment of aggressive psychiatric inpatients, *Biol. Psychiatr.*, 28, 728, 1990.
67. Lauer, J. W., Inskip, W. M., Sernsohn, J., and Zeller, E. A., Observations of schizophrenic patients after iproniazid and tryptophan, *AMA Arch. Neurol. Psychiatr.*, 80, 122, 1958.
68. Rosse, R. B., Schwartz, B. L., Zlotolow, S., Banay-Schwartz, M., Trinidad, A. C., Peace, T. D., and Deutsch, S. I., Effect of a low-tryptophan diet as an adjuvant to conventional neuroleptic therapy in schizophrenia, *Clin. Neuropharmacol.*, 15, 129, 1992.
69. Sharma, R. P., Shapiro, L. E., Kamath, S. K., Soll, E. A., Watanabe, M. D., and Davis, J. M., Acute dietary tryptophan depletion: Effects on schizophrenic positive and negative symptoms, *Neuropsychobiology*, 35, 5, 1997.
70. Delgado, P. L., Price, L. H., Miller, H. L., Salomon, R. M., Aghajanian, G. K., Heninger, G. R., and Charney, D. S., Serotonin and the neurobiology of depression. Effects of tryptophan depletion in drug-free depressed patients, *Arch. Gen. Psychiatr.*, 51, 865, 1994.
71. Barr, L. C., Goodman, W. K., McDougle, C. J., Delgado, P. L., Heninger, G. R., Charney, D. S., and Price, L. H., Tryptophan depletion in patients with obsessive-compulsive disorder who respond to serotonin reuptake inhibitors, *Arch. Gen. Psychiatr.*, 51, 309, 1994.
72. Smeraldi, E., Diaferia, G., Erzegovesi, S., Lucca, A., Bellodi, L., and Moja, E. A., Tryptophan depletion in obsessive-compulsive patients, *Biol. Psychiatr.*, 40, 398, 1996.
73. Huwig-Poppe, C., Voderholzer, U., Backhaus, J., Riemann, D., Konig, A., and Hohagen, F., The tryptophan depletion test. Impact on sleep in healthy subjects and patients with obsessive-compulsive disorder, *Adv. Exp. Med. Biol.*, 467, 35, 1999.
74. Fernstrom, J. D., Effects on the diet on brain neurotransmitters, *Metab. Clin. Exp.*, 26, 207, 1977.
75. McDougle, C. J., Naylor, S. T., Goodman, W. K., Volkmar, F. R., Cohen, D. J., and Price, L. H., Acute tryptophan depletion in autistic disorder: A controlled case study, *Biol. Psychiatr.*, 33, 547, 1993.
76. McDougle, C. J., Naylor, S. T., Cohen, D. J., Aghajanian, G. K., Heninger, G. R., and Price, L. H., Effects of tryptophan depletion in drug-free adults with autistic disorder, *Arch. Gen. Psychiatr.*, 53, 993, 1996.
77. D'Eufemia, P., Finocchiaro, R., Celli, M., Viozzi, L., Monteleone, D., and Giardini, O., Low serum tryptophan to large neutral amino acids ratio in idiopathic infantile autism, *Biomed. Pharmacother.*, 49, 288, 1995.
78. Croonenberghs, J., Delmeire, L., Verkerk, R., Lin, A. H., Meskal, A., Neels, H., Van der Planken, M., Scharpe, S., Deboutte, D., Pison, G., and Maes, M., Peripheral markers of serotonergic and noradrenergic function in post-pubertal, caucasian males with autistic disorder, *Neuropsychopharmacology*, 22, 275, 2000.

79. Comings, D. E., Blood serotonin and tryptophan in Tourette's syndrome, *Am. J. Med. Genet.*, 36, 418, 1990.
80. Rasmusson, A. M., Anderson, G. M., Lynch, K. A., McSwiggan-Hardin, M., Scahill, L. D., Mazure, C. M., Goodman, W. K., Price, L. H., Cohen, D. J., and Leckman, J. F., A preliminary study of tryptophan depletion on tics, obsessive-compulsive symptoms, and mood in Tourette's syndrome, *Biol. Psychiatr.*, 41, 117, 1997.
81. Chandler, M. L., Barnhill, J. L., Gualtieri, C. T., and Patterson, D. R., Tryptophan antagonism of stimulant-induced tics, *J. Clin. Psychopharmacol.*, 9, 69, 1989.
82. Rickards, H., Dursun, S. M., Farrar, G., Betts, T., Corbett, J. A., and Handley, S. L., Increased plasma kynurenine and its relationship to neopterin and tryptophan in Tourette's syndrome, *Psychol. Med.*, 26, 857, 1996.
83. Goddard, A. W., Sholomskas, D. E., Walton, K. E., Augeri, F. M., Charney, D. S., Heninger, G. R., Goodman, W. K., and Price, L. H., Effects of tryptophan depletion in panic disorder, *Biol. Psychiatr.*, 36, 775, 1994.
84. Sandyk, R., L-tryptophan in neuropsychiatric disorders: A review, *Int. J. Neurosci.*, 67, 127, 1992.
85. Park, S. B., Coull, J. T., McShane, R. H., Young, A. H., Sahakian, B. J., Robbins, T. W., and Cowen, P. J., Tryptophan depletion in normal volunteers produces selective impairments in learning and memory, *Neuropharmacology*, 33, 575, 1994.
86. del Angel-Meza, A. R., Gonzalez-Burgos, I., Olvera-Cortes, E., and Feria-Velasco, A., Chronic tryptophan restriction disrupts grooming chain completion in the rat, *Physiol. Behav.*, 59, 1099, 1996.
87. Gonzalez-Burgos, I., Olvera-Cortes, E., del Angel-Meza, A. R., and Feria-Velasco, A., Serotonin involvement in the spontaneous alternation ability: A behavioral study on tryptopha-restricted rats, *Neurosci. Lett.*, 190, 143, 1995.
88. Giammanco, S., Ernandes, M., Lopez, D. O., and Paderni, M. A., Short-term diet of precooked corn meal almost lacking in tryptophan and interspecific rat-mouse aggressive behaviour, *Arch. Int. Physiol. Biochim.*, 98, 23, 1990.
89. Carruba, M. O., Picotti, G. B., Genovese, E., and Mantegazza, P., Stimulatory effect of a maize diet on sexual behaviour of male rats, *Life Sci.*, 20, 159, 1977.
90. Fratta, W., Biggio, G., and Gessa, G. L., Homosexual mounting behavior induced in male rats and rabbits by a tryptophan-free diet, *Life Sci.*, 21, 379, 1977.
91. Benedetti, F. and Moja, E. A., Failure of a tryptophan-free amino acid mixture to modify sexual behaviour in the female rat, *Physiol. Behav.*, 54, 1235, 1993.
92. Zieve, L., Hepatic encephalopathy: summary of present knowledge with an elaboration on recent developments, *Progr. Liver Dis.*, 6, 327, 1979.
93. Modlinger, R. S., Schonmuller, J. M., and Arora, S. P., Adrenocorticotropin release by tryptophan in man, *J. Clin. Endocrinol. Metab.*, 50, 360, 1980.
94. Hirayama, C., Tryptophan metabolism in liver disease, *Clin. Chim. Acta*, 32, 191, 1971.
95. Ogihara, K., Mozai, T., and Hirai, S., Tryptophan as cause of hepatic coma, *N. Engl. J. Med.*, 275, 1255, 1966.
96. Knell, A. J., Davidson, A. R., Williams, R., Kantamaneni, B. D., and Curzon, G., Dopamine and serotonin metabolism in hepatic encephalopathy, *BMJ*, 1, 549, 1974.
97. Sourkes, T. L., Tryptophan in hepatic coma, *J. Neural Trans.*, (Suppl.), 79, 1978.
98. Ono, J., Hutson, D. G., Dombro, R. S., Levi, J. U., Livingstone, A., and Zeppa, R., Tryptophan and hepatic coma, *Gastroenterology*, 74, 196, 1978.

99. Rao, V. L., Audet, R. M., and Butterworth, R. E., Selective alterations of extracellular brain amino acids in relation to function in experimental portal-systemic encephalopathy: Results of an *in vivo* microdialysis study, *J. Neurochem.*, 65, 1221, 1995.

100. Woolley, D. W., *The Biochemical Basis of Psychoses or the Serotonin Hypothesis about Mental Disease*, John Wiley & Sons, New York, 1962.

101. Fischer, J. E., Hepatic coma in cirrhosis, portal hypertension, and following portacaval shunt. Its etiologies and the current status of its treatment, *Arch. Surg.*, 108, 325, 1974.

102. Tagliamonte, A., Biggio, G., Vargiu, L., and Gessa, G. L., Free tryptophan in serum controls brain tryptophan level and serotonin synthesis, *Life Sci. Pt. 2 Biochem., Gen. Mol. Biol.*, 12, 277, 1973.

103. Knott, P. J. and Curzon, G., Free tryptophan in plasma and brain tryptophan metabolism, *Nature*, 239, 452, 1972.

104. Mortiaux, A. and Dawson A. M., Plasma free fatty acids in liver disease, *Gut*, 2, 304, 1961.

105. Curzon, G., Friedel, J., and Knott, P. J., The effect of fatty acids on the binding of tryptophan to plasma protein, *Nature*, 242, 198, 1973.

106. Fernstrom, J. D. and Wurtman, R. J., Brain serotonin content: Physiological regulation by plasma neutral amino acids, *Science*, 178, 414, 1972.

107. James, J. H., Hodgman, J. M., Funovics, J. M., Yoshimura, N., and Fischer, J. E., Brain tryptophan, plasma free tryptophan and distribution of plasma neutral amino acids, *Metab. Clin. Exp.*, 25, 471, 1976.

108. Fischer, J. E., Rosen, H. M., Ebeid, A. M., James, J. H., Keane, J. M., and Soeters, P. B., The effect of normalization of plasma amino acids on hepatic encephalopathy in man, *Surgery*, 80, 77, 1976.

109. Iob, V., Coon, W. W., and Sloan, M., Free amino acids in liver, plasma, and muscle of patients with cirrhosis of the liver, *J. Surg. Res.*, 7, 41–43, 1967.

110. Sato, Y., Eriksson, S., Hagenfeldt, L., and Wahren, J., Influence of branched-chain amino acid infusion on arterial concentrations and brain exchange of amino acids in patients with hepatic cirrhosis, *Clin. Physiol.*, 1, 151, 1981.

111. James, J. H., Escourrou, J., and Fischer, J. E., Blood–brain neutral amino acid transport activity is increased after portacaval anastomosis, *Science*, 200, 1395, 1978.

112. Zanchin, G., Rigotti, P., Dussini, N., Vassanelli, P., and Battistin, L., Cerebral amino acid levels and uptake in rats after portacaval anastomosis. II. Regional studies *in vivo, J. Neurosci. Res.*, 4, 301, 1979.

113. Fischer, J. E. and Baldessarini, R. J., Pathogensis and therapy of hepatic coma, in *Progress in Liver Diseases*, Vol. 5, Popper, H. and Schaffer, F., Eds., Grune and Stratton, New York, 1976, 363.

114. Freund, H., Yoshimura, N., and Fischer, J. E., Chronic hepatic encephalopathy. Long-term therapy with a branched-chain amino-acid-enriched elemental diet, *JAMA*, 242, 347, 1979.

115. Freund, H., Dienstag, J., Lehrich, J., Yoshimura, N., Bradford, R. R., Rosen, H., Atamian, S., Slemmer, E., Holroyde, J., and Fischer, J. E., Infusion of branched-chain enriched amino acid solution in patients with hepatic encephalopathy, *Ann. Surg.*, 196, 209, 1982.

116. Wahren, J., Denis, J., Desurmont, P., Eriksson, L. S., Escoffier, J. M., Gauthier, A. P., Hagenfeldt, L., Michel, H., Opolon, P., Paris, J. C., and Veyrac, M., Is intravenous administration of branched-chain amino acids effective in the treatment of hepatic encephalopathy? A multicenter study, *Hepatology*, 3, 475, 1983.

117. Kienzl, E., Riederer, P., Brucke, T., Kleinberger, G., and Jellinger, K., Changes in and modulation of receptor activity in hepatic encephalopathy, *Infusionsther. Klin. Ernahrung*, 12, 32, 1985.

118. Fischer, J. F. and Bower R. H., Amino acids in liver disease, in *The Kidney in Liver Disease*, 2nd ed., Epstein, M., Ed., Elsevier Biomedical, New York, 1983, 515–534.

119. Gullino, P., Winitz, M., Birnbaum, S. M., Cornfield, J., Otey, M. C., and Greenstein, J. P., Studies on the metabolism of amino acids and related compounds *in vivo*. I. Toxicity of essential amino acids individually, in mixtures and the protective effect of L-arginine, *Arch. Biochem. Biophys.*, 64, 319, 1956.

120. Smith, B. and Prockop, D. J., Central nervous system effects of ingestion of L-tryptophan by normal subjects, *N. Engl. J. Med.*, 267, 1338, 1962.

121. Montenero, A. S., Toxicity and tolerance of tryptophan and its metabolites, (Italian), *Acta Vitaminol. Enzymol.*, 32, 188, 1978.

122. Coppen, A., Shaw, D. M., and Farrell, J. P., Potentiation of the antidepressive effect of monoamine-oxidase inhibitor by tryptophan, *Lancet*, 1, 79, 1963.

123. Curzon, G., Kantamaneni, B. D., Winch, J., Rojas-Bueno, A., Murray-Lyon, I. M., and Williams, R., Plasma and brain tryptophan changes in experimental acute hepatic failure, *J. Neurochem.*, 21, 137, 1973.

124. Moroni, F., Lombardi, G., Carla, V., Lal, S., Etienne, P., and Nair, N. P., Increase in the content of quinolinic acid in cerebrospinal fluid and frontal cortex of patients with hepatic failure, *J. Neurochem.*, 47, 1667, 1986.

125. Jorgensen, A. J. and Majumdar, A. P., Bilateral adrenalectomy: Effect of tryptophan force-feeding on amino acid incorporation into ferritin, transferrin, and mixed proteins of liver, brain and kidneys *in vivo*, *Biochem. Med.*, 16, 37, 1976.

126. Nakhla, A. M. and Majumdar, A. P., Tryptophan force-feeding: Changes in the activities of acetylcholinesterase in various tissues of well-fed normal and adrenalectomized rats, *Biochem. Biophys. Res. Commun.*, 79, 96, 1977.

127. Blazek, R. and Shaw, D. M., Tryptophan availability and brain protein synthesis, *Neuropharmacology*, 17, 1065, 1978.

128. Cosgrove, J. W., Verney, E., Schwartz, A. M., and Sidransky, H., Tryptophan binding to nuclei of rat brain, *Exp. Mol. Pathol.*, 57, 180, 1992.

129. Kurl, R. N., Verney, E., and Sidransky, H., Tryptophan binding sites on nuclear envelopes of rat liver, *Nutr. Rep. Int.*, 36, 669, 1987.

130. Kurl, R. N., Verney, E., and Sidransky, H., Identification and immunohistochemical localization of a tryptophan binding protein in nuclear envelopes of rat liver, *Arch. Biochem. Biophys.*, 265, 286, 1988.

131. Majumdar, A. P., Effects of fasting and subsequent feeding of a complete or tryptophan-free diet on the activity of DNA-synthesizing enzymes and protein synthesis in gastric mucosa of rats, *Ann. Nutr. Metab.*, 26, 264, 1982.

132. Majumdar, A. P., Bilateral adrenalectomy: Effect of tryptophan on protein synthesis and pepsin activity in the stomach of rats, *Scand. J. Gastroenterol.*, 14, 949, 1979.

133. Majumdar, A. P., Effect of adrenalectomy and tryptophan force-feeding on the activity of intestinal disaccharidases in adult rats, *Scand. J. Gastroenterol.*, 15, 225, 1980.

134. Majumdar, A. P. N., Influence of dietary tryptophan on the activity of intestinal digestive enzymes, *Nutr. Rep. Int.*, 24, 1067, 1981.

135. Ponter, A. A., Cortamira, N. O., Seve, B., Salter, D. N., and Morgan, L. M., The effects of energy source and tryptophan on the rate of protein synthesis and on hormones of the entero-insular axis in the piglet, *Br. J. Nutr.*, 71, 661, 1994.

136. Gacad, G., Dickie, K., and Massaro, D., Protein synthesis in lung: Influence of starvation on amino acid incorporation into protein, *J. Appl. Physiol.*, 33, 381, 1972.

137. Lin, F. D., Smith, T. K., and Bayley, H. S., A role for tryptophan in regulation of protein synthesis in porcine muscle, *J. Nutr.*, 118, 445, 1988.

138. Cortamira, N. O., Seve, B., Lebreton, Y., and Ganier, P., Effect of dietary tryptophan on muscle, liver and whole-body protein synthesis in weaned piglets: Relationship to plasma insulin, *Br. J. Nutr.*, 66, 423, 1991.

8

Pharmacology and Selected Therapeutic Uses

8.1 Introduction

The use of L-tryptophan as a therapeutic agent probably began in the 1970s and early 1980s when reports in the medical literature suggested that it might be useful for the treatment of depression.[1-3] Since then, its efficacy for a variety of other conditions has been examined; these include chronic pain, insomnia, premenstrual syndrome, schizophrenia, affective disorders, and behavioral disorders.[4-16] The rationale for its therapeutic use in treatment of psychiatric and behavioral disorders came mainly from the observation that brain serotonin content could be altered by changes in plasma tryptophan levels.[17]

During the 1980s, consumers or customers were encouraged by the popular press to use L-tryptophan for therapeutic purposes for a variety of problems.[18] L-tryptophan was available without prescription, as an over-the-counter remedy, at natural food stores and drug stores. L-tryptophan was manufactured as a nutritional supplement and regulated as a foodstuff, yet it was sold and used as a drug. Although L-tryptophan was removed from the GRAS (Generally Regarded As Safe) list many years ago (1977),[19] it remained widely available and largely unregulated. Thus, popularity and sales of L-tryptophan increased in the 1980 to 1990 period. For example, a 1990 survey of tryptophan use in the Minneapolis–St. Paul area revealed that 4% of households had at least one person who had used tryptophan between 1980 and 1989.[20] The overall prevalence of use was not known, but its manufacture and distribution were a multimillion dollar industry with increasing sales, particularly between 1985 and 1989. Then, the eosinophilia myalgia syndrome was reported in 1989, and the FDA discontinued sales of L-tryptophan (see Chapter 11).

The rationale for the therapeutic uses of tryptophan depends mainly on the knowledge that alterations in brain tryptophan levels influence serotonin synthesis. In humans,[21] as in rats,[17] brain tryptophan hydroxylase is normally only about half saturated with its substrate. Therefore, increases in availability of tryptophan can double the rate of serotonin synthesis.[21] Although it is clear that serotonin synthesis increases with tryptophan ingestion, the extent of its release and, therefore, its function is unclear.

A number of reviews have described the important role that serotonin, a derivative of tryptophan, plays within the central nervous system.[22-24] Also, Chapter 7 reviewed the importance of serotonin in selected diseases of the central nervous system. Serotonin neurons participate in a wide range of behaviors, including sleep, feeding, aggression, locomotor activity, and pain sensitivity.[25] Dietary manipulations that alter brain tryptophan levels can, in animals and in humans, affect many of these behaviors. Several examples of these effects are cited.

8.2 Actions Related to Serotonin

8.2.1 Pain

One of the early therapeutic uses of L-tryptophan was for pain. Pain, particularly chronic pain, is a frequent and important complaint for which relief is sought by millions of individuals. The search for relief of pain opens a Pandora's box for agents that may offer relief. In the 1980s, L-tryptophan, which was widely available, gained popularity as an agent for pain relief. Although this was based mainly on press releases and advertisements to increase sales, it did have some support from experimental and clinical studies.

Early behavioral and neurochemical studies suggested the involvement of L-tryptophan in the mechanisms of analgesia. These studies were followed by many experiments on the possible involvement of serotonin in this phenomenon. At present, the physiological role of serotonin in pain and analgesia still remains to be fully explained. During the last decade, a number of studies have suggested that another route of metabolism of tryptophan, the kynurenine pathway, was involved in the control of neuronal activity. Some of the experimental studies are cited here.

Increased sensitivity to painful stimuli has been reported in animals subjected to dietary deprivation of tryptophan.[26–28] Rats maintained on a tryptophan-deficient diet showed increased sensitivity to painful electric foot shock.[27] Also, some studies have revealed that in humans tryptophan causes decreased pain perception.[25]

A number of studies have investigated the efficacy of tryptophan in relieving clinical pain. King[29] reported that tryptophan relieved the pain of patients in whom chronic pain had recurred after successful treatment by rhizotomy or cordotomy. In a controlled trial, Seltzer et al.[30] found that tryptophan decreased clinical pain in patients with chronic maxillofacial pain. Tryptophan has also been reported to reduce pain 24 h after endodontic surgery.[31] Lieberman et al.[32] reviewed studies on the effect of L-tryptophan in decreasing human pain sensitivity and thought that it acted in a more specific manner than certain analgesic drugs.

On the other hand, other clinical studies have failed to report therapeutic effects on certain patients in pain. Some examples follow:

1. In patients with spinal disc disease, no effect of tryptophan was found.[33]

2. In patients with fibrositis syndrome, tryptophan was also ineffective when given at bedtime.[34]

3. Tryptophan given pre- and post-operatively did not affect pain development or analgesic consumption after third molar surgery.[35]

4. For pain after abdominal surgery, intravenous tryptophan infusions failed to decrease pain or morphine requirements.[36,37]

The varying results obtained with tryptophan in different types of clinical pain probably reflect the fact that pain includes many physiological phenomena, which act through many different mechanisms. Tryptophan has been shown to have a therapeutic effect most frequently with chronic pain associated with deafferentation or neural damage.

For a number of years, the management of chronic pain in patients using dietary metabolic precursors to neurotransmitters has received much attention. As pain evolves from acute to chronic, different neuronal pathways are used, and diverse areas of the brain become involved in the perception and modulation of pain. The serotonergic system serves as a useful model for understanding the effect of metabolic precursors. L-tryptophan given orally often decreases the perception of pain and appears to act synergistically with the endorphins and enkephalins. Drugs that increase the serotonin level cause decreased pain perception with increased pain threshold. Ingestion of dietary tryptophan from a therapeutic standpoint merits serious consideration.[38]

Weil-Fugazza[38] reviewed some endogenous kynurenine derivatives (e.g., kynurenic acid and quinolinic acid) and their association with pain. They concluded that kynurenine derivatives may play an important role in the mechanisms of the transmission of nociceptive messages at the level of the spinal cord. They speculated that pharmacologic studies of drugs modulating the kynurenine metabolism initiated for the treatment of neurologic dysfunctions could also be useful for therapy of pain. Specifically, a number of studies support the hypothesis that the kynurenine pathway is involved in the modulation of the activity of the excitatory amino acid transmitters in the CNS.[40,41]

8.2.2   Sleep and Insomnia

Administration of L-tryptophan to humans has been reported to reduce sleep latency and waking time.[42-44] Similar results in reduction of sleep latency also have been observed in rats.[45] Since tryptophan is a precursor of serotonin, which has been implicated in the mediation of sleep,[46] it was assumed that tryptophan produces these effects by increasing the availability of serotonin at sites where serotonin naturally occurs in the brain. However, in addition to its action on brain serotonin, it was suggested that tryptophan may produce its hypnotic effects via a nonserotonergic mechanism.[42] The reduction in concentration of both dopamine and norepinephrine induced in various brain regions by the administration of L-tryptophan also correlates with reduction in sleep latency.[47]

Moja et al.[48] studied the effects of an acute administration of a tryptophan-free amino acid mixture on rats. They reported a decrease in REM sleep and an increase in non-REM sleep time. Also, Moja et al.[49] reported that the polygraphic sleep pattern of healthy volunteers following the ingestion of an amino acid mixture containing all essential amino acids compared to that of ingestion of a tryptophan-free mixture was different. The latter group had a decrease in stage 4 sleep latency and an increase in stage 4 sleep during the first 3 h of sleep compared with the control group.

Other more recent studies have also investigated the effects of tryptophan depletion (using a tryptophan-devoid amino acid mixture) on sleep electroencephalograms in healthy humans.[50,51] Using 11 healthy males, Bhatti et al.[50] reported a significantly decreased REM latency in treated subjects compared to baseline. Voderholzer et al.,[51] using 12 healthy subjects, reported significant effects on sleep EEG in terms of decreased nonrapid eye movement (non-REM) stage 2, increase of wake percentage, and increase of rapid eye movement (REM) density due to a tryptophan-devoid mixture compared with baseline. A placebo group did not show effects. These studies support the involvement of serotonin deficiency, induced by a tryptophan-devoid amino acid mixture, in EEG sleep maintenance and on REM sleep.

Since the 1960s, L-tryptophan has been used to treat sleep disorders as well as depression. L-tryptophan can help re-establish a physiological sleep pattern in patients with chronic sleep problems. Demisch et al.[52] treated 39 subjects with chronic insomnia with L-tryptophan in a double-blind, cross-over study and concluded that, on the basis of subjective ratings, L-tryptophan was effective in promoting sleep in cases of chronic insomnia. Schneider-Helmert and Spinweber[53] reviewed sleep laboratory and out-patient studies of the hypnotic efficacy of L-tryptophan, with particular emphasis on evaluating therapeutic effectiveness in the treatment of insomnia. They concluded that L-tryptophan was an effective therapeutic agent for insomnia. Also, they stressed the absence of side effects and lack of development of tolerance in long-term use of L-tryptophan.

Many studies have tested tryptophan as a hypnotic agent. While the results have been variable, the consensus of reviews is that under certain conditions tryptophan can be an effective hypnotic.[54-57] Although in severe insomnia tryptophan is not as effective as standard hypnotics, in mild insomnia it is able to decrease sleep latency by about one half. It can be useful at low doses (<4 g) without altering sleep architecture.[58]

8.2.3 Feeding Behavior and Bulimia

Experimentally, it has been demonstrated that injections of L-tryptophan can have an effect upon the feeding behavior of rats. In freely feeding rats, injections of L-tryptophan brought about a significant diminution in the 24-h food intake and significantly reduced meal size.[59] Also, in food-deprived rats, tryptophan reduced the size of the first large meal taken after the deprivation period and markedly extended the duration of the postmeal interval.[59] The latter findings differ from those of other investigators,[60,61] who reported that tryptophan administered to 18- to 24-h food-deprived rats failed to demonstrate a significant depression of food consumption during the first 2 h after injection. The differences have been attributed to methodological differences in experimental designs.[59] Although the action of tryptophan is generally considered to be via its effect on brain serotonin, the mechanisms by which the short-term administration of tryptophan leads to subtle adjustments in meal parameters are still unclear. Relative to the effect of tryptophan on reducing meal size in rats, Stephens et al.[62,63] have described a specific tryptophan receptor for inhibition of gastric emptying in the dog. As in the dog, tryptophan inhibited gastric emptying, which was independent of stimulation of acid secretion, in the cat.[64] Thus, this effect by tryptophan on the stomach may influence the quantity of diet consumed. In humans, tryptophan has been utilized to decrease appetite.[65]

Tryptophan, given for several weeks, has been tested against placebo in two clinical studies to determine whether it would decrease total calorie or carbohydrate intake of obese and/or carbohydrate-craving subjects.[66,67] In neither of these studies was there any effect on weight or food selection of the patients. In a single study, a mixture of L-tryptophan, DL-phenylalanine, L-glutamine, and pyridoxal phosphate helped weight loss in carbohydrate-craving subjects.[68] However, the open design and the mixture of compounds given make the results of this study difficult to interpret.

Bulimia nervosa is the most common eating disorder that occurs in women with eating disorders who maintain normal weight. The symptomology includes disturbances in appetite modulation, abnormal body image, dysphoric mood, and neuroendocrine abnormalities.

Although the pathophysiology of bulimia is poorly understood, one hypothesis holds that bingeing behavior is precipitated by a reduction in serotonin activity in the brain.[69,70] Experimental evidence for this view is based upon studies:

1. Reducing transmission across brain serotonin synapses by drugs is known to stimulate food intake.[71,72]

2. Several studies suggest that normal weight bulimic women have reduced serotonin activity.[73,74]

3. Drugs that enhance serotonin transmission are useful in controlling bingeing in bulimic patients.[75]

However, others have not found a clear link between serotonin function and bulimia.[76,77]

Weltzin et al.[78] investigated whether acute tryptophan depletion would affect bulimic patients. For bulimic women, the tryptophan-devoid amino acid mixture produced a significant increase in fatigue and a trend toward increased anxiety and indecisiveness in comparison to the findings with controls (patients or normal women receiving tryptophan-containing amino acid mixture). The tryptophan-deficient amino acid mixture produced a rapid and substantial reduction in plasma tryptophan-to-LNAA ratio in all subjects, which suggested that the treatment reduced brain tryptophan uptake and serotonin synthesis.

8.2.4   Premenstrual Syndrome (PMS)

The symptoms of premenstrual syndrome (PMS), also called premenstrual dysphoric disorder, include depressed mood, anxiety, affective lability, and anger or irritability.[79] Since low serotonin levels are thought to be involved in the etiology of depression, aggression, and impulsivity,[80] specific serotonin reuptake inhibitors have been tested in PMS. The SSRI fluoxetine was found to be better than placebo.[81] Since chronic treatment with SSRIs can influence many neuron systems other than serotonin,[82] Steinberg et al.[83] designed a study using tryptophan, relatively specific for its effect on serotonin, on the effects of symptoms of PMS. In a randomized controlled clinical trial, 37 patients with premenstrual dysphoric disorder were treated with L-tryptophan 6 g/day, and 34 were given placebo. The treatments were given under double-blind conditions for 17 days, from the time of ovulation to the third day of menstruation, during three consecutive cycles. Visual Analog Mood Scales revealed a significant therapeutic effect of L-tryptophan relative to placebo for the cluster of mood symptoms comprising the items of dysphoria, mood swings, tension, and irritability. These results suggest that increasing serotonin synthesis during the late luteal phase of the menstrual cycle is therapeutic in patients with premenstrual dysphoric disorder.

In general, the results of experimental studies in patients with PMS have given mixed results on whether there is lowered serotonin function in these patients. Menkes et al.[84] reported that acute tryptophan depletion aggravated symptoms, particularly irritability, for women with PMS compared to controls. Ellenbogen et al.[85] reported that tryptophan depletion caused a modest lowering of mood in healthy women without PMS and with no family history of depression. On the other hand, Benkelfat et al.[86] reported no lowering of mood in healthy male subjects with no history of depression.

Sundblad et al.[87] reported that both L-tryptophan and other antidepressants are effective when given during the luteal phase of the cycle. L-tryptophan has benefits over antidepressants in that it does not require a period of toleration for efficacy.[88] Also, L-tryptophan can be used at the time of peak presentation of PMS and need not be used in each cycle.

8.2.5 Hyperactivity and Attention Deficit Disorder

Many reports have linked childhood hyperactivity to impaired central serotonin functions.[89] In animals, the occurrence of a behavioral syndrome consisting of hyperactivity, stereotyped movements, and increase of temperature has been induced by L-tryptophan, as a serotonin precursor, by serotonin reuptake inhibitors, and by MAOIs.[90] Most of these manifestations can be blocked specifically by pretreatment with an inhibitor of serotonin synthesis. In humans, the association of myoclonus, diarrhea, confusion, hypomania, agitation, hyperreflexia, shivering, incoordination, fever, and diaphoresis, when patients are treated with serotoninergic agents, could constitute a "serotonin syndrome." Such cases of serotonin syndrome were reported after treatments with L-tryptophan, MAOIs, serotonin reuptake inhibitors, and tricyclics, alone or in association.

In recent years, much interest has been directed toward the increasing incidence in attention deficit disorder (ADD). This disorder affects children with symptoms consisting of distractibility, short attention span, hyperactivity, emotional lability, and impulsivity. A number of investigators have researched whether this disorder may be related to differences in the serotonin metabolism in children with ADD.

Early studies by Gibson et al.[91] indicated tryptophan decreases locomotor activity in rats. However, in 1985 Hoshino et al.[92] reported that while the mean plasma total tryptophan levels in children with ADD was not significantly different from that of normal children, the mean plasma free tryptophan level in ADD children was significantly higher. A positive correlation between plasma free tryptophan levels and the Werry-Weiss-Peters Activity Scale in children with ADD seemed to exist, suggesting that the more severe the hyperactivity of ADD, the higher the plasma free tryptophan levels. These results suggested that there might be some disturbance in the tryptophan–serotonin metabolism in the brain of a child with ADD.

Bornstein et al.[93] examined the levels of plasma amino acids (phenylalanine, tyrosine, tryptophan, histidine, and isoleucine) in 28 patients with ADD and in 20 controls. Lower levels were found in the ADD subjects, which suggested a general deficit in amino acid transport, absorption, or both. Specifically, plasma tryptophan levels (μmol/l) were 58.1 in ADD group and 104.2 in control group. These findings are consistent with the findings by Coleman[94] and Bhagavan et al.[95] that reported decreased levels of serotonin in serum or whole blood in ADD subjects.

Though many studies indicate that elevated tryptophan levels, particularly free tryptophan levels, are observed in hyperactivity states, some studies have not verified such findings. Ferguson et al.[96] reported no differences in total and free plasma tryptophan levels between hyperactive children and age-matched controls. Actually, the literature contains conflicting data as to whether high or low levels of serotonin are involved in ADD.[96–98]

Nemzer et al.[99] conducted a double-blind study in which they compared the effects of tryptophan (100 mg/kg/day) or placebo on 14 children with ADD with hyperactivity of 1-week trials. Tryptophan, while not significantly different from placebo on teachers' ratings, was significantly better by parents' ratings. This suggested that tryptophan may have some benefit in selected cases of ADD, primarily with home behavior problems.

In conclusion, the results of the effects of L-tryptophan on ADD are variable and confusing. At present, whether or not L-tryptophan may have a therapeutic role is questionable.

8.2.6 Fatigue

Since L-tryptophan is the precursor for serotonin, which is involved in fatigue, many studies have been directed toward an attempt to understand the relationship between L-tryptophan levels and fatigue. It has been considered that increases of plasma free tryptophan lead to an increased rate of entry of tryptophan into the brain, leading to higher levels of serotonin, which may cause central fatigue. Central fatigue is implicated in clinical conditions such as chronic fatigue syndrome and postoperative fatigue.

Increased plasma free tryptophan leads to an increase in the plasma concentration ratio of free tryptophan to the branched-chain amino acids (BCAA), which compete with tryptophan for entry into the brain through the blood–brain barrier. Therefore, the plasma concentrations of these amino acids were measured in chronic fatigue patients before and after exercise[100] and in patients undergoing major surgery.[101] In chronic fatigue patients, the pre-exercise concentration of plasma free tryptophan was higher than in controls but did not change during or after exercise. In controls, plasma free tryptophan became increased after maximal exercise and returned toward baseline levels 60 min later. The apparent failure of the chronic fatigue patients to change the plasma free tryptophan concentration or the free tryptophan to BCAA ratio during exercise may indicate increased sensitivity of brain serotonin receptors, as has been reported in other studies.[102]

After major surgery, the postoperative recovery plasma free tryptophan concentrations were markedly increased over baseline levels, and the plasma free tryptophan to BCAA concentration ratio was also increased after surgery.[101] Since plasma albumin concentrations were decreased after surgery, it was considered that this may account for the rise in plasma free tryptophan levels.

Blomstrand et al.[103,104] reported that provision of BCAA improved mental performance in athletes after endurance exercise, which could be attributed to counteracting the effects of the increase in plasma free tryptophan levels due to the exercise. However, the plasma concentration ratio of free tryptophan to BCAA remained unchanged or even decreased when BCAAs were ingested.

Cunliffe et al.[105] reported on the effect of L-tryptophan administration (30 mg/kg) on subjective and objective measures of fatigue in six healthy volunteers. Subjects were tested for central and peripheral fatigue using a visual analog scale, flicker fusion frequency, grip strength, reaction time, and wrist ergometry. They concluded that tryptophan ingestion led to increased subjective and central fatigue. Increases in work output observed following tryptophan were considered to be the result of a reduced perception of discomfort during ergometry.

Yamamoto and Newsholme[106] used Nagase genetically analbuminemic rats (NAR) that were run to fatigue. Administration of BCAA before exhaustive exercise resulted in a postfatigue decreased tryptophan uptake and 5-hydroxytryptophan (5-HTP) uptake into the synaptosomes isolated from the striatum when compared with saline-administered controls. At the same time, rats who received either BCAA or 2-aminobicyclo[2,2,1]heptane-2-carboxylic acid (BCH, a specific inhibitor for the L-system transporter) had a considerably prolonged run time to exhaustion (by two-fold), compared to those who received saline treatment. When classified by run time, it was of interest that, when the data for BCAA and BCH treatments for the longer run time NAR were combined, it gave rise to a significant decrease in synaptosomal tryptophan and 5-HTP of a similar magnitude to that observed with BCAA alone. These levels were lower than those observed in rats in the shorter run time group for all treatments. These results support the view that an activated serotonergic function may be involved in central fatigue, which can be diminished by inhibition of the L-system transporter.

8.2.7   Other Conditions

A single case report suggests a therapeutic effect of tryptophan in nonketotic hyperglycemia,[107] a rare genetic disorder. Tryptophan increased the levels of the tryptophan metabolite kynurenic acid in the CSF. The interesting aspect of this case report is that the therapeutic effect of tryptophan was attributed to the inhibitory effect of kynurenic acid on excitatory amino acid receptors, rather than to an increase in serotonin levels.

In Chapter 7, attention was directed toward a number of psychiatric conditions where serotonin plays a role. Experimentation with acute tryptophan depletion has been a valuable source for correlating the connection between specific psychiatric abnormalities and serotonin misfunction. The usefulness of L-tryptophan treatment has been raised in a number of these conditions.

8.3   Antioxidant Activities

Much attention has been paid recently to the action of dietary antioxidants in health and disease.[108–110] Many dietary components have been investigated for their antioxidation actions. It has been speculated that these actions have great biologic significance.

8.3.1   L-Tryptophan

A number of small molecules, such as certain vitamins and metabolites, are known to contribute to the defenses that higher organisms possess against oxidating damage.[111,112] The antioxidant activities of L-tryptophan and some of its oxidative metabolites have been investigated and reported.[113,114] Of interest is that some of the oxidative tryptophan metabolites of the kynurenine pathway are powerful antioxidants.[113] Christen et al.[113] measured how efficiently the antioxidant activities of tryptophan and some of its oxidative metabolites inhibited peroxyl radical-mediated oxidation of phosphatidylcholine liposomes and β-phycoerythrin. Low micromolar concentrations of 5-hydoxytryptophan, 3-hydroxykynurenine, xanthurenic acid, or 3-hydroxyanthranilic acid, but not their corresponding nonhydroxylated metabolic precursors, scavenged peroxyl radicals with high efficiency. 3-Hydroxykynurenine and 3-hydroxyanthranilic acid particularly protected β-phycoerythrin from peroxyl radical-mediated oxidative damage more effectively than equimolar amounts of either ascorbate or Trolox (a water-soluble analog of vitamin E). In another report, Cadenas et al.[115] described the antioxidant properties of 5-hydroxytryptophan.

Since it is well recognized that reactive oxygen species produced by activated phagocytes are involved in inflammatory processes and can contribute to cell and tissue damage either directly or through activation of proteases,[116]

Christen et al.[113] studied tissues of mice suffering from acute viral pneumonia, where the viruses directly activate appropriate cells to produce reactive oxygen species,[117] and measured enzyme activities involved or related to oxidation of tryptophan metabolism, as well as endogenous concentrations of tryptophan and its metabolites. Infection resulted in a 100-fold induction of pulmonary indoleamine 2,3-dioxygenase. Increases in the levels of lung kynurenine (16-fold) and 3-hydroxykynurenine (3-fold) occurred. In contrast, endogenous concentrations of tryptophan and xanthurenic acid did not increase, and 3-hydroxyanthranilic acid could not be detected. Their results, plus the known requirement of indoleamine 2,3-dioxygenase for superoxide anion for catalytic activation, suggested that viral pneumonia was accompanied by oxidative stress, and that the induction of indoleamine 2,3-dioxygenase probably represented a local antioxidant defense against viral pneumonia and possibly other types of inflammatory diseases.

Thomas and Stocker[118] recently reported on studies supporting the proposal that induction of tryptophan degradation along the kynurenine pathway in human monocytes and macrophages by interferon-γ represents a novel extracellular antioxidant defense that acts to prevent inadvertent oxidative damage to host tissue during inflammation.

In consideration of the mechanism of antioxidant activity of tryptophan metabolites, the importance of the phenolic moiety as the active entity should be stressed. The findings that all phenolic metabolites, but not their nonhydroxylated metabolic precursors, show antioxidant activities are consistent with this interpretation.

8.3.2 Indoles and Indole-3-Pyruvic Acid

Indole compounds constitute one of the most important classes of substances interacting with toxic oxygen derivatives. Due to their widespread presence in living cells, they may be thought of as the first defense systems developed during evolution.

Indole-3-pyruvic acid (IPA), the keto-analog of tryptophan, can be readily obtained from the amino acid by means of several aromatic aminotransferases or amino acid oxidases. It is being considered as a pre-eminent indole in living organisms since it replenishes cells with important biochemicals and behaves like a strong antioxidant.[119] As a strong free-radical scavenger, IPA has been found to inhibit radical damages in abiotic systems as well as in organ homogenates.[120]

Since IPA has been recognized for its strong antioxidant properties, it has been studied extensively in mice, rats, and humans. Review of some of its pharmacologic effects[119] include sedation and increased sleep, antidepressant, antialcohol analgesia, antistress, and anorectic.

IPA has a pivotal role in liver reducing tryptophan-2,3-dioxygenase and thereby increases free tryptophan availability to the brain. In brain, it can detoxify cells from free-radicals, reducing activity of excitatory amino acids and stimulating biosynthesis of melatonin.

8.3.3   Concluding Comments

Currently, the therapeutic use of L-tryptophan for its antioxidative ability has received little attention. Yet the antioxidative actions of L-tryptophan and its metabolites merit recognition and need to be viewed as one of many dietary components which may come into play in body defenses against cellular and tissue damage in disease states. Further studies on the direct effects of L-tryptophan as an antioxidant need to be conducted.

8.4   Concluding Remarks

8.4.1   General Remarks

Many of the therapeutic uses of L-tryptophan are directed toward its effect on neurotransmission. Actually, diet itself clearly influences neurotransmission. This can best be illustrated in grossly undernourished children. Investigations have reported that starvation can impair neuronal maturation and can have lasting effects upon intellectual and behavior performance. When gross malnutrition does not exist, subtle changes in diet may modulate brain function. L-tryptophan, as well as tyrosine and choline, in the diet are precursors for neuronal synthesis of serotonin, dopamine, and norepinephrine, and acetycholine, respectively. Thus, L-tryptophan may be useful under certain circumstances as a drug in treatment of humans.[121] On the other hand, in states of undernutrition, L-tryptophan therapy in itself is not curative, while proper nutrition may be the therapy of choice.

8.4.2   Specific Remarks

Young and Teff[122] have stressed that altered tryptophan levels will be more likely to influence brain function at higher levels of behavioral arousal. Their rationale is that tryptophan increases serotonin synthesis. However, the extent that tryptophan increases serotonin release and, therefore, serotonin function is not clear. They consider the possibility that increased serotonin levels will lead to increased serotonin release as enhanced when serotonin neurons are firing at higher rates. The rate of firing of serotonin neurons is generally increased as the level of behavioral arousal increases. This concept appears to apply in some cases of aggression, sleep, and pain. Thus, the effects of altered tryptophan levels depend greatly upon the circumstances or conditions in which it is administered.

Many experimental studies with the effects of L-tryptophan on metabolic events, mainly in liver, have suggested that the administration of L-tryptophan can have a beneficial effect during tissue or organ injury. For example, the enhancement of protein synthesis due to the administration of L-tryptophan in experimental animal studies may have beneficial effects in some conditions, as L-tryptophan reverses the ethanol-induced depression of albumin synthesis in rabbits[123] and also reverses some of the cirrhotic changes in the livers of rats treated intermittently with carbon tetrachloride.[124] These experimental studies have been reviewed in Chapter 6. It suffices to conclude, based upon these investigative studies, that L-tryptophan may prove to have a beneficial effect on certain disease states in humans. Indeed, there is need for investigative studies to determine whether L-tryptophan may have a beneficial effect on certain diseases in man, especially in liver diseases. Here the effects of L-tryptophan may be direct, involving protein synthesis, and not secondary to serotonin. Thus far, the pharmacologic actions ascribed to L-tryptophan have been monolithic in that it was mainly attributed to its increase of serotonin. Some recent studies have suggested that the kynurenine pathway and its metabolites may be important in control of neuronal activity. Further studies are needed. Newer, important actions of L-tryptophan merit investigation and clarification.

References

1. Coppen, A., Shaw, D. M., Herzberg, B., and Maggs, R., Tryptophan in the treatment of depression, *Lancet*, 2, 1178, 1967.
2. Hartmann, E., Chung, R., and Chien, C. P., Tryptophan and an MAOI(N-nialamide) in the treatment of depression. A double-blind study, *Int. Pharmacopsych.*, 6, 92, 1971.
3. Young, S. N., Chouinard, G., and Annable, L., Tryptophan in the treatment of depression, *Adv. Exp. Med. Biol.*, 133, 727, 1981.
4. Brewerton, T. D. and Reus, V. I., Lithium carbonate and L-tryptophan in the treatment of bipolar and schizoaffective disorders, *Am. J. Psychiatr.*, 140, 757, 1983.
5. Hartmann, E., Lindsley, J. G., and Spinweber, C., Chronic insomnia: Effects of tryptophan, flurazepam, secobarbital, and placebo, *Psychopharmacology*, 80, 138, 1983.
6. Morand, C., Young, S. N., and Ervin, F. R., Clinical response of aggressive schizophrenics to oral tryptophan, *Biol. Psychiatr.*, 18, 575, 1983.
7. Harrison, W. M., Endicott, J., Rabkin, J. G., and Nee, J., Treatment of premenstrual dysphoric changes: Clinical outcome and methodological implications, *Psychopharmacol. Bull.*, 20, 118, 1984.
8. Chouinard, G., Young, S. N., and Annable, L., A controlled clinical trial of L-tryptophan in acute mania, *Biol. Psychiatr.*, 20, 546, 1985.
9. Fitten, L. J., Profita, J., and Bidder, T. G., L-tryptophan as a hypnotic in special patients, *J. Am. Geriatr. Soc.*, 33, 294, 1985.
10. Selzer, S., Pain relief by dietary manipulation and tryptophan supplements, *J. Endodont.*, 11, 449, 1985.
11. Cole, W. and Lapierre, Y. D., The use of tryptophan in normal-weight bulimia, *Can. J. Psychiatr. Rev. Can. Psychiatrie*, 31, 755, 1986.
12. Mattes, J. A., A pilot study of combined trazodone and tryptophan in obsessive-compulsive disorder, *Int. Clin. Psychopharmacol.*, 1, 170, 1986.

13. Millinger, G. S., Neutral amino acid therapy for the management of chronic pain, *Cranio*, 4, 157, 1986.
14. Nemzer, E. D., Arnold, L. E., Votolato, N. A., and McConnell, H., Amino acid supplementation as therapy for attention deficit disorder, *J. Am. Acad. Child Psychiatr.*, 25, 509, 1986.
15. Demisch, K., Bauer, J., Georgi, K., and Demisch, L., Treatment of severe chronic insomnia with L-tryptophan: Results of a double-blind cross-over study, *Pharmacopsychiatry*, 20, 242, 1987.
16. Leyton, M., Young, S. N., and Benkelfat, C., Relapse of depression after rapid depletion of tryptophan, *Lancet*, 349, 1840, 1997.
17. Fernstrom, J. D. and Wurtman, R. J., Brain serotonin content: Physiological dependence on plasma tryptophan levels, *Science*, 173, 149, 1971.
18. Mazer, E., Tryptophan: The three-way misery reliever, *Prevention*, 135, May 1983.
19. Code of Federal Regulation (42FR56728), *Fed. Reg.*, October 1977.
20. Belongia, E. A., Hedberg, C. W., Gleich, G. J., White, K. E., Mayeno, A. N., Loegering, D. A., Dunnette, S. L., Pirie, P. L., MacDonald, K. L., and Osterholm, M. T., An investigation of the cause of the eosinophilia-myalgia syndrome associated with tryptophan use, *N. Engl. J. Med.*, 323, 357, 1990.
21. Young, S. N. and Gauthier, S., Effect of tryptophan administration on tryptophan, 5-hydroxyindoleacetic acid and indoleacetic acid in human lumbar and cisternal cerebrospinal fluid, *J. Neurol. Neurosurg. Psychiatr.*, 44, 323, 1981.
22. Fernstrom, J. D. and Wurtman, R. J., Nutrition and the brain, *Sci. Am.*, 230(2), 84, 1901.
23. Wurtman, R. J. and Fernstrom, J. D., Control of brain neurotransmitter synthesis by precursor availability and nutritional state, *Biochem. Pharmacol.*, 25(15), 1691, 1901.
24. Wurtman, R. J., Nutrients that modify brain function, *Sci. Am.*, 246(4), 50, 1901.
25. Kolata, G., Food affects human behavior, *Science*, 218, 1209, 1982.
26. Lytle, L. D., Messing, R. B., Fisher, L., and Phebus, L., Effects of long-term corn consumption on brain serotonin and the response to electric shock, *Science*, 190, 692, 1975.
27. Messing, R. B., Fisher, L. A., Phebus, L., and Lytle, L. D., Interaction of diet and drugs in the regulation of brain 5-hydroxyindoles and the response to painful electric shock, *Life Sci.*, 18, 707, 1976.
28. Fernstrom, J. D. and Lytle, L. D., Corn malnutrition, brain serotonin and behavior, *Nutr. Rev.*, 34, 257, 1976.
29. King, R. B., Pain and tryptophan, *J. Neurosurg.*, 53, 44, 1980.
30. Seltzer, S., Dewart, D., Pollack, R. L., and Jackson, E. J., The effects of dietary tryptophan on chronic maxillofacial pain and experimental pain tolerance, *J. Psychiatr. Res.*, 17, 181, 1983.
31. Shpeen, S. E., Morse, D. R., and Furst, M. L., The effect of tryptophan on postoperative endodontic pain, *Oral Surg. Oral Med. Oral Pathol.*, 58, 446, 1984.
32. Lieberman, H. R., Corkin, S., Spring, B. J., Growdon, J. H., and Wurtman, R. J., Mood, performance, and pain sensitivity: Changes induced by food constituents, *J. Psychiatr. Res.*, 17, 135, 1982.
33. Sternbach, R. A., Janowsky, D. S., Huey, L. Y., and Segal, D. S., Effects of altering brain serotonin activity on human chronic pain, *Advances in Pain Research and Therapy*, Bonica, J. J. and Albe-Fessard, D., Eds., Raven Press, New York, 1976, 601–606.

34. Moldofsky, H. and Lue, F. A., The relationship of alpha and delta EEG frequencies to pain and mood in 'fibrositis' patients treated with chlorpromazine and L-tryptophan, *Electroencephalogr. Clin. Neurophysiol.*, 50, 71, 1980.

35. Ekblom, A., Hansson, P., and Thomsson, M., L-tryptophan supplementation does not affect postoperative pain intensity or consumption of analgesics, *Pain*, 44, 249, 1991.

36. Franklin, K. B., Abbott, F. V., English, M. J., Jeans, M. E., Tasker, R. A., and Young, S. N., Tryptophan-morphine interactions and postoperative pain, *Pharmacol. Biochem. Behav.*, 35, 157, 1990.

37. Ceccherelli, F., Diani, M. M., Altafini, L., Varotto, E., Stefecius, A., Casale, R., Costola, A., and Giron, G. P., Postoperative pain treated by intravenous L-tryptophan: A double-blind study versus placebo in cholecystectomized patients, *Pain*, 47, 163, 1991.

38. Weil-Fugazza, J., Endogenous kynurenine derivatives and pain, *Adv. Exp. Med. Biol.*, 398, 83, 1996.

39. Haze, J. J., Toward an understanding of the rationale for the use of dietary supplementation for chronic pain management: The serotonin model, *Cranio*, 9, 339, 1991.

40. Moroni, F., Russi, P., Gallo-Mezo, M. A., Moneti, G., and Pellicciari, R., Modulation of quinolinic and kynurenic acid content in the rat brain: Effects of endotoxins and nicotinylalanine, *J. Neurochem.*, 57, 1630, 1991.

41. Swartz, K., During, M. T., Freese, A., and Beal, N. F., Cerebral synthesis and release of kynurenic acid: The endogenous antagonist of excitatory amino acid receptors, *J. Neurosci.*, 10, 2965, 1990.

42. Wyatt, R. J., Engelman, K., Kupfer, D. J., Fram, D. H., Sjoerdsma, A., and Snyder, F., Effects of L-tryptophan (a natural sedative) on human sleep, *Lancet*, 2, 842, 1970.

43. Griffiths, W. J., Lester, B. K., Coulter, J. D., and Williams, H. L., Tryptophan and sleep in young adults, *Psychophysiology*, 9, 345, 1972.

44. Hartmann, E. and Spinweber, C. L., Sleep induced by L-tryptophan. Effect of dosages within the normal dietary intake, *J. Nerv. Ment. Dis.*, 167, 497, 1979.

45. Hartmann, E. and Chung, R., Sleep-inducing effects of L-tryptophan, *J. Pharm. Pharmacol.*, 24, 252, 1972.

46. Jouvet, M., Biogenic amines and the states of sleep, *Science*, 163, 32, 1969.

47. Wojcik, W. J., Fornal, C., and Radulovacki, M., Effect of tryptophan on sleep in the rat, *Neuropharmacology*, 19, 163, 1980.

48. Moja, E. A., Mendelson, W. B., Stoff, D. M., Gillin, J. C., and Wyatt, R. J., Reduction of REM sleep by a tryptophan-free amino acid diet, *Life Sci.*, 24, 1467, 1979.

49. Moja, E. A., Antinoro, E., Cesa-Bianchi, M., and Gessa, G. L., Increase in stage 4 sleep after ingestion of a tryptophan-free diet in humans, *Pharmacol. Res. Commun.*, 16, 909, 1984.

50. Bhatti, T., Gillin, J. C., Seifritz, E., Moore, P., Clark, C., Golshan, S., Stahl, S., Rapaport, M., and Kelsoe, J., Effects of a tryptophan-free amino acid drink challenge on normal human sleep electroencephalogram and mood, *Biol. Psychiatr.*, 43(1), 52, 1998.

51. Voderholzer, U., Hornyak, M., Thiel, B., Huwig-Poppe, C., Kiemen, A., Konig, A., Backhaus, J., Riemann, D., Berger, M., and Hohagen, F., Impact of experimentally induced serotonin deficiency by tryptophan depletion on sleep EEG in healthy subjects, *Neuropsychopharmacology*, 18(2), 112, 1998.

52. Demisch, K., Bauer, J., and Georgi, K., Treatment of severe chronic insomnia with L-tryptophan and varying sleeping times, *Pharmacopsychiatry*, 20, 245, 1987.
53. Schneider-Helmert, D. and Spinweber, C. L., Evaluation of L-tryptophan for treatment of insomnia: A review, *Psychopharmacology*, 89(1), 1, 1986.
54. Cooper, A. J., Tryptophan antidepressant 'physiological sedative': Fact or fancy? *Psychopharmacology*, 61(1), 97, 1979.
55. Hartmann, E. and Greenwald, D., Tryptophan and human sleep: An analysis of 43 studies, in *Progress in Tryptophan and Serotonin Research*, Schlossberger, H. G., Kochen, W., Linzen, B., and Steinhart, H. C., Eds., Walter de Gruyter, Berlin, 1984, 297–304.
56. Young, S. N., The clinical psychopharmacology of tryptophan, in *Nutrition and the Brain. Food Constituents Affecting Normal and Abnormal Behaviours*, Wurtman, R. J. and Wurtman, J. J., Eds., Raven Press, New York, 1986, 49–88.
57. Boman, B., L-tryptophan: A rational anti-depressant and a natural hypnotic, *Aust. N. Z. J. Psychiatr.*, 22, 83, 1988.
58. Sainio, E. L., Pulkki, K., and Young, S. N., L-tryptophan: Biochemical, nutrition and pharmacological aspects, *Amino Acids*, 10, 21, 1996.
59. Latham, C. J. and Blundell, J. E., Evidence for the effect of tryptophan on the pattern of food consumption in free feeding and food deprived rats, *Life Sci.*, 24(21), 1971, 1901.
60. Barrett, A. M. and McSharry, L., Inhibition of drug-induced anorexia in rats by methysergide, *J. Pharm. Pharmacol.*, 27(12), 889, 1901.
61. Weinberger, S. B., Knapp, S., and Mandell, A. J., Failure of tryptophan load-induced increases in brain serotonin to alter food intake in the rat, *Life Sci.*, 22(18), 1595, 1978.
62. Stephens, J. R., Woolson, R. F., and Cooke, A. R., Effects of essential and nonessential amino acids on gastric emptying in the dog, *Gastroenterology*, 69, 920, 1975.
63. Stephens, J. R., Woolson, R. F., and Cooke, A. R., Osmoltye and tryptophan receptors controlling gastric emptying in the dog, *Am. J. Physiol.*, 231, 848, 1976.
64. Cooke, A. R., Gastric emptying in the cat in response to hypertonic solutions and tryptophan, *Am. J. Dig. Dis.*, 23, 312, 1978.
65. Blundell, J. E., Serotonin and skin diseases, in *Serotonin in Health and Disease*, Vol. 5, Essman, W. B., Ed., S.P. Medical and Scientific Books, New York, 1979, 403–450.
66. Wurtman, J. J., Wurtman, R. J., Growdon, J. H., Lipsscomb, A., and Zeisel, S. H., Carbohydrate craving in obese people: Suppression by treatments affecting serotoninergic transmission, *Int. J. Eating Dis.*, 1, 2, 1981.
67. Strain, G. W., Strain, J. J., and Zumoff, B. L-tryptophan does not increase weight loss in carbohydrate-craving obese subjects, *Int. J. Obesity*, 9, 375, 1985.
68. Blum, K., Trachtenberg, M. C., and Cook, D. W., Neuronutrient effects on weight loss in carbohydrate bingers: An open clinical trial, *Curr. Ther. Res.*, 48, 217, 1990.
69. Kaye, W. H., Gwirtsman, H. E., Brewerton, T. D., George, D. T., and Wurtman, R. J., Bingeing behavior and plasma amino acids: A possible involvement of brain serotonin in bulimia nervosa, *Psychiatr. Res.*, 23, 31, 1988.
70. Jimerson, D. C., Lesem, M. D., Kaye, W. H., Hegg, A. P., and Brewerton, T. D., Eating disorders and depression: Is there a serotonin connection? *Biol. Psychiatr.*, 28, 443, 1990.

71. Blundell, J. E., Serotonin and appetite, *Neuropharmacology*, 23, 1537, 1984.
72. Fernstrom, J. D., *The Science of Food Regulation*, Vol. 2, LSU Press, Baton Rouge, LA, 1992.
73. Brewerton, T. D., *Serotonin in Major Psychiatric Disorders*, AP Press, New York, 1990, 153–184.
74. Goldbloom, D. S., Hicks, L. K., and Garfinkel, P. E., Platelet serotonin uptake in bulimia nervosa, *Biol. Psychiatr.*, 28, 644, 1990.
75. Fluoxetine Bulimia Collaborative Study Group, Fluoxetine in the treatment of bulimia nervosa: A multicenter, placebo-controlled, double-blind trial, *Arch. Gen. Psychiatr.*, 49, 139, 1992.
76. Jimerson, D. C., Lesem, M. D., Kaye, W. H., and Brewerton, T. D., Low serotonin and dopamine metabolite concentrations in cerebrospinal fluid from bulimic patients with frequent binge episodes, *Arch. Gen. Psychiatr.*, 49, 132, 1992.
77. Kaye, W. H., Ballenger, J. C., Lydiard, R. B., Stuart, G. W., Laraia, M. T., O'Neil, P., Fossey, M. D., Stevens, V., Lesser, S., and Hsu, G., CSF monoamine levels in normal-weight bulimia: Evidence for abnormal noradrenergic activity, *Am. J. Psychiatr.*, 147, 225, 1990.
78. Weltzin, T. E., Fernstrom, J. D., McConaha, C., and Kaye, W. H., Acute tryptophan depletion in bulimia: Effects on large neutral amino acids, *Biol. Psychiatr.*, 35, 388, 1994.
79. American Psychiatric Association, *Diagnostic and Statistical Manual of Mental Disorders*, 4th ed., American Psychiatric Association, Washington, D.C., 1994.
80. Heninger, G. R., *Psychopharmacology*, Bloom, E. and Kupfer, J., Eds., Raven Press, New York, 1995, 471–482.
81. Steiner, M., Steinberg, S., Stewart, D., Carter, D., Berger, C., Reid, R., Grover, D. (Canadian Fluoxetine/Premenstrual Dysphoria Collaborative Study Group), and Streiner, D., Fluoxetine in the treatment of premenstrual dysphoria, *N. Engl. J. Med.*, 332, 1529, 1995.
82. Tollefson, G. D., Serotonin uptake inhibitors, in *Textbook of Psychopharmacology*, Schatzberg, A. F. and Nemeroff, C. B., American Psychiatry Press, Washington, D.C., 1995.
83. Steinberg, S., Annable, L., Young, S. N., and Liyanage, N., A placebo-controlled clinical trial of L-tryptophan in premenstrual dysphoria, *Biol. Psychiatr.*, 45, 313, 1999.
84. Menkes, D. B., Coates, D. C., and Fawcett, J. P., Acute tryptophan depletion aggravates premenstrual syndrome, *J. Affective Dis.*, 32, 37, 1994.
85. Ellenbogen, M. A., Young, S. N., Dean, P., Palmour, R. M., and Benkelfat, C., Mood response to acute tryptophan depletion in healthy volunteers: Sex differences and temporal stability, *Neuropsychopharmacology*, 15, 465, 1996.
86. Benkelfat, C., Ellenbogen, M. A., Dean, P., Palmour, R. M., and Young, S. N., Mood-lowering effect of tryptophan depletion. Enhanced susceptibility in young men at genetic risk for major affective disorders, *Arch. Gen. Psychiatr.*, 51(9), 687, 1994.
87. Sundblad, C., Hedberg, M. A., and Eriksson, E., Clomipramine administered during the luteal phase reduces the symptoms of premenstrual syndrome: A placebo-controlled trial, *Neuropsychopharmacology*, 9(2), 133, 1993.
88. Steinberg, S., Annable, L., Young, S. N., and Belanger, M. C., Tryptophan in the treatment of late luteal phase dysphoric disorder: A pilot study, *J. Psychiatr. Neurosci.*, 114, 1994, 1994.

89. Sandyk, R., L-tryptophan in neuropsychiatric disorders: A review, *Int. J. Neurosci.*, 67(1–4), 127, 1992.

90. Lejoyeux, M., Rouillon, F., Leon, E., and Ades, J., The serotonin syndrome: Review of the literature and description of an original study, *Encephale*, 21(5), 537, 1995.

91. Gibson, C. J., Deikel, S. M., Young, S. N., and Binik, Y. M., Behavioural and biochemical effects of tryptophan, tyrosine and phenylalanine in mice, *Psychopharmacology*, 76(2), 118, 1981.

92. Hoshino, Y., Ohno, Y., Yamamoto, T., Kaneko, M., and Kumashiro, H., Plasma free tryptophan concentration in children with attention deficit disorder, *Folia Psychiatr. Neurol. Japonica*, 39(4), 531, 1985.

93. Bornstein, R. A., Baker, G. B., Carroll, A., King, G., Wong, J. T., and Douglass, A. B., Plasma amino acids in attention deficit disorder, *Psychiatry Res.*, 33(3), 301, 1990.

94. Coleman, M., Serotonin concentrations in whole blood of hyperactive children, *J. Pediatr.*, 78(6), 985, 1971.

95. Bhagavan, H. N., Coleman, M., and Coursin, D. B., The effect of pyridoxine hydrochloride on blood serotonin and pyridoxal phosphate contents in hyperactive children, *Pediatrics*, 55(3), 437, 1975.

96. Ferguson, H. B., Pappas, B. A., Trites, R. L., Peters, D. A., and Taub, H., Plasma free and total tryptophan, blood serotonin, and the hyperactivity syndrome: No evidence for the serotonin deficiency hypothesis, *Biol. Psychiatr.*, 16(3), 231, 1981.

97. Greenberg, A. S. and Coleman, M., Depressed 5-hydroxyindole levels associated with hyperactive and aggressive behavior. Relationship to drug response, *Arch. Gen. Psychiatr.*, 33(3), 331, 1976.

98. Irwin, M., Diagnosis of anorexia nervosa in children and the validity of DSM-III, *Am. J. Psychiatr.*, 138(10), 1382, 1981.

99. Nemzer, E. D., Arnold, L. E., Votolato, N. A., and McConnell, H., Amino acid supplementation as therapy for attention deficit disorder, *J. Am. Acad. Child Psychiatr.*, 25(4), 509, 1986.

100. Castell, L. M., Yamamoto, T., Phoenix, J., and Newsholme, E. A., The role of tryptophan in different conditions of stress, *Adv. Exp. Med. Biol.*, 467, 697, 1999.

101. Yamamoto, T., Castell, L. M., Botella, J., Powell, H., Hall, G. M., Young, A., and Newsholme, E. A., Changes in the albumin binding of tryptophan during postoperative recovery: a possible link with central fatigue? *Brain Res. Bull.*, 43, 43, 1997.

102. Cleare, A. J., Bearn, J., Allain, T., McGregor, A., Wessely, S., Murray, R. M., and O'Keane, V., Contrasting neuroendocrine responses in depression and chronic fatigue syndrome, *J. Affective Dis.*, 34(4), 283, 1995.

103. Blomstrand, E., Andersson, S., Hassmen, P., Ekblom, B., and Newsholme, E. A., Effect of branched-chain amino acid and carbohydrate supplementation on the exercise-induced change in plasma and muscle concentration of amino acids in human subjects, *Acta Physiol. Scand.*, 153, 87, 1995.

104. Blomstrand, E., Hassmen, P., Ek, S., Ekblom, B., and Newsholme, E. A., Influence of ingesting a solution of branched-chain amino acids on perceived exertion during exercise, *Acta Physiol. Scand.*, 159, 41, 1997.

105. Cunliffe, A., Obeid, O. A., and Powell-Tuck, J., A placebo controlled investigation of the effects of tryptophan or placebo on subjective and objective measures of fatigue, *Eur. J. Clin. Nutr.*, 52(6), 425, 1998.

106. Yamamoto, T. and Newsholme, E. A., Diminished central fatigue inhibition of the L-system transporter for the uptake of tryptophan, *Brain Res. Bull.*, 52, 35, 2000.

107. Matsuo, S., Inoue, F., Takeuchi, Y., Yoshioka, H., Kinugasa, A., and Sawada, T., Efficacy of tryptophan for the treatment of nonketotic hyperglycinemia: A new therapeutic approach for modulating the N-methyl-D-aspartate receptor, *Pediatrics*, 95(1), 142, 1995.

108. Delanty, N. and Dichter, M. A., Antioxidant therapy in neurologic disease, *Arch. Neurol.*, 57(9), 1265, 2000,

109. Gutteridge, J. M. and Halliwell, B., Free radicals and antioxidants in the year 2000. A historical look to the future, *Ann. N.Y. Acad. Sci.*, 899, 136, 2000.

110. McCord, J. M., The evolution of free radicals and oxidative stress, *Am. J. Med.*, 108(8), 652, 2000.

111. Stocker, R. and Ames, B. N., Potential role of conjugated bilirubin and copper in the metabolism of lipid peroxides in bile, *Proc. Natl. Acad. Sci. U.S.A.*, 84(22), 8130, 1987.

112. Frei, B., Stocker, R., and Ames, B. N., Antioxidant defenses and lipid peroxidation in human blood plasma, *Proc. Natl. Acad. Sci. U.S.A.*, 85(24), 9748, 1988.

113. Christen, S., Peterhans, E., and Stocker, R., Antioxidant activities of some tryptophan metabolites: Possible implication for inflammatory diseases, *Proc. Natl. Acad. Sci. U.S.A.*, 87(7), 2506, 1990.

114. Chan, T. Y. and Tang, P. L., Characterization of the antioxidant effects of melatonin and related indoleamines *in vitro*, *J. Pineal Res.*, 20(4), 187, 1996.

115. Cadenas, E., Simic, M. G., and Sies, H., Antioxidant activity of 5-hydroxytryptophan, 5-hydroxyindole, and DOPA against microsomal lipid peroxidation and its dependence on vitamin E, *Free Radical Res. Commun.*, 6(1), 11, 1989.

116. Weiss, S. J., Tissue destruction by neutrophils, *N. Engl. J. Med.*, 320(6), 365, 1989.

117. Peterhans, E., Chemiluminescence: An early event in the interaction of Sendai and influenza viruses with mouse spleen cells. I. The role of the envelope glycoproteins in the stimulation of chemiluminescence, *Virology*, 105(2), 445, 1980.

118. Thomas, S. R. and Stocker, R. Antioxidant activities and redox regulation of interferon-gamma-induced tryptophan metabolism in human monocytes and macrophages, *Adv. Exp. Med. Biol.*, 467, 541, 1999.

119. Politi, V., D'Alessio, S., Di Stazio, G., and De Luca, G., Antioxidant properties of indole-3-pyruvic acid, *Adv. Exp. Med. Biol.*, 398, 291, 1996.

120. Politi, V., *Kynurenine and Serotonin Pathway*, Plenum Press, New York, 1991, 515–518.

121. Zeisel, S. H., Dietary influences on neurotransmission, *Adv. Pediatr.*, 33, 23, 1986.

122. Young, S. N. and Teff, K. L., Tryptophan availability, 5HT synthesis and 5HT function, *Progr. Neuro-Psychopharmacol. Biol. Psychiatr.*, 13(3-4), 373, 1989.

123. Rothschild, M. A., Oratz, M., Mongelli, J., and Schreiber, S. S., Alcohol-induced depression of albumin synthesis: reversal by tryptophan, *J. Clin. Invest.*, 50(9), 1812, 1971.

124. Sidransky, H., Verney, E., Kurl, R. N., and Razavi, T., Effect of tryptophan on toxic cirrhosis induced by intermittent carbon tetrachloride intoxication in the rat, *Exp. Mol. Pathol.*, 49, 102, 1988.

9

Toxicity

CONTENTS

9.1 Humans

In humans, few adverse effects have been reported with L-tryptophan, even when taken in large doses (up to 9 g/day) for extended periods of time. The few adverse effects that have been reported include ataxia, tremor, diaphoresis, blurred vision, dry mouth, muscle stiffness, palpitations, and urticaria.[1] Overall, tryptophan was considered to be quite safe in clinical use prior to late 1989 when the epidemic of eosinophilia myalgia syndrome (EMS) occurred.[2-4]

Even though tryptophan was used clinically for over 20 years, the literature had few reports of adverse effects when pure tryptophan supplements were given to humans.[5] Thomson et al.[6] reported that tryptophan alone (3 g/day) produced no more side effects than did placebos. In studies using higher doses of tryptophan (9.6 g/day) in affective disorder patients[7] and 20 g/day in schizophrenic patients,[8] no side effects were reported. In other studies where side effects were found, they were mild (most common being nausea and lightheadedness).[5]

The most common adverse effect reported when tryptophan is given to humans is the serotonin syndrome. Two reviews[9,10] describe such cases (most were associated with a combination of tryptophan and a monoamine oxidase inhibitor). The main symptoms reported were changes in mental status, including confusion and hypomania, restlessness, myoclonus, hyperreflexia, diaphoresis, shivering, and tremor. Although the incidence of the serotonin syndrome in patients is unknown, Sternbach[9] believes that it is probably underreported because it is not recognized. The serotonin syndrome usually resolves within 24 h of cessation of tryptophan treatment, with no residual syndromes.

9.2   Animals

9.2.1   Rats

9.2.1.1 LD_{50}

In rats, tryptophan has the lowest LD_{50} of any amino acid. Its LD_{50} is 1.6 g/kg IP.[11] There was a 7-fold difference in toxicity between the least toxic amino acid, L-isoleucine, and the most toxic amino acid, L-tryptophan. Symptoms of toxicity appeared between 10 min and 2 h after ingestion of L-tryptophan; these consisted of dyspnea, hypothermia, and extreme prostration. Deaths occurred between 5 h and 3 days. Surviving rats (10 days after LD_{50} dose) when autopsied revealed no gross or microscopic abnormalities. Equating this LD_{50} dose of 1.6 g/kg in the rat to humans, a 70-kg man would need to ingest over 100 g tryptophan. Since lower doses when taken orally induce vomiting in humans, it is unlikely that tryptophan ingestion could be used for suicide attempts.

A drastic increase in acute toxicity due to L-tryptophan occurred when rats were subjected to adrenalectomy or after a blockade of corticosteroid production by metyrapone, causing a 50% decrease in plasma corticosterone level. The LD_{50} was reduced to 11.4 mg/kg after adrenalectomy and to 24.9 mg/kg after metyrapone administration.[12,13] The cause of the high lethality was considered to be due to excessive formation of tryptamine with an increase in blood pressure and cardiovascular dysfunction due to loss of tryptophan 2,3-dioxygenase activity.

9.2.1.2   Effect on Food Intake and Growth

Using levels of L-tryptophan below the LD_{50} levels, fed long-term to rats, led to reduced food intake and growth of rats. However, such effects have been described with many diets in which there is an imbalance of any amino acid; therefore, the effects cannot be attributed specifically to tryptophan.

9.2.1.3   Fatty liver

Hirata et al.[14] and Ramakrishna Rao et al.[15] first reported that the administration of high levels (0.5 to 2 g/kg) of L-tryptophan to fasted (20 h) rats induced a fatty liver within 2.5 to 4 h. However, Sakurai et al.[16,17] and Fears and Murrell,[18] using lower doses of L-tryptophan (0.05 to 0.5 g/kg), reported no changes in hepatic total lipids. Trulson and Sampson[19] reported fatty liver and ultrastructural hepatic changes due to tryptophan, but Matthies and Jacobs[20] did not find a fatty liver after tryptophan administration.

In consideration of an explanation for the fatty liver due to tryptophan observed by some workers, it has been attributed to an increased mobilization of free fatty acids as reflected in the elevated levels of plasma free fatty acids and to increased hepatic fatty acid synthesis.[15] A number of investigators[15,17,18,21] have reported that hepatic fatty acid synthesis is increased following low (5 mg per 100 g body weight) or high (75 mg per 100 g body weight) doses of L-tryptophan in both fasted and fed rats. In attempting to explain the enhanced hepatic fatty acid synthesis, the following mechanisms have been considered: Miyazawa et al.[21] proposed the activation of the lipogenic enzyme acetyl-CoA carboxylase (EC 6.4.1.2) by citrate, and Fears and Murrell[18] proposed that the stimulation of insulin secretion by tryptophan increases the activities of hepatic fatty acid synthetase and adipose tissue lipoprotein lipase.

Concerning the fatty livers due to tryptophan described by some investigators, Hirata et al.[14] reported a decrease in the level of adenosine triphosphate (ATP) in the liver caused by tryptophan administration that they considered to play a role in the induction of the fatty liver. However, Sakurai et al.[17] failed to observe a change in the hepatic ATP level caused by tryptophan. Dianzani[22] speculated that the fatty liver provoked by treatment with tryptophan was due to impaired synthesis of apolipoprotein, possibly related to a diversion of synthesis directed to other proteins. Aviram et al.[23] reported enhancement of plasma lipid peroxidation in rats due to tryptophan.[24] Thus, currently, the mechanism whereby tryptophan affects lipid metabolism in the liver is not clear. The need for very high doses of L-tryptophan to induce fatty liver in the rat suggests that it may be related to toxicity. Indeed, Gullino et al.[11] reported that the LD_{50} level for L-tryptophan in the rat is 162 mg per 100 g body weight.

9.2.1.4   Muscle and Lung Fibrosis

In general, animal studies regarding the effects of increased L-tryptophan ingestion and tissue fibrosis have been controversial. Ronen et al.[25] reported that excessive dietary tryptophan (1%) (casein at 10% in diet for 3 weeks) resulted in the appearance of increased fibrosis of muscle, of lungs, and an increase in tumor necrosis factor-α (TNFα)-positive cells of female rats. However, these pathologic changes were described only in a few rats and in only those that received 1% tryptophan plus injections of p-chlorophenylalanine, an inhibitor of tryptophan hydroxylase. No mention is made of pathologic findings in rats fed the 1% tryptophan added to diet alone.

Gross et al.[26] fed female rats for 3, 6, and 12 weeks on a diet containing 20% casein with added 1, 2, or 5% L-tryptophan. The results based upon a small number of rats in each group revealed that in gastrocremius muscle there were mild inflammatory infiltration and moderate hyperplasia of fibroblasts in endomysial septa of some rats, especially in rats fed the 5% tryptophan diet for 12 weeks. In lungs, focal areas of inflammation accompanied by increased fibrosis were reported in the experimental groups. However, documentation in the paper was poor, and the number of rats involved was not given. Especially in light of many other experimental rat studies dealing with experimental eosinophilia myalgia syndrome where implicated L-tryptophan was used, the question of whether tryptophan provoked myofascial fibrosis in rats is questionable (see Chapter 11).

9.2.1.5   Pancreatic Changes

Love et al.[27] reported fibrosis and acinar changes in the pancreas due to high levels of administered tryptophan. Whether this may be related to high levels of tryptophan in the pancreas is not known, but Sainio et al.[28] reported that tryptophan levels in the pancreas were five times higher than in mouse liver.

9.2.1.6   Serotonin Syndrome

As mentioned earlier, the most common adverse effect reported when tryptophan is given to humans is the serotonin syndrome. However, this syndrome was first described in rats. When rats were given tryptophan plus a monoamine oxidase inhibitor, or various other drugs such as high doses of 5-hydroxytryptophan with a peripheral decarboxylase inhibitor, or serotonin receptor agonists, the rats show tremor, hypertonicity, rigidity, rigidly arched tail, lateral head shaking, hind-limb abduction, hyperreactivity, myoclonus, treading movements of the forelimbs, and even generalized seizures.[29] Such animal model studies suggested that serotonin antagonists may be a useful treatment.

9.2.2   Mice and Rabbits

Reports on LD_{50} of L-tryptophan in mice and rabbits and by different routes of administration have been reviewed.[30] By I.V. or I.P., the dose in all animals was about 2 g/kg, while by oral route it was 5 to 16 g/kg. Thus, in the rat, mouse, or rabbit, tryptophan is generally considered to be of low acute toxicity or to be essentially nontoxic.

9.2.3 Hamsters

Madara and Carlson[31] reported that high levels of tryptophan elicited cytoskeletal and macromolecular permeability alterations in hamster small intestinal epithelium *in vitro*.

9.2.4 Ponies

Acute hemolytic anemia has been reported in ponies by Paradis et al.[32] by oral administration of tryptophan.

9.2.5 Ruminants (Cattle, Goats)

Oral tryptophan causes marked pulmonary edema and emphysema. This appears to be due to the bacterial conversion of tryptophan to skatole (3-methylindole), which causes the same type of lung lesion.[33]

9.2.6 Species Differences

Badawy and Evans[34] speculated that certain species of animals were more sensitive to tryptophan toxicity than were others. This speculation was based upon studies on liver tryptophan 2,3-dioxygenase activity in different species: Group 1 (rat, mouse, pig, turkey, and chicken) and Group 2 (cat, frog, guinea pigs, hamster, gerbil, ox, sheep, and rabbit). Group 2 species lacked the apoenzyme or the hormonal induction mechanism and have a deficient kynurenine pathway. Some of the species of Group 2 showed a far more sensitive toxicity reaction than those of Group 1 in that they displayed marked lethality at doses to which the species of Group 1 were resistant. Humans behaved like the Group 1 species. Human liver tryptophan 2,3-dioxygenase most likely exists in both forms, holoenzyme and apoenzyme, and can be induced by cortisol administration.[35] Humans are able to survive repeated high doses of tryptophan during treatment for neuropsychiatric diseases. Using male adult animals, some species of Group 2 (frog and hamster) showed deaths and signs of toxicity symptoms due to tryptophan administration, which suggested that others of Group 2 also have increased toxicity effects due to tryptophan.[34] Indeed, consistent findings have been reported in earlier studies with guinea pigs,[36] gerbil,[37] and bovines (steer).[38] In general, Group 1 species appeared to be much less sensitive to tryptophan toxicity. Herbst[30] reviewed L-tryptophan toxicity in rats, mice, and rabbits. The above information is important for anyone planning experiments relating to tryptophan toxicity and in attempting to extrapolate the findings to humans.

9.2.7 Overview

Review of the literature appears to indicate that L-tryptophan itself is generally not toxic in humans, or if it is toxic, very high levels are needed. However, it does appear that under certain conditions, as with certain contaminants or impurities (as in eosinophilia myalgia syndrome), it may contribute to the toxicity of the toxic compounds.

9.3 Toxicity of Tryptophan in Food

The chemistry of tryptophan in food was considered to some extent in an earlier chapter (Chapter 4). Friedman and Cuq[39] have reviewed the topic of toxicity of tryptophan in food in detail. Here attention focuses on toxicity derived from breakdown products of tryptophan present in food proteins.

9.3.1 Toxicity of Derivatives

Among oxidation products resulting from photooxidation or from the oxidation of tryptophan by strong oxidizing agents such as hydrogen peroxide or peroxidizing lipids are N-formylkyrurenine, kynurenine, dioxindole-3-alanine, β-carboline, quinazoline, and hexahydropyrroloindole derivatives.[40-45] These compounds do not possess any nutritional value, and some exhibit toxicity for bacteria, isolated mammalian cells, and animals.[46,47]

When protein reacts with oxidizing lipids, extensive loss of available tryptophan is observed. This loss is due to the destruction of this amino acid and to the general decrease in protein digestibility.[46,48]

9.3.2 Toxicology of Carbolines

Carboline formation occurs when free or bound tryptophan is heated at high temperature. These derivatives also have been found in foods such as commercial beef extracts and fried hamburger,[49,50] heated milk,[51] and beer and wine.[52] Among these compounds, two γ-carbolines (Trp-P-1, Trp-P-2) and two α-carbolines (A-α-C, Me-A-α-C) show significant mutagenic activity in *Salmonella tryphimurium* tester strains after metabolic activation. Although not mutagenic themselves, the β-carbolines (harmane and norharmane) enhance the activity of the mutagenic α- or γ-carbolines. There is an abundance of scientific information on the *Salmonella* mutagenicity of these compounds, and some important reviews by Sugimura have been written on this topic.[53,54] Feeding mice a diet containing Trp-P-1, Trp-P-2, or other carbolines demonstrated the hepatocarcinogenicity of these compounds. This was discussed in Chapter 6.

9.3.3 Comment

The occurrence of heat- and chemical-induced transformations of tryptophan and the nutritional and toxicologic consequences suggest a need for additional research to define possible approaches to prevent or minimize the formation of antinutritional and toxic tryptophan condensation and oxidation products in foods. The possible beneficial effects of antioxidants such as vitamins C and E, carotenes, flavonoids, indole derivatives, selenium compounds, and sulfur amino acids in enhancing the stability of tryptophan in foods need to be investigated.

9.4 Conclusions

Much information is available about the toxicity of L-tryptophan in humans and in animals. Generally, in humans the toxicity of L-tryptophan alone appears to be minimal. In animals, certain species appear to be more sensitive than others to L-tryptophan toxicity. Overall, these differences appear to be related to the animal's ability to metabolize tryptophan via tryptophan 2,3-dioxygenase; species with high enzyme levels are less toxic in response to L-tryptophan administration.

In relation to food intake, pyrolysis products of L-tryptophan in which highly mutagenic γ-carboline, tryptophan-P-1 (3-amino-1, 4-dimethyl-5H-pyrido[4,3-b] indole and tryptophan-P-2 (3-amino-1-methyl-5H-pyrido[4,3-b] indole are formed and can be activated to mutagens in liver. Implications of such events in liver carcinogenesis are discussed in Chapter 6.

Because of the high increase in toxicity of L-tryptophan in animals with adrenalectomy or induced adrenal insufficiency, administration of high doses must be avoided in certain humans, patients with adrenal insufficiency, in neonates, and in pregnant women.

The occurrence of the eosinophilia myalgia syndrome discussed in Chapter 11 suggests that L-tryptophan containing minute amounts of impurities or contaminants may be causative of a disease state in certain individuals. The role of L-tryptophan itself in this syndrome is not defined. Conceivably, it plays a supportive role to toxic contaminants in selected, susceptible individuals to induce the syndrome.

References

1. Pakes, G. E., L-tryptophan in psychiatric practice, *Drug Intell. Clin. Pharm.*, 13, 391, 1979.
2. Belongia, E. A., Hedberg, C. W., Gleich, G. J., White, K. E., Mayeno, A. N., Loegering, D. A., Dunnette, S. L., Pirie, P. L., MacDonald, K. L., and Osterholm, M. T., An investigation of the cause of the eosinophilia-myalgia syndrome associated with tryptophan use, *N. Engl. J. Med.*, 323, 357, 1990.
3. Eidson, M., Philen, R. M., Sewell, C. M., Voorhes, R., and Kilbourne, E. M., L-tryptophan and eosinophilia-myalgia syndrome in New Mexico, *Lancet*, 335, 645, 1990.
4. Belongia, E. A., Mayeno, A. N., and Osterholm, M. T., The eosinophilia-myalgia syndrome and tryptophan, *Annu. Rev. Nutr.*, 12, 235, 1992.
5. Young, S. N., The clinical psychopharmacology of tryptophan, in *Nutrition and the Brain. Food Constituents Affecting Normal and Abnormal Behavior*, Vol. 7, Wurtman, R. J. and Wurtman, J. J., Eds., Raven Press, New York, 1986, 49–88.
6. Thomson, J., Rankin, H., Ashcroft, G. W., Yates, C. M., McQueen, J. K., and Cummings, S. W., The treatment of depression in general practice: A comparison of L-tryptophan, amitriptyline, and a combination of L-tryptophan and amitriptyline with placebo, *Psychol. Med.*, 12, 741, 1982.
7. Murphy, D. L., Baker, M., Goodwin, F. K., Miller, H., Kotin, J., and Bunney, W. E., Jr., L-tryptophan in affective disorders: Indoleamine changes and differential clinical effects, *Psychopharmacologia*, 34, 11, 1974.
8. Gillin, J. C., Kaplan, J. A., and Wyatt, R. J., Clinical effects of tryptophan in chronic schizophrenic patients, *Biol. Psychiatr.*, 11, 635, 1976.
9. Sternbach, H., The serotonin syndrome, *Am. J. Psychiatr.*, 148, 705, 1991.
10. Lejoyeux, M., Rouillon, F., Leon, E., and Ades, J., The serotonin syndrome: Review of the literature and description of an original study, *Encephale*, 21(5), 537, 1995.
11. Gullino, P., Winitz, M., Birnbaum, S. M., Cornfield, J., Otey, M. C., and Greenstein, J. P., Studies on the metabolism of amino acids and related compounds *in vivo*. I. Toxicity of essential amino acids individually, in mixtures and the protective effect of L-arginine, *Arch. Biochem. Biophys.*, 64, 319, 1956.
12. Curzon, G. and Knott, P. J., Environmental, toxicological and related aspects of tryptophan metabolism with particular reference to the central nervous system, *CRC Crit. Rev. Toxicol.*, 5, 145, 1977.
13. Trulson, M. E. and Ulissey, M. J., Low doses of L-tryptophan are lethal in rats with adrenal insufficiency, *Life Sci.*, 41, 349, 1987.
14. Hirata, Y., Kawachi, T., and Sugimura, T., Fatty liver induced by injection of L-tryptophan, *Biochim. Biophys. Acta*, 144, 233, 1967.
15. Ramakrishna Rao, P., Bhaskar Rao, A., and Ramakrishnan, S., Biochemical mechanism of induction of fatty liver by tryptophan, *Ind. J. Exp. Biol.*, 18, 1335, 1980.
16. Sakurai, T., Miyazawa S., and Hashimoto, T., Effect of tryptophan on fatty acid synthesis in rat liver, *FEBS Lett.*, 36, 96, 1973.
17. Sakurai, T., Miyazawea, S., Shindo, Y., and Hashimoto, T., The effect of tryptophan administration on fatty acid synthesis in the liver of the fasted normal rat, *Biochim. Biopys. Acta*, 360, 275, 1974.

18. Fears, R. and Murrell, E. A., Tryptophan and the control of triglyceride and carbohydrate metabolism in the rat, *Br. J. Nutr.*, 43, 349, 1980.
19. Trulson, M. E. and Sampson, H. W., Ultrastructural changes of the liver following L-tryptophan ingestion in rats, *J. Nutr.*, 116, 1109, 1986.
20. Matthies, D. L. and Jacobs, F. A., Rat liver is not damaged by high dose tryptophan treatment, *J. Nutr.*, 123, 852, 1993.
21. Miyazawa, S., Sakurai, T., Shindo, Y., Imura, M., and Hashimoto, T., The effect of tryptophan administration on fatty acid synthesis in the livers of rats under various nutritional conditions, *J. Biochem.*, 78, 139, 1975.
22. Dianzani, M. U., Biochemical aspects of fatty liver, *Biochem. Soc. Trans.*, 14, 903, 1973.
23. Aviram, M., Cogan, U., and Mokady, S., Excessive dietary tryptophan enhances plasma lipid peroxidation in rats, *Atherosclerosis*, 88, 29, 1991.
24. Christen, S., Peterhans, E., and Stocker, R., Antioxidant activities of some tryptophan metabolites: Possible implication for inflammatory diseases, *Proc. Natl. Acad. Sci. U.S.A.*, 87, 2506, 1990.
25. Ronen, N., Gross, B., Ben-Shachar, D., and Livne, E. The effects of induced kynurenine pathway on immunocytochemical changes in rat tissues following excessive L-tryptophan consumption, *Adv. Exp. Med. Biol.*, 398, 177, 1996.
26. Gross, B., Ronen, N., Honigman, S., and Livne, E., Tryptophan toxicity — time and dose response in rats, *Adv. Exp. Med. Biol.*, 467, 507, 1999.
27. Love, L. A., Rader, J. I., Crofford, L. J., Raybourne, R. B., Principato, M. A., Page, S. W., Trucksess, M. W., Smith, M. J., Dugan, E. M., and Turner, M. L., Pathological and immunological effects of ingesting L-tryptophan and 1,1'-ethylidenebis (L-tryptophan) in Lewis rats, *J. Clin. Invest.*, 91, 804, 1993.
28. Sainio, E. L., Narvanen, S., Sainio, P., and Tuohimaa, P., Distribution of tryptophan in normal and glucose loaded mice, *Amino Acids*, 1, 160, 1991.
29. Gerson, S. C. and Baldessarini, R. J., Motor effects of serotonin in the central nervous system, *Life Sci.*, 27, 1435, 1980.
30. Herbst, M., L-tryptophan toxicity: A review, in *Current Progress in Medicine and Drug Safety*, Kochen, W. and Steinhart, H., Eds., de Gruyton, Berlin, 1994, 200–212.
31. Madara, J. L. and Carlson, S., Supraphysiologic L-tryptophan elicits cytoskeletal and macromolecular permeability alterations in hamster small intestinal epithelium *in vitro*, *J. Clin. Invest.*, 87(2), 454, 1991.
32. Paradis, M. R., Breeze, R. G., Bayly, W. M., Counts, D. F., and Laegreid, W. W., Acute hemolytic anemia after oral administration of L-tryptophan in ponies, *Am. J. Vet. Res.*, 52, 742, 1991.
33. Carlson, J. R., Yokoyama, M. T., and Dickinson, E. O., Induction of pulmonary edema and emphysema in cattle and goats with 3-methylindole, *Science*, 176, 298, 1972.
34. Badawy, A. A. and Evans, M., Animal liver tryptophan pyrrolases: Absence of apoenzyme and of hormonal induction mechanism from species sensitive to tryptophan toxicity, *Biochem. J.*, 158, 79, 1976.
35. Altman, K. and Greengard, O., Correlation of kynurenine excretion with liver tryptophan pyrrolase levels in disease and after hydrocortisone induction, *J. Clin. Invest.*, 45, 1525, 1966.
36. Hvitefelt, J. and Santti, R. S., Tryptophan pyrrolase in the liver of guinea pig: The absence of hydrocortisone induction, *Biochim. Biophys. Acta*, 258(2), 358, 1972.

37. Baughman, K. L. and Franz, J. M., Control of tryptophan oxygenase and formamidase activity in the gerbil, *Int. J. Biochem.*, 2, 201, 1971.
38. Johnson, R. J. and Dyer, I. A., Effect of orally administered tryptophan on tryptophan pyrrolase activity in ovine and bovine, *Life Sci.*, 5, 1121, 1966.
39. Friedman, M. and Cuq, J. L., Chemistry, analysis, nutritional value, and toxicology of tryptophan in food. A review, *J. Agric. Food Chem.*, 36, 1079, 1988.
40. Walrant, P. and Santus, R., N-formyl-kynurenine, a tryptophan photooxidation product, as a photodynamic sensitizer, *Photochem. Photobiol.*, 411, 1974, 1974.
41. Savige, W. E., New oxidation products of tryptophan, *Aust. J. Chem.*, 28, 2275, 1975.
42. Nakagawa, M. and Hino, T., Photosensitized indole derivatives, *Heterocycles*, 6, 1575, 1977.
43. Sun, M. and Zigman, S., Isolation and identification of tryptophan photoproducts from aqueous solution of tryptophan exposed to near UV-light, *Photochem. Photobiol.*, 29, 893, 1979.
44. Young, S. H., Lau, S., Hsieh, Y., and Karel, M., Degradation products of L-tryptophan reacted with peroxidizing methyl linoleate, in *Autooxidation in Food and Biological Systems*, Simic, M. and Karel, G., Eds., Plenum Press, New York, 1980, 237.
45. Kanner, J. D. and Fennema, O., Photooxidation of tryptophan in the presence of riboflavin, *J. Agric. Food Chem.*, 35, 71, 1987.
46. Steinhart, H. and Kirchgessner, M., Toxicity of tryptophan oxidation products in chickens, *Z. Tierphysiol. Tierernahr. Futtermittelkd.*, 40, 332, 1978.
47. de Weck, D., Nielsen, H. K., and Finot, P. A., Oxidation rate of free and protein-bound tryptophan by hydrogen peroxide and the bioavailability of the oxidation products, *J. Sci. Food Agric.*, 41, 179, 1987.
48. Nielsen, H. K., Finot, P. A., and Hurrell, R. F., Reactions of proteins with oxidizing lipids. 1. Influence of protein quality on the bioavailability of lysine, methionine, cysteine, and tryptophan as measured in rat assays, *Br. J. Nutr.*, 53, 75, 1985.
49. Felton, J. S., Bjeldaness L. F., and Hatch, F. T., Mutagens in cooked foods — metabolism and genetic toxicity, in *Nutritional and Toxicological Aspects of Food Safety*, Friedman, M., Ed., Plenum Press, New York, 1984, 555.
50. Bjeldanes, L. F., Felton, J. S., and Hatch, F. T., Mutagens in cooked food: Chemical aspects, *Adv. Exp. Med. Biol.*, 177, 545, 1984.
51. Rogers, A. M. and Shibamoto, T., Mutagenicity of the products obtained from heated milk systems, *Food Chem. Toxicol.*, 20, 259, 1982.
52. Bosin, T., Krogh S., and Mais, D., Indentification and quantification of 1,2,3,4-tetrahydro-beta-carboline-3-carboxylic acid and 1-methyl-1,2,3,4-tetrahydro-beta-arboline-3-carboxylic acid in beer and wine, *J. Agric. Food Chem.*, 34, 843, 1986.
53. Sugimura, T., Carcinogenicity of mutagenic heterocyclic amines formed during the cooking process, *Mutat. Res.*, 150, 33, 1985.
54. Sugimura, T., Studies on environmental chemical carcinogenesis in Japan, *Science*, 233, 312, 1986.

10

Serotonin and Melatonin

CONTENTS

10.1 Introduction

This book is primarily concerned with L-tryptophan. However, two major derivatives of tryptophan, serotonin and melatonin, have gained prominence in recent years and appear to have overshadowed L-tryptophan. For example, during the last 35 years (1965 to 2000) the total citations on the Medline database were as follows: tryptophan, 17,106; serotonin, 44,841; and melatonin, 8,130. In Medline literature citations, serotonin has by far (2- to 3.5-fold) outnumbered L-tryptophan continuously from 1961 until the present time (Figure 10.1). Also, it is interesting to note that melatonin citations have gradually climbed from 1961 to the present and now equal those of tryptophan (Figure 10.1). The citations refer to total citations, which include all subcategories of each of the three categories.

In this chapter, a brief review of serotonin and melatonin is included. However, detailed coverage of these two important topics is beyond the scope of this book. Nonetheless, a number of reviews on these topics are cited in this brief, limited review.

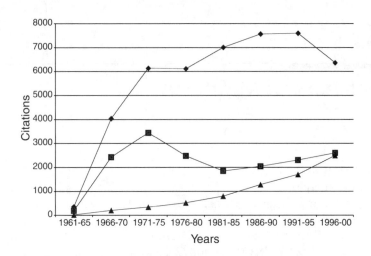

FIGURE 10.1
Total citations on Medline for 5-year periods from 1961 to 2000. L-tryptophan = ■; serotonin = ♦; and melatonin = ▲.

10.2 Serotonin

Whenever the actions or effects of L-tryptophan are considered or evaluated, it is usual that serotonin, an important derivative of L-tryptophan, is brought into the picture. Throughout the earlier chapters, many of the effects of L-tryptophan depletion or excess by dietary means have been explained in terms of actions of serotonin, which is synthesized directly from L-tryptophan. The formation of serotonin and its dependency upon L-tryptophan is a vital process that has gained recognition and attention over many years. The literature involving serotonin is extensive and is often cited in earlier chapters where serotonin has been considered to come into play in explaining certain actions of L-tryptophan. A number of reviews have described the role that serotonin plays within the central nervous system.[1-4]

The neurotransmitter serotonin has been implicated in many physiologic functions and in pathophysiological disorders. Hydroxylation of tryptophan is rate-limiting in the synthesis of serotonin, and the rate-limiting enzyme, tryptophan hydroxylase (TPH), determines the *in vivo* concentration of serotonin. Relative concentrations of serotonin are important in neural transmission. The low levels of TPH in tissues and its instability have hindered identification of the mechanisms regulating TPH activity. New avenues of research for identifying TPH regulatory mechanisms have been developed; these involve recombinant DNA technology, enabling synthesis of TPH deletions, chimeras, and point mutations that have served as tools for identifying structural and functional domains within TPH. New findings have also revealed regulation of TPH activity by post-translational phosphorylation, kinetic inhibitions, and covalent modification. These approaches have been reviewed by Mockus and Vrana.[5]

Serotonin has been reported to function as a local antioxidant. The antioxidative properties of serotonin as well as of melatonin have been well documented.[6-10] A discussion of the antioxidative actions of L-tryptophan and its metabolites is included in Chapter 9.

10.3 Melatonin

Although serotonin has gained much recognition over the years, more recently another tryptophan-related compound, melatonin, has been gaining notoriety. L-tryptophan is the precursor and serotonin an intermediary product for melatonin synthesis in the pineal gland.[11] In the following section on melatonin, a brief review of its actions and relationships to L-tryptophan and melatonin is given.

Melatonin, a molecule widely produced in both the plant and animal kingdom, has been considered for many years to function exclusively as a synchronizer of seasonal reproductions, i.e., that it adjusts the biological clock, and is a sleep-inducing agent and immune system stimulator. Some of these roles are briefly described in the following sections. In recent years, melatonin has also been found to be a free-radical scavenger and antioxidant. Many recent studies have stressed the possible significance of this important property.[9]

Melatonin is a hormone secreted mainly by the pineal gland but also by the retina. It is synthesized from L-tryptophan. Its characteristic circadian rhythm is ruled by light through the control of two limiting enzymatic activities of N-acetyl-transferase and hydroxyindole-O-methyl-transferase. In all species studied including humans, its maximal plasma concentration occurs at night. It is considered as a signal transducing information on solar light in the organism and provides a temporal framework upon which metabolic pathways are organized. It has been implicated as being involved in aging[12] and has been considered to have a role in the treatment of circadian rhythm-associated sleep disorders, in jet lag, in immunological functions, etc.[13]

The ability of melatonin to cross biological (lipid membrane) barriers and to diffuse into compartments within cells is probably related to its lipophilic ability in nature. The rhythm in melatonin secretion is generated endogenously by the circadian pacemaker(s) in the suprachiasmatic nuclei (SCN) and is regulated by the environmental light-to-dark cycle. Melatonin, through its action in the SCN, synchronizes disrupted or free-running circadian rhythms and regulates a variety of daily and seasonal changes in the physiology and behavior of animals.

10.3.1 Specific Actions of Melatonin

10.3.1.1 Reproduction

In photoperiodic nonhuman mammals, the secretion of melatonin from the pineal gland plays a major role in regulating reproductive physiology. Unfortunately, in humans these relationships are less clear. The melatonin rhythm has been reported to change throughout life, with the first substantial change in nocturnal melatonin secretion occurring with puberty. Sexual maturation is considered to be associated with a reduction in nocturnal melatonin levels, but cause-and-effect relativity still needs to be established. At high latitudes, the amount of melatonin produced by the pineal gland varies with the season (light–dark cycle changes), which suggests that this changes reproductive efficiency. In humans, correlations between melatonin and the status of the reproductive system have been observed, but whether they are functionally related needs to be established. This subject has been reviewed by Reiter.[14]

10.3.1.2 Immune System Stimulator

Recent evidence suggests that melatonin has an immuno-hematopoetic role.[15] In studies with animals, it has been reported to prevent stress-induced immunodepression, provide protection against Gram-negative septic shock, and restore immune functions after hemorrhage shock. In studies with humans, it amplified the antihumoral activity of interleukin-2.

10.3.1.3 Rhythm Disorders

One of the most popular uses of melatonin has been in the treatment of rhythm disorders, such as those occurring with jet lag, shift work, or blindness.

10.3.1.4 Sleep

It has been known for years that L-tryptophan plays a role in certain sleep disorders.[16] Acute tryptophan depletion can lead to impairment of sleep continuity. In certain patients with chronic sleep problems, tryptophan can help reestablish a physiological sleep pattern.

The role that melatonin may play as a consequence of tryptophan intake in sleep merits consideration. Improvement in sleep latency, increasing sleep efficiency, and raising sleep quality scores in elderly, melatonin-deficient insomniacs occur with low doses of melatonin.

10.3.1.5 Antioxidant and Radical Scavengers

Melatonin has a variety of seemingly unrelated functions in organisms. Recently, it was found to be an effective antioxidant.[9,17,18] It detoxifies a variety of free radicals and reactive oxygen intermediates, including hydroxyl radical, peroxynitrite anion, singlet oxygen, and nitric oxide. Also, it reportedly stimulates several antioxidative enzymes, including glutathione peroxidase, glutathione reductase, glucose-6-phosphate dehydrogenase, and superoxide dimutase, and conversely it inhibits a proxidative enzyme, nitric oxide synthase. Since it crosses many morphologic and physiologic barriers (blood–brain barrier, placenta) and distributes throughout cells, the increased efficacy of melatonin as an antioxidant is evident. The importance of this property has been stressed as potentially protective in a variety of age-associated degenerative diseases where toxic free radicals have been implicated.[19,20]

10.3.2 Concluding Remarks

Melatonin has been conserved evolutionarily in almost all groups of organisms from plants to protozoa to humans. It is derived from dietary sources of the amino acid tryptophan in vertebrates. It has numerous actions and functions. Increased interest in this hormone molecule has occurred in recent years, and it has been described as a master hormone and candidate for universal panacea.[13] However, caution should be exercised before going overboard in regard to the overall significance of the many important activities and actions attributed to melatonin. In observing its overall and specific importance, further studies and documentation are needed. Often, such detailed analyses temper early overenthusiasm.

References

1. Fernstrom, J. D. and Wurtman, R. J., Nutrition and the brain, *Sci. Am.*, 230, 83, 1974.
2. Wurtman, R. J. and Fernstrom, J. D., Control of brain neurotransmitter synthesis by precursor availability and nutritional state, *Biochem. Pharmacol.*, 25(15), 1691, 1976.
3. Wurtman, R. J., Nutrients that modify brain function, *Sci. Am.*, 246(4), 50, 1982.
4. Fernstrom, J. D., Can nutrient supplements modify brain function? *Am. J. Clin. Nutr.*, 71(6 Suppl.), 1669S, 2000.
5. Mockus, S. M. and Vrana, K. E., Advances in the molecular characterization of tryptophan hydroxylase, *J. Mol. Neurosci.*, 10(3), 163, 1998.
6. Schuff-Werner, P., Splettstosser, W., Schmidt, F., and Huether, G., Serotonin acts as a radical scavenger and is oxidized to a dimer during the respiratory burst of human mononuclear and polymorphonuclear phagocytes, *Eur. J. Clin. Invest.*, 25(7), 477, 1901.
7. Wrona, M. Z. and Dryhurst, G., Interactions of 5-hydroxytryptamine with oxidative enzymes, *Biochem. Pharmacol.*, 41(8), 1145, 1991.
8. Huether, G. and Schuff-Werner, P., Platelet serotonin acts as a locally releasable antioxidant, *Adv. Exp. Med. Biol.*, 398, 299, 1996.
9. Reiter, R. J., Tan, D. X., Cabrera, J., D'Arpa, D., Sainz, R. M., Mayo, J. C., and Ramos, S., The oxidant/antioxidant network: Role of melatonin, *Biol. Signals Receptors*, 8(1–2), 56, 1999.

10. Reiter, R. J., Tan, D. X., Cabrera, J., and D'Arpa, D., Melatonin and tryptophan derivatives as free radical scavengers and antioxidants, *Adv. Exp. Med. Biol.*, 467, 379, 1999.
11. Cardinali, D. P., Melatonin. A mammalian pineal hormone, *Endocrine Rev.*, 2(3), 327, 1981.
12. Touitou, Y., Bogdan, A., Auzeby, A., and Selmaoui, B., Melatonin and aging, *Therapie*, 53(5), 473, 1998.
13. Kumar, V., Melatonin: A master hormone and a candidate for universal panacea, *Ind. J. Exp. Biol.*, 34(5), 391, 1996.
14. Reiter, R. J., Melatonin and human reproduction, *Ann. Med.*, 30(1), 103, 1998.
15. Bubenik, G. A., Blask, D. E., Brown, G. M., Maestroni, G. J., Pang, S. F., Reiter, R. J., Viswanathan, M., and Zisapel, N., Prospects of the clinical utilization of melatonin, *Biol. Signals Receptors*, 7(4), 195, 1998.
16. Riemann, D. and Vorderholzer, U., Treatment of depression and sleep disorders. Significance of serotonin and L-tryptophan in pathophysiology and therapy, *Fortschr. Med.*, 116(32), 40, 1998.
17. Chan, T. Y. and Tang, P. L., Characterization of the antioxidant effects of melatonin and related indoleamines *in vitro*, *J. Pineal Res.*, 20(4), 187, 1996.
18. Reiter, R. J., Carneiro, R. C., and Oh, C. S., Melatonin in relation to cellular antioxidative defense mechanisms, *Horm. Metab. Res.*, 29(8), 363, 1997.
19. Reiter, R. J., Cytoprotective properties of melatonin: Presumed association with oxidative damage and aging, *Nutrition*, 14(9), 691, 1997.
20. Reiter, R. J., Oxidative damage in the central nervous system: Protection by melatonin, *Progr. Neurobiol.*, 56(3), 359, 1998.

11

The Eosinophilia Myalgia Syndrome: A Tryptophan Tragedy

CONTENTS

11.1　Introduction

Since tryptophan was first described some 100 years ago, continuous progress has been made in our understanding of the importance and actions of this vital amino acid. Therefore, it was most disturbing that in the winter of 1989 an incident occurred that flagged L-tryptophan as possibly being a hazardous substance. This occurrence identified L-tryptophan as being responsible for a new disease entity, the eosinophilia myalgia syndrome (EMS). Thus, L-tryptophan, an important nutrient, which was considered to be indispensable and also beneficial in many ways, became implicated in a tragic event. This chapter reviews how L-tryptophan became accused of causing a disease entity, EMS. Also, it reviews the current state of knowledge about EMS and considers the complex lesson that may be learned in regard to its occurrence. Such a lesson may be of value in alerting scientists (nutritionists, biochemists, molecular biologists, pathologists, clinicians, epidemiologists, and geneticists) to become aware of the potential threat of new diseases or syndromes similar to EMS that may appear in years to come. The tryptophan tragedy may offer information that may be utilized to become better prepared to confront new challenging diseases or syndromes.

Since EMS is the only disease that has been attributed directly to or related to the ingestion of L-tryptophan, it merits a detailed review. Extensive data have been collected about EMS, yet its cause and pathogenesis remain a puzzle. However, this syndrome has disclosed how limited or deficient our knowledge has been about how L-tryptophan acts normally or may act abnormally under certain circumstances. In searching for answers relating to this interesting and intriguing syndrome, much additional basic information concerning L-tryptophan has been gained, and the need for further probing and investigations has become apparent.

11.2 Etiology

Based upon epidemiological data, it was concluded rapidly that EMS was related directly to the ingestion of L-tryptophan. This indispensable amino acid has been used widely for many years as a readily obtainable natural agent for relieving depression, pain, insomnia, hyperactivity, and eating disorders. It was available over the counter in drug stores and in natural food stores. In November 1989, the Food and Drug Administration terminated the distribution and availability of L-tryptophan in response to the epidemiological evidence gathered that related the amino acid to the onset of EMS. The incidence of new cases of EMS rapidly diminished thereafter.

Epidemiological investigations revealed that EMS was related to the ingestion of L-tryptophan from a single manufacturer in Japan.[1-4] Further probes revealed that the manufacturer had modified some of its manufacturing processes during the time before its product became implicated in the onset of EMS. High-performance liquid chromatography (HPLC) analysis revealed that the manufacturer's L-tryptophan was highly pure (99.6%), with only some minor contaminants or impurities (ranging from 50 to 200 ppm). Three HPLC peaks, peak 97 (or peak E), peak UV-5, and peak 200, have been considered as possibly having etiological significance.[5-11] On chemical analysis, peak 97 (or peak E) has been determined to be 1,1'-ethylidenebis(L-tryptophan; EBT);[5,6] peak UV-5 is 3-anilino-L-alanine (PAA);[7,8] and peak 200 is 2(3-indolymethyl)-L-tryptophan.[10] A brief review of studies relating to these contaminants follows.

11.2.1 Contaminants

11.2.1.1 1,1'-Ethylidenebis(Tryptophan) (EBT)

The first contaminant identified in L-tryptophan implicated in EMS was EBT. Based upon HPLC analysis, preparations of such L-tryptophan revealed a distinct peak, initially called peak E[1,5,10] or peak 97,[12,13] that is a dimeric form of L-tryptophan.[5,13] Thus, early on, the presence of EBT became associated with EMS.[2,6] Ito et al.[14] studied EBT, purified by using HPLC, for its behavior in an acid environment. EBT is unstable in such an environment and decomposes to form L-tryptophan and compounds that were named peak X/X' substances. Peak Y/Y′ substances were observed as intermediary products between EBT and peak X/X′. Investigations designed to determine how EBT may be involved in EMS are described in Section 11.10.

11.2.1.2   3-Phenylamino-L-Alanine (PAA)

The presence of another contaminant peak in L-tryptophan implicated in EMS was detected upon HPLC with both UV and FL analyses by Toyo'oka et al.[9] and was characterized as PAA by Goda et al.[7] Adachi et al.[15] studied the metabolism of PAA in rats and described four metabolites of PAA in the urine (N-(hydroxyphenyl)glycine, N-phenylglycine, 3-(phenylamino)lactic acid, and 3-(hydroxy-phenylamino)-lactic acid). The results suggested that the degradation pathway of PAA was similar to that of phenylalanine. Other studies with PAA are described in Section 11.10.

11.2.1.3   2(3-Indolymethyl)-L-Tryptophan (Peak 200)

Peak 200 is one of the four HPLC peaks that marks lots produced by Showa Denko KK. Its structure has been determined by Muller et al.[16] as 2(3-indolymethyl)-L-tryptophan.[10] It has not been tested on animals.

11.2.1.4   Other Contaminants

Detailed analyses by HPLC revealed that there were more than 60 minor contaminants in the implicated L-tryptophan from Showa Denko.[10] Of these contaminants, six were considered to be associated with EMS. The structures of the three contaminants are known and have been described previously, but the full identities of the other three contaminants are unknown. Simat et al.[17] used single reversed-phase high-performance liquid chromatography run using UV and fluorescence detection on implicated L-tryptophan and observed 17 contaminants. Most of these contaminants were classified as tryptophan metabolites, nonphysiological oxidation, or carbonyl condensation compounds of tryptophan.

Using the powerful structural elucidation technique of tandem mass spectrometry coupled with on-line HPLC (LC-ESI-MS/MS), the structural characterization of a number of additional contaminants of L-tryptophan associated with EMS has been performed.[18] The identity of the contaminants were as follows. Peaks UV-5 included 3-phenylamino-L-alanine (PAA); 1,1′-ethylidenebis(tryptophan) (EBT); 2-(3-indolymethyl)-L-tryptophan (200) (all identified as case related). Peaks 1,3-carboxyl-1,2,3,4-tetrahydro-β-carboline; 2,3-carboxy-1-methyl-1,2,3,4-tetrahydro-β-carboline; 2-(2,3 dihydroxy-1-[3-indolyl]-propyl)-L-tryptophan (100); and diastereomers of 3-carboxy-1-[3-indolyl-methyl]-1,2,3,4 tetrahydro-β-carboline (300 and 400), were confirmed by this technique. Peak P31, previously unresolved from peak 200, a case-related compound, has been tentatively identified as 2-(3-indolyl)-L-tryptophan. Thus, progress on structural analyses of contaminants has progressed far beyond studies evaluating their toxicologic and physiologic potentials.

Although much data have been derived about contaminants in implicated L-tryptophan, the causative etiologic agent, if there is only one, of EMS is still unknown.[19] Epidemiologic studies thus far indicate a lack of statistical significance for the association of EMS with the single peaks of EBT, PAA, or Peak 200.[10,11]

11.3   Incidence and Prevalence

In the United States, more than 1500 cases of EMS have been reported since November 1989, of which some 38 were fatal.[20,21] Based upon a 1990 survey of use of L-tryptophan in the Minneapolis–St. Paul area, 4% of households had at least one person who had used L-tryptophan between 1980 and 1989.[1] The prevalence of use increased markedly between 1985 and 1989 and was highest in women. Overall, the incidence of EMS in the general population was low. Even among frequent users of L-tryptophan, the attack rate was estimated to be probably less than 2 per 1000.[1,2,22,23]

Certain residents of the western United States (white, non-Hispanic women predominantly with a median age of 48 years) were primarily afflicted.[4,20,24] Reports abroad also were documented. Germany ranked second in the number of cases of EMS (105 cases).[25] As for the United States, all cases of EMS were associated with implicated L-tryptophan obtained from Showa Denko of Japan.

Overall, the exact incidence and prevalence of EMS were difficult to evaluate and characterize. These were dependent upon the criteria used for diagnosis of the disease. The two major types of criteria were classification criteria and diagnostic criteria.[26] Classification criteria were designed to ascertain a group of patients who were the same from series to series, regardless of location or country. They assisted in differentiating one disorder from another. However, they were not designed to diagnose individual cases. Diagnostic criteria were formulated to identify individual cases specifically. In retrospect, the EMS case definition developed early by the Centers for Disease Control (CDC) was deficient in that their criteria lacked sufficient sensitivity. Therefore, much confusion has arisen relating to the true incidence and prevalence of EMS.

11.4   Clinical Features of Eosinophilia Myalgia Syndrome

The clinical signs and symptoms of EMS have been described and established based upon review of many clinical reports in the literature.[27,28] In general, the clinical course of EMS may be divided into two phases. The acute phase (weeks or months) was characterized by signs and symptoms of intense myalgia, cough and dypsnea, paresthesia, and peripheral blood eosinophilia. The chronic phase followed and was characterized by varying degrees of sclerosis (dermal and subcutaneous), persistent myalgia, and muscle cramps, neuropathy, and neurocognitive symptoms.[29]

Though most information about the clinical course of patients with EMS comes from reports in the United States, it is of interest that cases have also been reported abroad. Cases with similar findings to those in the United States have been reported from Japan,[30,31] Germany,[25] and Italy.[32]

11.4.1　Acute Phase

The onset of EMS is typically explosive, being swift and severe, and causing great anguish.[27] Frequent findings at onset (within the first 2 to 3 months) include generalized, severe myalgias; a "flu-like" illness with malaise and fatigue; cutaneous involvement (generalized pruritis, nonspecific erythema); and respiratory symptoms or pneumonitis. The most significant laboratory finding is eosinophilia.

11.4.2　Chronic Phase

The most common objective clinical components of the chronic phase of EMS involve the skin, muscle, and nerves.[33] Several reports have focused attention on long-term follow-up studies of EMS.[34-36] Most of the patients continued to have symptomatic disease with the following clinical manifestations: fatigue, myalgia, paresthesias, articular symptoms, scleroderma-like skin changes, and muscle weakness.[35] Cognitive symptoms were new findings that were observed frequently.[35,37,38]

11.4.3　Intermediate Stage

Some investigators have described an intermediate stage (approximately 2 months after onset).[27] Additional clinical manifestations in this stage are edema (extremities and torso) in half of cases. Following diuresis, the edematous soft tissue becomes rock hard and becomes bound to underlying structures, changes typical of eosinophilia fasciitis. Neurologic dysfunction, which evolve primarily from subjective paresthesias and dysesthesias to frank sensorimotor peripheral neuropathies, are present in about one third of the cases. Myopathy with proximal weakness is commonplace.

11.5　Pathology

The pathologic lesions in patients with EMS consist primarily of widespread inflammatory cells (monocytes, lymphocytes, macrophages, plasma cells), mainly scattered in skin, muscle, and connective tissue. Endothelial cells reveal swelling, degeneration, and necrosis. Fibroblast proliferation and fibrosis are frequent findings. In many patients, the condition becomes a chronic process.[39]

The pathologic lesions described in the literature are derived from numerous case report findings.[27,40,41] Detailed reports describing the pathologic lesions in specific organs are available.

11.5.1 Skin and Subcutaneous Tissue

The pathologic changes in skin and subcutaneous tissue are similar to those of scleroderma.[42] Skin biopsy specimens show infiltration of inflammatory cells, extensive collagen deposition, and collagen-encased ectatic sweat glands. The inflammatory infiltrates (mainly lymphocytes and monocytes, with some eosinophils and plasma cells) are located around small blood vessels, hair follicles, eccrine glands, and nerves. The subcutaneous connective tissue shows replacement of fat cells by collagen and thickened and fibrotic septa. The superficial fascia also reveal inflammatory infiltrates.[42]

11.5.2 Fascia

In addition to pathologic changes involving skin and subcutaneous tissue, a number of reports describe pathologic changes of deeper involvement of the fascia.[42,43] The inflammatory changes are often seen in the superficial fascia and in the epimysial-fascial areas.[42,43]

11.5.3 Muscles and Nerves

Among the pathologic lesions of skeletal muscle and peripheral nerves of patients with EMS, the following changes are frequently described: perimyositis (with eosinophils, T-helper cells, mast cells, and activated macrophages), type 2 myofiber atrophy, epineural inflammation, and fasciitis.[44] Histoenzymatic features in muscle biopsies of patients with EMS reveal a preferential epimysial-perimysial noneosinophilia infiltration characterized by acid phosphatase reactive histiocytosis, non-necrotizing venulitis, perineural inflammation within dermis and perimysium, type II fiber atrophy with superimposed denervation features, and perifascicular alkaline phosphatase reactivity representing early neofibroplasia.[43]

According to Verity et al.,[43] the described pathologic changes in skin, fascia, and muscle, along with the defined clinical syndrome of EMS, allow for an accurate differentiation from related syndromes, including eosinophilia polymyositis, scleroderma, idiopathic polymyositic/dermatomyositis, polyarteritis nodosa, and toxic oil syndrome.[43] A few reports have considered the comparison of the histopathologic features of Shulman's syndrome (diffuse fasciitis with eosinophilia) and the fasciitis associated with EMS.[43]

Feldman et al.[45] described that in both cases inflammatory changes were present in the subcutaneous fat, septa, and fascia, but the cutaneous changes were more prominent in EMS. In general, Shulman's syndrome tends to involve the subcutis alone, and EMS tends to be a pancutaneous-subcutaneous process.[45]

11.5.4　Lungs

Lung tissue of patients with EMS reveals interstitial pneumonitis, small-to-medium vessel mixed-cell (primarily lymphocytes and eosinophils), vasculitis, and alveolar exudates of histiocytes and eosinophils.[46] Others have also reported on similar pathologic findings in the lungs of EMS patients.[47,48]

11.5.5　Heart

Pathologic findings in the heart have been described.[49,50] Pathologic lesions are present in the coronary arteries, neural structures, and conduction system of the heart.[50] James et al.[51] reported that the cardiac abnormalities in the toxic oil syndrome resemble those described in EMS.

11.6　Treatment

Although there have been many reports describing how patients with EMS have been treated, results were not successful in the majority of patients. Basically, the treatment of EMS has consisted of discontinuation of L-tryptophan and administration of corticosteroids, nonsteroidal anti-inflammatory drugs, and several other drugs, such as D-penicillamine and colchicine, cyclophosphamide, AZA (azathioprine), methotrexate, amitriptyline, acetaminophen, aspirin, naproxen, diphenhydramine, cyclobenzaprine, and fluoxetine.[21,52–56] In general, it was concluded that prednisone was helpful in the acute phase of the disease. Slow improvement was reported in 79% of the 193 patients. However, no treatment was clearly valuable in the management of the later phase of the syndrome.[55]

11.7　Pathophysiology of EMS

As is the case with most rheumatic and connective tissue diseases, the pathophysiology of EMS has been highly speculative. Therefore, one can only offer speculation regarding the pathophysiology of EMS. The pathophysiology of the nonspecific constitutional symptoms of EMS is uncertain. However, they have been considered probably to be related to immunologic and inflammatory events that occur during the acute phase of EMS. Cytokines capable of inducing many of the relevant signs and symptoms have been thought to play a role, but available data have not been conclusive. Some evidence reveals that certain cytokines are present in increased amounts in the serum of some patients with EMS,[29] and a few findings merit description. IFN-γ and neopterin, a surrogate marker for IFN-γ, were elevated in patients with active disease.[42,57,58] Elevated serum and CSF levels of kynurenine and quinolinic acid were probably due to IFN-γ induction of the rate-limiting enzyme, indoleamine-2,3-dioxygenase. Serum-soluble IL-2 receptor levels are reported to be elevated in patients with EMS.[59] Also, serum IL-4 has been reported to be increased in some patients with EMS.[60] Serum IL-5 activity is reported to be increased in some patients with EMS.[61] Transforming growth factor-β (TGF-β), a fibrogenic cytokine, has been found to show increased expression in the epidermis, dermis, fascia, and fibrous tissue in and around muscle and nerve tissue in EMS.[62,63]

Overall, much evidence suggests that a cell-mediated immune response occurs in patients with EMS that culminates in fibrosis of connective tissue in muscles, nerves, and other organs and of the skin. Possibly chemical contaminants may form protein adducts or may be incorporated into host proteins and thereby induce an immune response. A few experimental studies with EBT, one important contaminant of implicated L-tryptophan, have reported that EBT becomes incorporated into proteins of liver and blood (reticulocytes).[64,65] EBT has also been reported to enhance IL-5 production by splenic T lymphocytes.[66]

The immune response occurring in EMS is thought to induce considerable microangiopathy and cytokine production. Fibrogenic cytokines stimulate fibroblasts to proliferate and make extracellular proteins in dermis, subcutaneous tissue, and many organs. These changes may induce many signs and symptoms associated with EMS.

11.8 Factors Modifying Risk

The following factors have been considered in modifying the risk of developing EMS.

11.8.1 Dose

The dose of implicated L-tryptophan ingested strongly affects the risk of illness. The findings from a study of patients in a South Carolina psychiatric practice[23] clearly indicated that an increasing dose-response curve was evident (range of doses from 0.250 to 4.0 or more g). These findings (statistically significant) strongly suggested that the severity of illness depended on the amount of contaminated L-tryptophan ingested. Another study from New York confirmed the dose-response relationship.[67] In these studies, it was considered that the L-tryptophan dose may serve as a surrogate measure of the amount of the contaminant ingested. L-tryptophan itself may have been a necessary cofactor, required along with the contaminant(s), for EMS to develop. Other experimental studies have indicated that the dose of the L-tryptophan vehicle ingested was an important factor contributing to EMS risk and perhaps also was related to disease severity.

11.8.2   Age

Older age increased the risk of developing EMS, with persons ≥ 50 years of age being about twice as likely to have developed EMS as were younger persons.[67]

11.8.3   Sex

Initially, a predominance of female patients was reported.[20] However, other later studies have not established that the female sex was an independent factor for the development of EMS.[23] The increased rate of EMS reported for women may have been due to greater use of L-tryptophan.[20] Furthermore, only women used L-tryptophan for treatment of premenstrual syndrome, a frequently cited indication for usage. Also, women used benzodiazepines more than men to treat anxiety and/or insomnia.

11.8.4   Concurrent Use of Other Medications

Many attempts have been made to determine whether medications were influential as a risk factor. Although use of a prescription or nonprescription medication did not differ substantially between case patients and controls, it appeared that the use of an antidepressant or psychotropic medication (any antipsychotic, antidepressant, benzodiazepines, and/or other anxiolytic) could increase the risk of developing EMS.[22,67]

It is of interest that a number of medications, such as corticosteroids, oral contraceptives, and estrogen, which can alter tryptophan metabolism, have not been determined to have an effect on the development of EMS. Actually, some clinicians have postulated that EMS itself may be caused by or related to abnormal tryptophan metabolism.[42,68]

11.9 Possible Relationship between Eosiniophilia Myalgia Syndrome and Toxic Oil Syndrome

In 1981, another poorly understood epidemic, the toxic oil syndrome (TOS), occurred in Spain.[69-71] It was associated with ingestion of adulterated rapeseed oil.[120] The pathology of TOS has been described.[72] It is of interest that many of the clinical and histopathologic features of TOS resemble those of EMS.[36,73]

A number of reports have attempted to investigate whether the similarities between the two syndromes may be related to common features:

1. Possible similarities in contaminants associated with EMS and TOS; 3-(phenylamino)alanine (PAA) was found to be one of a number of contaminants in L-tryptophan implicated in EMS. PAA is chemically similar to 3-phenylamino-1,2-propanediol, an aniline derivative that was isolated from samples of denatured rapeseed oil that had been consumed by persons in whom TOS developed.[74] Mayeno et al.[8] first raised the issue that the above evidence could possibly link EMS with TOS. Whether this speculation is valid has not been confirmed.

2. Silver et al.[75] considered whether patients with EMS and TOS might share similar alterations in L-tryptophan metabolism, i.e., elevated levels of L-kynurenine and quinolinic acid, which might mediate some of the clinical and pathophysiological features of each of the syndromes. They reported that patients with EMS or TOS had significantly higher levels of L-kynurenine and quinolinic acid than control subjects. Likewise, neopterin, a product of cell-mediated immune activation and marker of interferon-gamma (IFN-γ), a potent inducer of indoleamino-2,3-dioxygenase, the rate-limiting enzyme in the kynurenine pathway of L-tryptophan metabolism, was elevated in blood of EMS and TOS patients.

3. In searching for other similarities, Carreira et al.[76] reported on antiphospholipid antibodies in patients with EMS and TOS and found that such antibodies with a different specificity than in controls were present in a high percentage of EMS and TOS patients. Kaufman et al.[63] studied whether growth factors of potential pathogenetic significance were deposited in the skin, muscle, and peripheral nerve lesions of EMS and TOS.

These studies implicated transforming growth factor-β and platelet growth factor as potential important cytokines in EMS and suggested that the pathogenesis of tissue fibrosis in EMS and TOS may be dependent on different growth factors.

11.10 Experimental Models of Eosinophilia Myalgia Syndrome

11.10.1 *In Vivo* Studies

Shortly after the establishment of the EMS as a disease entity in humans who had ingested L-tryptophan from a Japanese manufacturer, Showa Denko, animal studies were undertaken in an attempt to establish the precise etiologic agent responsible for EMS. Scores of studies were undertaken,[77] but only a few have been published.[78–81] A brief review of the published studies follows.

Crofford et al.[78] were the first to report a potential animal model of EMS. Using female Lewis rats, they tube administered implicated (Showa Denko) or control L-tryptophan (1600 mg/kg per day) for 38 days. Their findings in rats fed the implicated L-tryptophan revealed increased thickness of the fascia and inflammatory foci in the perimycial region. The gastrointestinal tract of these animals revealed increased perivascular inflammation (mast cells, eosinophils, and monocytes) in the lamina propria.[82] Love et al.[80] expanded on the preceding findings by also using EBT alone or together with nonimplicated L-tryptophan. Lewis rats were used and were lavaged daily with test compounds. At 6 weeks, all groups treated with either form of L-tryptophan (implicated or nonimplicated) or EBT showed increased fascial thickness, which was most marked in animals treated with implicated L-tryptophan or EBT.

Emslie-Smith et al.[81] treated female Lewis rats with EBT and nonimplicated L-tryptophan intraperitoneally and studied muscle. They reported based upon only a few rats that EBT-treated rats had a few necrotic muscle fibers and some revealed thickened perimysium and fascia with inflammation (lymphocytes, macrophages, and sparse eosinophils).

Silver et al.[79] studied female C57B1/6 mice that received intraperitoneal injections of saline, nonimplicated L-tryptophan without or with EBT, or EBT alone. The doses used were much lower than in the preceding rat studies. Their principal findings were that mice treated with EBT developed inflammation (mononuclear and mast cells) of the fascia as well as fascial thickening and fibrosis. These developed by 3 days and progressed at 6 and 21 days. Mice receiving L-tryptophan alone showed some increases in fascial thickening. Concurrent administration of L-tryptophan and EBT had less effect than EBT alone.

In view of these four reported experimental animal studies, it became apparent that a useful or acceptable experimental model of EMS had not been established. Also, a detailed review of other animal studies, which remains unpublished or only in abstracts, stressed negative data or data which refuted earlier observations.[77] Also, in an attempt to conduct a comparative evaluation and review of the histopathologic findings in experimental studies with mice from four different laboratories, Brown[83] reported that the findings were inconsistent, nonreproducible, and did not support a conclusion that implicated L-tryptophan, EBT, PAA, or combinations thereof, under the conditions of the studies, induced lesions of skin or muscle in C57Black, Ball/c, SJL, or B10.s strains of mice.

In view of the inability to develop or establish a satisfactory experimental model in animals of the EMS, other studies have focused on selected specific aspects of the actions of implication L-tryptophan or its contaminants. The following studies were directed in this manner.

11.10.2   *In Vitro* Studies

In view of the complexity of the variables in experimental animals studies concerned with establishing models of EMS, a number of investigators have attempted to gain some insight into the pathogenesis of EMS by conducting defined *in vitro* studies. Some of these studies are reviewed below.

11.10.2.1   In Vitro *³H-Tryptophan Binding Assay with Nuclei and Nuclear Envelopes*

Utilizing an *in vitro* ³H-tryptophan binding assay with rat hepatic nuclei or nuclear envelopes developed for other studies,[84,85] Sidransky et al.[86] investigated whether EMS-implicated L-tryptophan from Showa Denko would affect such binding differently than that obtained using nonimplicated L-tryptophan from another source. Using equimolar concentrations of excess, unlabeled L-tryptophan, the implicated L-tryptophan revealed significantly less ³H-tryptophan binding to hepatic nuclear envelopes than did the nonimplicated L-tryptophan. This suggested that there may be abnormalities (contaminants or impurities) in the implicated L-tryptophan which could be responsible for the differences in binding. Next, *in vitro* binding assay studies revealed that the addition of PAA but not of EBT to nonimplicated L-tryptophan revealed effects similar to those detected with implicated L-tryptophan.[64,86] These studies indicated that the implicated L-tryptophan and a contaminant (PAA) affected a biological system as determined by assaying *in vitro* ³H-tryptophan binding to hepatic nuclei. The possible significance of such an altered response is unknown and, indeed, may or may not have any direct relationship to the pathogenesis of EMS. Nonetheless, the *in vitro* assay system was utilized in other experimental studies. By utilizing information or association(s) obtained from clinical observations of patients with EMS, studies were designed to probe for the effects of selected variables.

Since the use of antidepressant or psychotropic medications along with implicated L-tryptophan was often reported in patients with EMS, these drugs were considered as possible risk factors.[22,67] Therefore, studies were conducted to determine whether drugs, such as benzodiazepines[87,88] or metyrapone, an inhibitor of endogenous adrenal corticoid synthesis,[89] would affect *in vitro* ³H-tryptophan binding to rat hepatic nuclei or nuclear envelopes. The drugs alone did not appear to influence tryptophan receptor binding. However, each drug demonstrated an interactive effect with unlabeled L-tryptophan to diminish specific binding when compared to the effect of excess unlabeled L-tryptophan alone. Experiments using implicated L-tryptophan instead of nonimplicated L-tryptophan revealed similar responses to each drug as indicated above.

Based upon the above-cited experimental studies with benzodiazepines, it appeared that they could bind to certain nuclear receptors. Therefore, this raised the question whether L-tryptophan might interfere with benzodiazepine (BDZ) receptors.[90] Using a peripheral benzodiazepine(PBDZ) receptor ligand, PK11195 (1-(2-chlorophenyl)-*N*-methyl-*N*-(1-methyl-propyl)-3-isoquinoline-carboxamide), it was determined that a receptor existed for PBDZ in nuclei of rat hepatocytes and macrophages (WLGS). Using [³H]-PK11195 and assaying *in vitro* for specific binding to rat liver and WLGS nuclei, studies revealed that nuclei incubated with known $PBDZ_R$ (mixed) ligands, diazepam, and demoxepam revealed marked inhibition of binding, but no inhibition was observed on incubation with the central benzodiazepine ligand, flumazenil. Using the above *in vitro* assay system with added L-tryptophan revealed that nonimplicated L-tryptophan had little effect on *in vitro* [³H]-PK11195 binding to nuclear (rat liver, murine macrophages) preparations, but that the addition of implicated L-tryptophan did have an appreciable inhibitory effect on binding.[90,91] Also, the addition of PAA alone, but not of EBT alone, appeared to act as did implicated L-tryptophan when added to the *in vitro* assay system.[92] The above findings with liver cells and macrophages suggested that peripheral-type benzodiazepine receptors may become affected by implicated L-tryptophan, or even by a contaminant such as PAA. One might, thereby, speculate that such alterations possibly involving leukocytes could affect immunologic responses as suggested by others,[93-95] who have stressed the possible importance of peripheral benzodiazepine receptors on leukocytes in relation to immunological responses. Conceivably, implicated L-tryptophan alone or with benzodiazepines (frequently used by patients with EMS) might induce disturbances in immunomodulary actions that may be involved in the pathogenesis of EMS.

11.10.3   Studies Relating to Possible Immunological Responses in Eosinophilia Myalgia Syndrome

It has been suggested that contaminants of implicated L-tryptophan form abnormal proteins.

11.10.3.1   EBT

In vitro studies with EBT revealed that EBT did not affect ¹⁴C-leucine incorporation into hepatic proteins.[64] Also, EBT addition to an *in vitro* system for hepatic protein synthesis, in which ³H-tryptophan incorporation into proteins (acid-precipitable) was measured, revealed that EBT competed in a manner similar to that observed with equimolar concentrations of unlabeled L-tryptophan.[64] ^{14}C-EBT became incorporated *in vitro* into proteins (acid-precipitable), and this incorporation was diminished in the presence of equimolar concentrations of unlabeled EBT or L-tryptophan.[64] This latter finding with ^{14}C-EBT has been confirmed by others.[65]

Kurihara et al.[96] reported that polyclonal anti-EBT antibodies were generated by immunizing rabbits with EBT alone or as EBT-BSA conjugate. Yamaoka et al.[97] raised the possibility that EBT induces T cells to produce IL-5. Subsequently, Yamaoka et al.[66] showed that EBT but not nonimplicated L-tryptophan elicited the release of excessive amounts of eosinophil cationic protein from normo-dense eosinophils and upregulated IL-5 receptor (IL-5R) levels in normo-dense eosinophils.

11.10.3.2 PAA

Addition of PAA to an *in vitro* system for protein synthesis, in which [3H]-tryptophan or [3H]alanine incorporation into acid-precipitable hepatic proteins was measured, revealed that PAA competed similarly, but somewhat less, than did equimolar concentrations of unlabeled L-tryptophan or L-alanine.[98] These findings suggested that PAA or a breakdown compound may become incorporated into proteins.

11.10.4   Other Experimental Studies

11.10.4.1   EBT

Takagi et al.,[99] using fibroblast (human dermal) cultures, studied the effects of EBT on fibroblast-DNA and collagen synthesis. They reported that EBT was a potent stimulant for fibroblast activation and collagen synthesis and may possibly provide a mechanism for the development of fibrosis in EMS.

Zangrilli et al.[100] investigated the effects of EBT on normal human fibroblast function *in vitro*. Incubation of confluent fibroblasts with EBT, but not its hydrolysis product 1-methyl-tetrahydro-β-carboline-3-carboxylic acid, caused a dose-dependent increase in collagen synthesis and in type I collagen mRNA levels independent of its effect on proliferation. In contrast, expression mRNA for fibrorectin was not affected. Takagi et al.[101] also reported results similar to the above. In regard to these findings, it is of interest that Li et al.[102] have reported that L-tryptophan alone induces expression of collagenase gene in human fibroblasts. Thus, it appears the L-tryptophan alone, as well as EBT, can affect fibroblast responses.

11.10.4.2   PAA

Adachi et al.[103] studied the distribution and elimination of PAA in Lewis rats after a single tube-feeding of PAA. PAA concentrations in blood, brain, kidney, and liver were substantial after 5 h and decreased after 16 h. Also, administration for 4 days or feeding in diet for 6 weeks revealed appreciable accumulation of PAA in all of the above organs. PAA tissue levels declined to trace concentrations within 3 days after discontinuing administration but were still detectable for at least 12 days.

Mayeno et al.[8] reported that PAA could become metabolized to 3-phenyl-amino-1,2-propane-diol (PAP), a compound that was found to be contaminating the rapeseed oil consumed by individuals who developed the toxic oil syndrome in Spain in 1981.[74]

11.11 Overview

In considering the discovery and pathogenesis of a new disease entity, the EMS, many basic and interesting questions have arisen. Although the etiology of the disease has focused on the ingestion of L-tryptophan containing impurities or contaminants supplied from a single manufacturer, its significance is not entirely clear. Although many individuals ingested the implicated L-tryptophan, only a few developed the syndrome. Thus, host susceptibility must play an important and vital role. In reviewing series of patients who developed EMS, other complex and confusing points became apparent. Among them were as follows:

1. Many patients were on medications that may have played an influential role on their altered host susceptibility, as well as the underlying condition that existed for which the medications were taken.

2. Some studies have attempted to evaluate whether the levels of L-tryptophan intake would be of importance. Increasing dosage of implicated L-tryptophan did seem to influence the severity of EMS.

3. Women more than men developed EMS, possibly because women more than men took L-tryptophan.

Subsequently, a number of questions have been raised which cast many doubts about EMS. Some epidemiologists have questioned the etiology of EMS in regard to epidemiologic evidence alone.[104–106] Others have raised questions about the criteria for disease classification and diagnostic criteria, for case definition of EMS.[107] Failure of reproducible or definitive findings with experimental models of EMS[77] cast doubt on the toxicity of the impurities or contaminants within the implicated L-tryptophan in EMS. Some of these cautious views appear to be rational. Yet a critical review of the pros and cons appears to justify the establishment of EMS as a new important clinical syndrome.[108] Although other forms of eosinophilia and fibromyalgia have existed for years and do have overlapping clinical manifestations, EMS merits its own designation as a new clinical entity, one which is related to the ingestion of implicated L-tryptophan manufactured by Showa Denko of Japan. However, the pathogenesis of the disease remains unclear. Its cause or etiology appears to be multifactorial[109] and, therefore, efforts to clarify the process have been elusive.

Review of the current understanding of some of the multifactorial aspects involved in EMS is appropriate. A brief consideration of some of these aspects follows.

11.11.1 Host Susceptibility

It is clear that only a few individuals who ingested implicated L-tryptophan from Showa Denko developed EMS. Most consumers did not. Attempts thus far to categorize susceptible individuals have failed. Yet, some leads have developed that merit further investigation. Some of these are as follows.

11.11.1.1 Altered Metabolism of L-Tryptophan

Silver et al.[58] have reported that during the active phase of EMS tryptophan metabolism via the kynurenine pathway was accentuated, probably secondary to induction of the enzyme indoleamine-2,3-dioxygenase. Indeed, patients with EMS generally have low plasma L-tryptophan and high plasma L-kynurenine and quinolinic acid levels.

11.11.1.2 Altered Xenobiotic Metabolism

Flockhart et al.[110] reported a study that tested the hypothesis that patterns of xenobiotic metabolism in patients with EMS may differ from healthy control subjects. In studies for the cytochrome P450 CYP2D6 polymorphism, they studied metabolic phenotypes of patients with EMS for 5-mephenytoin hydroxylation and dapsome acetylation and compared these with healthy control subjects. The incidence of the CYP2D6 post-metabolizer genotype (mutant/mutant) was 0.185 in patients with EMS and 0.061 in control subjects. The mephenytoin S:R ratios were 0.39 with EMS vs. 0.18 in controls, with no difference in dapsome acetylation between the two groups. The significance of the differences of xenobiotic metabolism in the pathogenesis of EMS remains unclear.

Whether the altered metabolic parameters described above are related to cause or effect in EMS is not clear. However, based upon animal studies where species and strain differences in response to L-tryptophan have been reported,[111-113] such differences probably also exist in humans. Thus, it is important to establish whether differences in tryptophan metabolism exist in humans and then possibly to relate the changes to altered host susceptibility to diseases.

11.11.1.3   Autoimmune Response

Individuals who are prone to develop autoimmune responses may be susceptible to the development of EMS due to implicated L-tryptophan. Many investigators who reviewed cases of EMS have suggested that an autoimmune mechanism was involved in EMS.[50,114–116] Some experimental studies with contaminants or impurities of implicated L-tryptophan have proposed mechanisms whereby abnormal proteins may be formed that may elicit an autoimmune response, with major consequences thereof.[64,65,98] Patients with EMS have increased levels of plasma neopterin, a marker of immune activation.[58]

11.11.2   Toxicity of L-Tryptophan Itself or of Related Compounds

Whether very high levels of L-tryptophan intake may be toxic to humans is not known. However, in animal studies, ingestion of high levels of nonimplicated L-tryptophan can be lethal. The LD_{50} level of L-tryptophan for rats is 1.62 g/kg.[117] Similar levels are effective in mice and rabbits. Guidelines for the upper limits of L-tryptophan ingestion in humans need to be established.

11.11.3   Variability (Species and Strains) in Response to L-Tryptophan

A number of studies have revealed that differences exist in the response of different species or strains of animals to the administration of L-tryptophan.[111–113] Such variations may also exist in humans and may be of importance as to how certain individuals handle high, ingested levels of L-tryptophan alone or together with related impurities or contaminants, as occurs with intake of implicated Showa Denko L-tryptophan.

Animal studies with different species have revealed differences in hepatic tryptophan 2-3 dioxygenase activities which affect tryptophan metabolism (see Chapter 4).

11.11.4   Intake of Other Medications and Interaction with Ingested Drugs

The use of antidepressant or psychotropic medications has been reported to be common among many of the patients who developed EMS. This has been considered as a possible risk factor for the development of the syndrome.[22,67] Although certain drugs used simultaneously with the ingestion of implicated L-tryptophan have been described in the case of EMS, no definitive correlation between the two has been unraveled based upon epidemiologic studies. Yet, based upon experimental studies with selected drugs, it appears that certain drugs, especially benzodiazepines, may influence the effects of L-tryptophan, such as dealing with nuclear L-tryptophan receptor binding.[87,88] Findings with liver cells and macrophages suggest that peripheral-type benzodiazepine receptors may become affected by implicated L-tryptophan or by a contaminant such as PAA. Such alterations, possibly involving leukocytes, could affect immunologic responses as suggested by others.[93-95] Investigation into this possible relationship is merited.

Whether the experimental findings reported earlier offer any insight into the pathogenesis of EMS is speculative and problematic. Yet they stress that the interactions with or within cells and tissues of L-tryptophan alone or together with other selected compounds (i.e., medications) need elucidation and clarification. As a detailed (basic and fundamental) understanding of how L-tryptophan acts normally becomes unraveled, a better understanding of the pathogenesis of the tryptophan-related disease, EMS, may then become available.

It is generally considered that most or even all chronic diseases have a genetic component. Genes define susceptibility to disease, and environmental factors determine those among the susceptible individuals who might develop disease. Nutrition is considered to be one of the most important environmental factors. Thus, it is vital to gain knowledge of gene differences relating to susceptibility of certain humans to EMS. Such knowledge will help identify those who were at higher risk for the disease, as well as their response to high intake of L-tryptophan alone or plus contaminants.

11.11.5   Concluding Comments

It is important to acknowledge that the occurrence of new diseases or syndromes such as EMS may first be detected in patients, and only thereafter may searches, epidemiological and otherwise, be undertaken. As for EMS, credit must be given to primary physicians who, by practicing high-quality medicine that includes good history taking, were able to trigger epidemiologic investigation. This led to clear evidence of the involvement of the crucial factor, L-tryptophan and its specific source, and then to the prompt halting by the FDA of the sale of L-tryptophan. The rapid detective action prevented the occurrence of additional cases of EMS, alleviated much pain and debility, and saved lives. Thus, vigilance at many levels is necessary for the early detection of new diseases or syndromes. When a new disease arises, it is necessary to mobilize whatever expertise exists in an attempt to determine its pathogenesis. New challenges lie ahead, and scientists must be prepared to recognize diseases or syndromes as they arise and attempt to contribute to a comprehensive understanding.

References

1. Belongia, E. A., Hedberg, C. W., Gleich, G. J., White, K. E., Mayeno, A. N., Loegering, D. A., Dunnette, S. L., Pirie, P. L., MacDonald, K. L., and Osterholm, M. T., An investigation of the cause of the eosinophilia-myalgia syndrome associated with tryptophan use, *N. Engl. J. Med.*, 323, 357, 1990.

2. Slutsker, L., Hoesly, F. C., Miller, L., Williams, L. P., Watson, J. C., and Fleming, D. W., Eosinophilia-myalgia syndrome associated with exposure to tryptophan from a single manufacturer, *JAMA*, 264, 213, 1990.

3. Varga, J., Uitto, J., and Jimenez, S. A., The cause and pathogenesis of the eosinophilia-myalgia syndrome, *Ann. Int. Med.*, 116, 140, 1992.

4. Belongia, E. A., Mayeno, A. N., and Osterholm, M. T., The eosinophilia-myalgia syndrome and tryptophan, *Annu. Rev. Nutr.*, 12, 235, 1992.

5. Mayeno, A. N., Lin, F., Foote, C. S., Loegering, D. A., Ames, M. M., Hedberg, C. W., and Gleich, G. J., Characterization of "peak E," a novel amino acid associated with eosinophilia-myalgia syndrome, *Science*, 250, 1707, 1990.

6. Smith, M. J., Mazzola, E. P., Farrell, T. J., Page, S. W., Ashley, D., Sirimanne, S. R., and Hill, R. H., 1,1'-ethylideenebis(tryptophan) structure determination of contaminant "97"-implicated in the eosinophilia-myalgia syndrome (EMS), *Tetrahedron Lett.*, 32, 991, 1991.

7. Goda, Y., Suzuki, J., Maitani, T., Yoshihira, K., Takeda, M., and Uchiyama, M., 3-anilino-L-alanine, structural determination of UV-5, a contaminant in EMS-associated L-tryptophan samples, *Chem. Pharm. Bull.*, 40, 2236, 1992.

8. Mayeno, A. N., Belongia, E. A., Lin, F., Lundy, S. K., and Gleich, G. J., 3-(Phenyl-amino)alanine, a novel aniline-derived amino acid associated with the eosino-philia-myalgia syndrome: A link to the toxic oil syndrome? *Mayo Clin. Proc.*, 67, 1134, 1992.

9. Toyo'oka, T., Yamazaki, T., Tanimoto, T., Sato, K., Sato, M., Toyoda, M., Ishibashi, M., Yoshihira, K., and Uchiyama, M., Characterization of contami-nants in EMS-associated L-tryptophan samples by high-performance liquid chromatography, *Chem. Pharm. Bull.*, 39, 820, 1991.

10. Hill, R. H., Caudill, S. P., Philen, R. M., Bailey, S. L., Flanders, W. D., Driskell, W. J., Kamb, M. L., Needham, L. L., and Sampson, E. J., Contaminants in L-tryp-tophan associated with eosinophilia myalgia syndrome, *Arch. Environ. Contam-ination Toxicol.*, 25, 134, 1993.

11. Philen, R. M., Hill, R. H., Flanders, W. D., Caudill, S. P., Needham, L., Sewell, L., Sampson, E. J., Falk, H., and Kilbourne, E. M., Tryptophan contaminants associated with eosinophilia-myalgia syndrome. The Eosinophilia-Myalgia Studies of Oregon, New York and New Mexico, *Am. J. Epidemiol.*, 138, 154, 1993.

12. Centers for Disease Control, Analysis of L-tryptophan for the etiology of eosi-nophilia-myalgia syndrome, *Morb. Mort. Wkly. Rep.*, 39, 589, 1990.

13. Centers for Disease Control. Update: Analysis of L-tryptophan for the etiology of eosinophilia-myalgia syndrome, *Morb. Mort. Wkly. Rep.*, 39, 789, 1990.

14. Ito, J., Hosaki, Y., Torigoe, Y., and Sakimoto, K., Identification of substances formed by decomposition of peak E substance in tryptophan, *Food Chem. Tox-icol.*, 30, 71, 1992.

15. Adachi, J., Mio, T., Ueno, Y., Naito, T., Nishimura, A., Fujiwara, S., Sumino, K., and Tatsuno, Y., Identification of four metabolites of 3-(phenylamino)alanine, a constituent in L-tryptophan products implicated in eosinophilia-myalgia syn-drome, in rats, *Arch. Toxicol.*, 68, 500, 1994.

16. Muller, A., Busker, E., Gunther, K., and Hoppe, B., Characterization of byprod-ucts in L-tryptophan, *Bioforum*, 14, 350, 1991.

17. Simat, T., van Wickern, B., Eulitz, K., and Steinhart, E. H., Contaminants in biotechnologically manufactured L-tryptophan, *J. Chromatogr. B Biomed. Appl.*, 685, 41, 1996.

18. Williamson, B. L., Benson, L. M., Tomlinson, A. J., Mayeno, A. N., Gleich, G. J., and Naylor, S., On-line HPLC-tandem mass spectrometry analysis of contaminants of L-tryptophan associated with the onset of the eosinophilia-myalgia syndrome, *Toxicol. Lett.*, 92, 139, 1997.
19. Mayeno, A. N. and Gleich, G. J., Eosinophilia-myalgia syndrome and tryptophan production: A cautionary tale, *Trends Biotechnol.*, 12, 346, 1994.
20. Swygert, L. A., Maes, E. F., Sewell, L. E., Miller, L., Falk, H., and Kilbourne, E. M., Eosinophilia-myalgia syndrome. Results of national surveillance, *JAMA*, 264, 1698, 1990.
21. Kilbourne, E. M., Eosinophilia-myalgia syndrome: Coming to grips with a new illness, *Epidemiol. Rev.*, 14, 16, 1992.
22. Henning, K. J., Jean-Baptiste, E., Singh, T., Hill, R. H., and Friedman, S. M., Eosinophilia-myalgia syndrome in patients ingesting a single source of L-tryptophan, *J. Rheumatol.*, 20, 273, 1993.
23. Kamb, M. L., Murphy, J. J., Jones, J. L., Caston, J. C., Nederlof, K., Horney, L. F., Swygert, L. A., Falk, H., and Kilbourne, E. M., Eosinophilia-myalgia syndrome in L-tryptophan-exposed patients, *JAMA*, 267, 77, 1992.
24. Centers for Disease Control. Eosinophilia-myalgia syndrome and L-tryptophan-containing products — New Mexico, Minnesota, Oregon, and New York, *Morb. Mort. Wkly. Rep.*, 38, 785, 1989.
25. Carr, L., Ruther, E., Berg, P. A., and Lehnert, H., Eosinophilia-myalgia syndrome in Germany: An epidemiologic review, *Mayo Clin. Proc.*, 69, 620, 1994.
26. Medsger, T. A., Clinical issues in eosinophilia-myalgia syndrome, *J. Rheumatol.*, 23(Suppl. 46), 1, 1996.
27. Duffy, J., The lessons of eosinophilia-myalgia syndrome, *Hosp. Pract.*, 27, 65, 1901.
28. Martin, R. W., Duffy, J., Engel, A. G., Lie, J. T., Bowles, C. A., Moyer, T. P., and Gleich, G. J., The clinical spectrum of the eosinophilia-myalgia syndrome associated with L-tryptophan ingestion. Clinical features in 20 patients and aspects of pathophysiology, *Ann. Int. Med.*, 113, 124, 1990.
29. Silver, R. M., Pathophysiology of the eosinophilia-myalgia syndrome, *J. Rheumatol. Suppl.*, 46, 26, 1996.
30. Tsutsui, K., Taniuchi, K., Mori, T., and Takehara, K., Eosinophilia-myalgia syndrome: A report of two cases in Japan, *Eur. J. Dermatol.*, 6, 113, 1996.
31. Mizutani, T., Mizutani, H., Hashimoto, K., Nakamura, Y., Kishida, M., Taniguchi, H., Murata, M., Kuzuhara, S., and Shimizu, M., Simultaneous development of two cases of eosinophilia-myalgia syndrome with the same lot of L-tryptophan in Japan, *J. Am. Acad. Dermatol.*, 25, 512, 1991.
32. Priori, R., Conti, F., Luan, F. L., Arpino, C., and Valesini, G., Chronic fatigue: A peculiar evolution of eosinophilia myalgia syndrome following treatment with L-tryptophan in four Italian adolescents, *Eur. J. Pediatr.*, 153, 344, 1994.
33. Hertzman, P., Falk, H., Kilbourne, E. M., Page, S., and Shulman, L. E., The eosinophilia-myalgia syndrome: The Los Alamos Conference, *J. Rheumatol.*, 18, 867, 1991.
34. Campbell, D. S., Morris, P. D., and Silver, R. M., Eosinophilia-myalgia syndrome: A long-term follow-up study, *Southern Med. J.*, 88, 953, 1995.
35. Kaufman, L. D., Chronicity of the eosinophilia-myalgia syndrome. A reassessment after three years, *Arthritis Rheum.*, 37, 84, 1994.
36. Sack, K. E. and Criswell, L. A., Eosinophilia-myalgia syndrome: The aftermath, *Southern Med. J.*, 85, 878, 1992.

37. Krupp, L. B., Masur, D. M., and Kaufman, L. D., Neurocognitive dysfunction in the eosinophilia-myalgia syndrome, *Neurology,* 43, 931, 1993.
38. Armstrong, C., Lewis, T., D'Esposito, M., and Freundlich, B., Eosinophilia-myalgia syndrome: Selective cognitive impairment, longitudinal effects, and neuroimaging findings, *J. Neurol. Neurosurg. Psychiatr.,* 63, 633, 1997.
39. Sidransky, H. and Bills, N. D., Malnutritional deprivation diseases, in *Anderson's Pathology,* 10th ed., Damjanov, I. and Linder, J., Eds., C. V. Mosby, St. Louis, 1996, 1, 712–740.
40. Herrick, M. K., Chang, Y., Horoupian, D. S., Lombard, C. M., and Adornato, B. T., L-tryptophan and the eosinophilia-myalgia syndrome: pathologic findings in eight patients, *Hum. Pathol.,* 22, 12, 1991.
41. Burns, S. M., Lange, D. J., Jaffe, I., and Hays, A. P., Axonal neuropathy in eosinophilia-myalgia syndrome, *Muscle Nerves,* 17, 293, 1994.
42. Silver, R. S., Heye, M. P., Maize, J. C., Quearry, B., Viooonnet-Fousset, M., and Sternberg, E. M., Sclerodrma, faciitis, and eosinophilia associated with the ingestion of tryptophan, *N. Engl. J. Med.,* 322, 874, 1990.
43. Verity, M. A., Bulpitt, K. J., and Paulus, H. E., Neuromuscular manifestations of L-tryptophan-associated eosinophilia-myalgia syndrome: A histomorphologic analysis of 14 patients, *Hum. Pathol.,* 22, 3, 1991.
44. Seidman, R. J., Kaufman, L. D., Sokoloff, L., Miller, F., Iliya, A., and Peress, N. S., The neuromuscular pathology of the eosinophilia-myalgia syndrome, *J. Neuropathol. Exp. Neurol.,* 50, 49, 1991.
45. Feldman, S. R., Silver, R. M., and Maize, J. C., A histopathologic comparison of Shulman's syndrome (diffuse fasciitis with eosinophilia) and the fasciitis associated with the eosinophilia-myalgia syndrome, *J. Am. Acad. Dermatol.,* 26, 95, 1992.
46. Strumpf, I. J., Drucker, R. D., Anders, K. H., Cohen, S., and Fajolu, O., Acute eosinophilic pulmonary disease associated with the ingestion of L-tryptophan-containing products, *Chest,* 99, 8, 1991.
47. Travis, W. D., Kalafer, M. E., Robin, H. S., and Luibel, F. J., Hypersensitivity pneumonitis and pulmonary vasculitis with eosinophilia in a patient taking an L-tryptophan preparation, *Ann. Int. Med.,* 112, 301, 1990.
48. Tazelaar, H. D., Myers, J. L., Drage, C. W., King, T. E. J., Aguayo, S., and Colby, T. V., Pulmonary disease associated with L-tryptophan-induced eosinophilic myalgia syndrome. Clinical and pathologic features, *Chest,* 97, 1032, 1990.
49. Berger, P. B., Duffy, J., Reeder, G. S., Karon, B. L., and Edwards, W. D., Restrictive cardiomyopathy associated with the eosinophilia-myalgia syndrome, *Mayo Clin. Proc.,* 69, 162, 1994.
50. James, T. N., Kamb, M. L., Sandberg, G. A., Silver, R. M., and Kilbourne, E. M., Postmortem studies of the heart in three fatal cases of the eosinophilia-myalgia syndrome, *Ann. Int. Med.,* 115, 102, 1991.
51. James, T. N., Gomez-Sanchez, M. A., Martinez-Tello, F. J., Posada-de la Paz, M., Abaitua-Borda, I., and Soldevilla, L. B., Cardiac abnormalities in the toxic oil syndrome, with comparative observations on the eosinophilia-myalgia syndrome, *J. Am. Coll. Cardiol.,* 18, 1367, 1991.
52. Kaufman, L. D., Seidman, R. J., and Gruber, B. L., L-tryptophan-associated eosinophilic perimyositis, neuritis, and fasciitis. A clinicopathologic and laboratory study of 25 patients, *Medicine,* 69, 187, 1990.
53. Clauw, D. J. and Katz P., Treatment of the eosinophilia-myalgia syndrome, *N. Engl. J. Med.,* 323, 417, 1990.

54. Martinez-Osuna, P., Wallach, P. M., Seleznick, M. J., Levin, R. W., Silveira, L. H., Jara, L. J., and Espinoza, L. R., Treatment of the eosinophilia-myalgia syndrome, *Sem. Arthritis Rheum.*, 21, 110, 1991.
55. Hertzman, P. A., Clauw, D. J., Kaufman, L. D., Varga, J., Silver, R. M., Thacker, H. L., Mease, P., Espinoza, L. R., and Pincus, T., The eosinophilia-myalgia syndrome: Status of 205 patients and results of treatment 2 years after onset, *Ann. Int. Med.*, 122, 851, 1995.
56. Kilbourne, E. M., Swygert, L. A., Philen, R. M., Sun, R. K., Auerbach, S. B., Miller, L., Nelson, D. E., and Falk, H., Interim guidance on the eosinophilia-myalgia syndrome, *Ann. Int. Med.*, 112, 85, 1990.
57. Clauw, D. J., Zackrison, L. H., and Katz, P., Serum cytokines and the eosinophilia myalgia syndrome, *Ann. Int. Med.*, 117, 344, 1992.
58. Silver, R. M., McKinley, K., Smith, E. A., Quearry, B., Harati, Y., Sternberg, E. M., and Heyes, M. P., Tryptophan metabolism via the kynurenine pathway in patients with the eosinophilia-myalgia syndrome, *Arthritis Rheum.*, 35, 1097, 1992.
59. McKinley, K. L., Harati, Y., and Schneider, L. W., Chronic immune activation in the eosinophilia-myalgia syndrome, *Muscle Nerve*, 16, 947, 1993.
60. Kaufman, L. D., Gruber, B. L., and Needleman, B. W., Interleukin-4 levels in the eosinophilia-myalgia syndrome, *Am. J. Med.*, 91, 664, 1991.
61. Owen, W. F., Petersen, J., Sheff, D. M., Folkerth, R. D., Anderson, R. J., Corson, J. M., Sheffer, A. L., and Austen, K. F., Hypodense eosinophils and interleukin-5 activity in the blood of patients with the eosinophilia-myalgia syndrome, *Proc. Natl. Acad. Sci. U.S.A.*, 87, 8647, 1990.
62. Peltonen, J., Varga, J., Sollberg, S., Uitto, J., and Jimenez, S. A., Elevated expression of the genes for transforming growth factor-beta 1 and type VI collagen in diffuse fasciitis associated with the eosinophilia-myalgia syndrome, *J. Invest. Dermatol.*, 96, 20, 1991.
63. Kaufman, L. D., Gruber, B. L., Gomez-Reino, J. J., and Miller, F., Fibrogenic growth factors in the eosinophilia-myalgia syndrome and the toxic oil syndrome, *Arch. Dermatol.*, 130, 41, 1994.
64. Sidransky, H., Verney, E., Cosgrove, J. W., Latham, P. S., and Mayeno, A. N., Studies with 1,1'-ethylidenebis (tryptophan), a contaminant associated with L-tryptophan implicated in the eosinophilia-myalgia syndrome, *Toxicol. Appl. Pharmacol.*, 126, 108, 1994.
65. Buss, W. C., Stepanek, J., Bankhurst, A. D., Mayeno, A. N., Pastuszyn, A., and Peabody, D., EBT, a tryptophan contaminant associated with eosinophilia myalgia syndrome, is incorporated into proteins during translation as an amino acid analog, *Autoimmunity*, 25, 33, 1996.
66. Yamaoka, K. A., Miyasaka, N., Inuo, G., Saito, I., Kolb, J. P., Fujita, K., and Kashiwazaki, S., 1,1'-Ethylidenebis(tryptophan)(peak E) induces functional activation of human eosinophils and interleukin 5 production from T lymphocytes: Association of eosinophilia-myalgia syndrome with a L-tryptophan contaminant, *J. Clin. Invest.*, 14, 50, 1994.
67. Back, E. E., Henning, K. J., Kallenbach, L. R., Brix, K. A., Gunn, R. A., and Melius, J. M., Risk factors for developing eosinophilia myalgia syndrome among L-tryptophan users in New York, *J. Rheumatol.*, 20, 666, 1993.
68. Clauw, D. J., Nashel, D. J., Umhau, A., and Katz, P., Tryptophan-associated eosinophilic connective-tissue disease. A new clinical entity? *JAMA*, 263, 1502, 1990.

69. Toxic Epidemic Syndrome Study Group. Toxic epidemic syndrome, Spain, 1981, *Lancet*, 2, 697, 1982.
70. Kilbourne, E. M., Rigau-Perez, J. G., Heath, C. W. J., Zack, M. M., Falk, H., Martin-Marcos, M., and de Carlos, A., Clinical epidemiology of toxic-oil syndrome. Manifestations of a new illness, *N. Engl. J. Med.*, 309, 1408, 1983.
71. Posada-de la Paz, M., Abaitua, B. I., Kilbourne, E. M., Tabuenca, O. J., Diaz, D. R., and Castro, G. M., Late cases of toxic oil syndrome: Evidence that the aetiological agent persisted in oil stored for up to one year, *Food Chem. Toxicol.*, 27, 517, 1989.
72. Martinez Tello, F. J., Navas Palacios, J. J., Ricoy, J. R. et al., Pathology of a new toxic syndrome caused by ingestion of adulterated oil in Spain, *Virchows Arch. (Pathol. Anat.)*, 397, 261, 1982.
73. Shulman, L. E., The eosinophilia-myalgia syndrome associated with ingestion of L-tryptophan, *Arthritis Rheum.*, 33, 913, 1990.
74. Vazquez, R. A., Janer, D. V., Maestro, D. R., and Graciani, C. E., New aniline derivatives in cooking oils associated with toxic oil syndrome, *Lancet*, 2, 1024, 1983.
75. Silver, R. M., Sutherland, S. E., Carreira, P., and Heyes, M. P., Alterations in tryptophan metabolism in the toxic oil syndrome and in the eosinophilia-myalgia syndrome, *J. Rheumatol.*, 19, 69, 1992.
76. Carreira, P. E., Montalvo, M. G., Kaufman, L. D., Silver, R. M., Izquierdo, M., and Gomez-Reino, J. J., Antiphospholipid antibodies in patients with eosinophilia myalgia and toxic oil syndrome, *J. Rheumatol.*, 24, 69, 1997.
77. Clauw, D. J., Animal models of the eosinophilia-myalgia syndrome, *J. Rheumatol.*, 23(Suppl. 46), 93, 1996.
78. Crofford, L. J., Rader, J. I., Dalakas, M. C., Hill, R. H. J., Page, S. W., Needham, L. L., Brady, L. S., Heyes, M. P., Wilder, R. L., and Gold, P. W., L-tryptophan implicated in human eosinophilia-myalgia syndrome causes fasciitis and perimyositis in the Lewis rat, *J. Clin. Invest.*, 86, 1757, 1990.
79. Silver, R. M., Ludwicka, A., Hampton, M., Ohba, T., Bingel, S. A., Smith, T., Harley, R. A., Maize, J., and Heyes, M. P., A murine model of the eosinophilia-myalgia syndrome induced by 1,1'-ethylidenebis (L-tryptophan), *J. Clin. Invest.*, 93, 1473, 1994.
80. Love, L. A., Rader, J. I., Crofford, L. J., Raybourne, R. B., Principato, M. A., Page, S. W., Trucksess, M. W., Smith, M. J., Dugan, E. M., and Turner, M. L., Pathological and immunological effects of ingesting L-tryptophan and 1,1'-ethylidenebis (L-tryptophan) in Lewis rats, *J. Clin. Invest.*, 91, 804, 1993.
81. Emslie-Smith, A. M., Mayeno, A. N., Nakano, S., Gleich, G. J., and Engel, A. G., 1,1'-Ethylidenebis[tryptophan] induces pathologic alterations in muscle similar to those observed in the eosinophilia-myalgia syndrome, *Neurology*, 44, 2390, 1994.
82. DeSchryver-Kecskrmrti, K., Gramlich, T. L., Crofford, L. J., Rader, J. I., Needham, L. L., Hill, R. H., and Eternberg, E. M., Mast cell and eosinophil infiltration in intestinal mucosa of Lewis rats treated with L-tryptophan implicated in human eosinophilia-myalgia syndrome, *Mod. Pathol.*, 4, 354, 1991.
83. Brown, W. R., Comparative histopatholic evaluation of animal studies: Murine studies with L-tryptophan and constituents, *J. Rhreumatol.*, 23(Suppl. 46), 99, 1996.
84. Kurl, R. N., Verney, E., and Sidransky, H., Tryptophan binding sites on nuclear envelopes of rat liver, *Nutr. Rep. Int.*, 36, 669, 1987.

85. Kurl, R. N., Verney, E., and Sidransky, H., Identification and immunohistochemical localization of a tryptophan binding protein in nuclear envelopes of rat liver, *Arch. Biochem. Biophys.*, 265, 286, 1988.
86. Sidransky, H., Verney, E., and Cosgrove, J. W., Competitive studies relating to tryptophan binding to rat hepatic nuclear envelopes as a sensitive assay for unknown compounds, *Toxicology*, 76, 89, 1992.
87. Sidransky, H., Verney, E., Cosgrove, J. W., and Schwartz, A. M., Effect of benzodiazepines on tryptophan binding to rat hepatic nuclei, *Toxicol. Pathol.*, 20, 350, 1992.
88. Sidransky, H., Verney, E., Cosgrove, J. W., and Schwartz, A. M., Inhibitory effect of demoxepam on tryptophan binding to rat hepatic nuclei, *Biochem. Med. Metab. Biol.*, 47, 270, 1992.
89. Verney, E. and Sidransky, H., Effect of metyrapone on tryptophan binding to rat hepatic nuclei, *Metab. Clin. Exp.*, 43, 79, 1994.
90. Latham, P. S., Verney, E., and Sidransky, H., A high-affinity peripheral benzodiazepine receptor is expressed on nuclei of rat liver cells and a macrophage cell line, *Hepatology*, 22, 445a, 1995.
91. Latham, P. S., Verney, E., and Sidransky, H., High-affinity peripheral benzodiazepine receptors are expressed on nuclei of liver cells and a murine macrophage cell line, *FASEB J.*, 10, A145, 1996.
92. Sidransky, H., Verney, E., Latham, P., and Schwartz, A., Effects of tryptophan related compounds on nuclear regulatory control. Possible role in the eosinophilia-myalgia syndrome, *Adv. Exp. Med. Biol.*, 398, 343, 1996.
93. Drugan, R. C., Are the nonmitochondrial peripheral benzodiazepine receptors on leukocytes a novel intermediary of brain, behavior, and immunity? *Lab. Invest.*, 70, 1, 1994.
94. Cahard, D., Canat, X., Carayon, P., Roque, C., Casellas, P., and Le Fur, G., Subcellular localization of peripheral benzodiazepine receptors on human leukocytes, *Lab. Invest.*, 70, 23, 1994.
95. Rocca, P., Bellone, G., Benna, P., Bergamasco, B., Ravizza, L., and Ferrero, P., Peripheral-type benzodiazepine receptors and diazepam binding inhibitor-like immunoreactivity distribution in human peripheral blood mononuclear cells, *Immunopharmacology*, 25, 163, 1993.
96. Kurihara, N., Yanagisawa, H., Jin, Z., and Wada, O., Production of polyclonal antibodies against 1,1'-ethyliden bis[L-tryptophan] (EBT), a potential contaminant causing eosinophilia-myalgia syndrome (EMS), *Toxicol. Lett.*, 66, 231, 1993.
97. Yamaoka, K. A., Miyazaki, N., and Kashiwazaki, S., L-tryptophan contaminant "Peak E" and interleukin-5 production from T cells, *Lancet*, 338, 1468, 1991.
98. Sidransky, H., Verney, E., Cosgrove, J. W., and Latham, P. S., Effect of 3-phenyl-amino-L-alanine on tryptophan binding to rat hepatic nuclear envelopes, *Toxicology*, 86, 135, 1994.
99. Takagi, H., Ochoa, M.S., Zhou, L., Helfman, T., Murata, H., and Falanga, V., Enhanced collagen synthesis and transcription by peak E, a contaminant of L-tryptophan preparations associated with the eosinophilia myalgia syndrome epidemic, *J. Clin. Invest.*, 96, 2120, 1995.
100. Zangrilli, J. G., Mayeno, A. N., Vining, V., and Varga, J., 1,1'-Ethylidene-bis[L-tryptophan], an impurity in L-tryptophan associated with eosinophilia-myalgia syndrome, stimulates type I collagen gene expression in human fibroblasts *in vitro*, *Biochem. Mol. Biol. Int.*, 37, 925, 1995.

101. Takagi, T., Zhou, L., Ochoa, S., and Falanga, V., Increased collagen synthesis and transcription by peak E, a contaminant of L-tryptophan preparations associated with the EMS epidemic, *J. Invest. Dermatol.*, 104, 581, 1995.

102. Li, L., Gotta, S., Mauviel, A., and Varga, J., L-tryptophan induces expression of collagenase gene in human fibroblasts: Demonstration of enhanced AP-1 binding and AP-1 binding site-driven promoter activity, *Cell. Mol. Biol. Res.*, 41, 361, 1995.

103. Adachi, J., Gomez, M., Smith, C. C., and Sternberg, E. M., Accumulation of 3-(phenylamino)alanine, a constituent in L-tryptophan products implicated in eosinophilia-myalgia syndrome, in blood and organs of the Lewis rats, *Arch. Toxicol.*, 69, 266, 1995.

104. Daniels, S. R., Hudson, J. I., and Horwitz, R. I., Epidemiology of potential association between L-tryptophan ingestion and eosinophilia-myalgia syndrome, *J. Clin. Epidemiol.*, 48, 1413, 1995.

105. Horowitz, R. I. and Daniels, S. R., Bias or biology: Evaluating the epidemiologic studies of L-tryptophan and the eosinophilia-myalgia syndrome, *J. Rheumatol.*, 23(Suppl. 46), 60, 1996.

106. Shapiro, S., Epidemiologic studies of the association of L-tryptophan with the eosinophilia-myalgia syndrome: A critique, *J. Rheumatol.*, 23(Suppl. 46), 44, 1996.

107. Hertzman, P. A., Criteria for the definition of the eosinophilia-myalgia syndrome, *J. Rheumatol.*, 23(Suppl. 46), 7, 1996.

108. Kilbourne, E. M., Philen, R. M., Kamb, M. L., and Falk, H., Tryptophan produced by Showa Denko and epidemic eosinophilia-myalgia syndrome, *J. Rheumatol.*, 23(Suppl. 46), 81, 1996.

109. Sidransky, H., Eosinophilia-myalgia syndrome: A recent syndrome serving as an alert to new diseases ahead, *Mod. Pathol.*, 7, 806, 1994.

110. Flockhart, D. A., Clauw, D. J., Sale, E. B., Hewett, J., and Woosley, R. L., Pharmacogenetic characteristics of the eosinophilia-myalgia syndrome, *Clin. Pharmacol. Ther.*, 56, 398, 1994.

111. Sidransky, H. and Verney, E., L-tryptophan binding to hepatic nuclei: Age and species differences, *Amino Acids*, 12, 77, 1997.

112. Sidransky, H. and Verney, E., Differences in tryptophan binding to hepatic nuclei of NZBWF1 and Swiss mice: Insight into mechanism of tryptophan's effects, *J. Nutr.*, 127, 270, 1997.

113. Sidransky, H. and Verney, E., Comparative studies on tryptophan binding to hepatic nuclear envelopes in Sprague-Dawley and Lewis rats, *Am. J. Physiol.*, 267, R502, 1994.

114. Sale, G. E., Eosinophilia-myalgia syndrome, *Lancet*, 1, 420, 1990.

115. Kaufman, L. D., Gruber, B. L., and Gregersen, P. K., Clinical follow-up and immunogenetic studies of 32 patients with eosinophilia-myalgia syndrome, *Lancet*, 337, 1071, 1991.

116. Varga, J., Jimenez, S. A., and Uitto, J., L-tryptophan and the eosinophilia-myalgia syndrome: Current understanding of the etiology and pathogenesis, *J. Invest. Dermatol.*, 100, 97S, 1993.

117. Gullino, P., Winitz, M., Birnbaum, S. M., Cornfield, J., Otey, M. C., and Greenstein, J. P., Studies on the metabolism of amino acids and related compounds *in vivo*. I. Toxicity of essential amino acids individually, in mixtures and the protective effect of L-arginine, *Arch. Biochem. Biophys.*, 64, 319, 1956.

12

Tryptophan: Past and Future Directions

CONTENTS

In this concluding chapter, it is appropriate to briefly summarize some of the major points reviewed in the earlier chapters and to propose some direction for future investigations dealing with L-tryptophan.

12.1 The Past

The existence of tryptophan was recognized some 100 years ago. First, it was discovered to be a vital foodstuff, an essential building block for proteins in animals. Then, it was chemically identified. Its presence in proteins was quantified, and its degradative pathways were investigated. Gradually, its major metabolic pathway, as well as its minor pathways, were unraveled. The enzymes involved in these pathways and the hormones that affected the enzymes became the subject and interest of many investigations. Early on, it became apparent that tryptophan was the precursor of a number of important compounds, particularly serotonin. Interest in serotonin and its biologic importance rapidly overshadowed the interest in tryptophan itself. More recently, melatonin, another metabolite of tryptophan, has gained much attention and prominence for its biologic actions. Other less known metabolites have been investigated, such as quinolinic and kynurenic acid, but their actions or functions are still somewhat speculative at the present time. Perhaps there are still other jewels among the many metabolites with important biologic significance that need to be uncovered and defined.

Early investigative studies recognized the importance of the metabolism of tryptophan and of its metabolites in many organs and tissues, predominantly in liver and brain. The discovery of the action of the enzyme tryptophan dioxygenase in the kynurenine–niacin pathway led to many important studies.

The more recent discovery that the enzyme indolamine dioxygenase (IDO) also is involved in the kynurenine–niacin pathway in nonhepatic tissues, such as lung, intestine, and epididymis, or in cells, such as monocytes, macrophages, and eosinophils, has been a major breakthrough. It has expanded the information about the utilization and involvement of tryptophan in cells considered to be active in immunologic reactivity and responses.

In addition to being an indispensable amino acid that is present in proteins of animals and humans and that becomes incorporated into proteins during protein synthesis, tryptophan itself has been found to have a regulatory effect on protein synthesis. Tryptophan can stimulate hepatic protein synthesis. Although the mechanism for this regulatory action appears to be complex, it is apparent that this action involves a specific nuclear envelope receptor to which it binds, followed by enhanced nucleocytoplasmic translocation of mRNA, and subsequent increased cytoplasmic protein synthesis.

The ability of L-tryptophan to bind to plasma proteins of the blood and circulate as free and bound tryptophan is a unique feature for an amino acid. This binding is affected by and competes with other compounds that bind plasma proteins, such as nonesterified fatty acids (NEFA) and certain drugs. This relationship in blood affects its transport from the blood to the brain because only the free tryptophan is transplanted through the blood–brain barrier. Free tryptophan's concentration in blood in relation to other amino acids, particularly branched-chain amino acids (BCAA), affects its transport to the brain.

The common finding that blood tryptophan levels are altered, usually decreased, in many disease states is of great interest and raises a number of questions. In most cases, the findings have been verified but are as yet unexplained. Their possible significance to the underlying disease states is not clear. Answers are needed. These alterations may be due to one or more of the following:

1. Altered metabolism of tryptophan due to enzymes involved in catabolism
2. Genetic influence on the enzyme levels and actions
3. Hormonal influences on the enzymes
4. Alteration in free blood tryptophan levels due to influences on bound blood tryptophan
5. Imbalanced states with other circulating amino acids in blood
6. Divergence to selected organs or tissues
7. Altered immunological state

These are some of the questions that need to be assessed.

In recent times compounds with antioxidant activity have gained much attention. This has occurred in conjunction with the concept that antioxidants play a major scavenging role in many biologic proccesses in health and disease. L-tryptophan and related compounds (mainly related to the indole radical) have been reported to exert antioxidant activity. Whether and to what extent this activity may have biologic significance still need to be established.

One fascinating aspect of tryptophan is that it has been known for years as a remedy for pain (simple, menstrual, migraine, etc.) and for sleep. Also, it has been used for depression and certain other mental disturbances. While in the United States it has not been used as a prescription drug and was available over-the-counter until 1989, in a number of European countries physicians prescribed it as a therapeutic agent. In general, it has been assumed that it acts mainly by becoming converted to serotonin, which is known to have many effects on the central nervous system. Its use in a variety of mental disturbances has been investigated, with some studies suggesting beneficial effects while other studies were equivocal or questionable. More studies are needed to relate to the therapeutic benefits of L-tryptophan alone or in combination with other drugs.

Interest in certain nutrients or special compounds often is stimulated by unexpected events or occurrences. Such was the case with the discovery of the eosinophilia-myalgia syndrome in 1989. The rapid development and documentation of a new disease syndrome traced epidemiologically to a single manufacturer of L-tryptophan in Japan popularized L-tryptophan and acknowledged its widespread use by the general population throughout the United States and abroad. Tryptophan's uses for pain, sleep, and depression were widely acknowledged. It had become a multimillion dollar over-the-counter therapeutic agent. The Japanese manufacturer who was the prime supplier of L-tryptophan decided to use genetic engineering in its microbiologic fermentation process to enhance its yield of L-tryptophan. This act seemed to initiate the occurrence of the eosinophilia-myalgia syndrome. Minute amounts of new contaminants or impurities were introduced into the relatively highly purified L-tryptophan. This new product appears to have caused the development of the eosinophilia-myalgia syndrome in a small fraction of the public who consumed this product. The consequences have been described in Chapter 11. This new syndrome has served a useful purpose in requiring regulatory agencies to act promptly to stop the sale of L-tryptophan. It raised the issue of the many dangers that exist in the availability of unregulated consumer products over-the-counter. It raised questions about problems that may be introduced with genetic engineering of consumable products. It also stimulated interest in the basic understanding of how L-tryptophan itself or in combination with other compounds may affect humans. New studies relating to L-tryptophan and its involvement in immunologic responses and its relationship to fibrogenesis and collagen synthesis have been reported (see Chapter 11). This resurgence of interest in

L-tryptophan will contribute much to our understanding of the many actions of this important nutrient in health and disease.

The existence of nutrient imbalances has been promulgated for many years. Imbalances among amino acids, fats, carbohydrates, vitamins, and minerals have been reported. Thus, it was not surprising that imbalances between L-tryptophan and other amino acids, carbohydrates, vitamins, and minerals have been observed. Some of these have been described in earlier chapters. The significance of these subtle or marked imbalances, which also occur with certain hormones and drugs, is difficult to assess. Yet their occurrences suggest that they may have significance and need to be assessed and evaluated. These disturbances in the homeostatic balanced state (established as the normal or ideal state) may become involved in tilting the normal state into the abnormal state. L-tryptophan may have a special vital role in many important metabolic interrelationships.

Table 12.1 summarizes the major actions (direct and indirect) of L-tryptophan. It is apparent that this amino acid has unique characteristics, and its importance as an amino acid is probably not equalled or surpassed by any other single amino acid. It appears to have a physiologic role in many important processes within cells, tissues, and organs. Also, it and its metabolites are involved in pharmacologic actions, some of which may prove to be beneficial in a number of diseases. In view of its many capabilities, it is not surprising that many studies have been directed toward its influence on a variety of diseases, particularly chronic diseases, such as aging, cancer, liver disease, cardiovascular disease, etc. In relation to immunologic diseases, its metabolism through IDO by certain cells and tissues has raised many questions regarding its importance thereof. The actions of serotonin and melatonin, two major metabolites, have gained increasing prominence in controlling vital processes within the nervous system.

TABLE 12.1

Actions of L-Tryptophan

Direct Action	Indirect Action or via Precursors for
1. Building block for proteins	1. NAD
2. Stimulates protein synthesis	2. Serotonin
3. Binds to plasma proteins	3. Melatonin
4. Antioxidant	4. Indolic compounds (antioxidants)
	5. Immunomodulary events

12.2 The Future

Many studies have demonstrated that certain nutrients control gene expression, leading to changes in cell metabolism, growth, or differentiation. These studies suggest that in the future additional mechanisms for nutrient control of gene expression will be discovered. Specifically, defining the molecular basis for L-tryptophan's involvement in cell metabolism and function may provide further insight into the action(s) of L-tryptophan in both normal and pathophysiologic states. This may provide novel approaches to influencing certain chronic disease, such as fibromyalgia and others. Such an approach has already been the case in extensive investigations into disturbance in cholesterol or lipid homeostasis, i.e., coronary artery disease, hypertension, and obesity. The future directions of research involving L-tryptophan and its metabolites and their biologic effects will certainly be rewarding.

In an attempt to practice good medicine, the student of disease states should consider L-tryptophan as a vital compound whose many actions need to be clarified and understood. Such understanding will lead to major advances that will contribute to the practice of good medicine.

12.3 Conclusion

The book may serve as a travelogue for L-tryptophan. It has attempted to cover the current terrain, with stopovers at selected sites considered to be important and informative. It becomes apparent that some sites or areas have much historical significance and are quite developed. On the other hand, some areas are primitive or poorly explored. Yet others may still be completely unexplored. Much about L-tryptophan is known and well established. Yet it is apparent that more still needs to be explained. The unknown, and those still poorly investigated, areas beckon for inquiry. Indeed, such studies will offer significant rewards and treasures. They will provide vital links and better understanding of many important biologic processes. The author hopes that this book will stimulate interest and progress in research pertaining to the unique amino acid, L-tryptophan.

Index